Emerging Infections in Asia

Emerging Infections in Asia

Edited by

Yichen Lu
Harvard School of Public Health, Boston, MA, USA

M. Essex
Harvard School of Public Health, Boston, MA, USA

Bryan Roberts
Cambridge, MA, USA

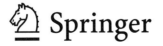 Springer

Editors:
Yichen Lu, PhD
Director General
Haikou VTI Biological Institute
Haikou, Hainan, China

Principal Research Scientist, Harvard
  School of Public AIDS Initiative
Harvard School of Public Health
Boston, Massachusetts, USA

Special Professor
Nankai University Vaccine Laboratory
Nankai University
Tianjin, China

M. Essex, DVM, PhD
Chairman, Harvard School of Public Health
  AIDS Initiative
Mary Woodard Lasker Professor of Health
  Sciences,
Harvard School of Public Health
Boston, Massachusetts, USA

Bryan Roberts, DPhil
President
Apex Consulting Group
Cambridge, Massachusetts USA

Managing Editor:
Chris Chanyasulkit, MPH
Harvard School of Public Health AIDS
  Initiative
Harvard School of Public Health
Boston, Massachusetts, USA

Assistant Managing Editor:
June Chanyasulkit, B.A.
Georgetown University
Washington, District of Columbia, USA

ISBN: 978-0-387-75721-6   e-ISBN: 978-0-387-75722-3
DOI: 10.1007/978-0-387-75722-3

Library of Congress Control Number: 2008921388

Cover illustration: Photo courtesy of Alex Zhang of The Hong Kong Polytechnic University & James Song of Toronto University

Printed on acid-free paper

9 8 7 6 5 4 3 2 1

springer.com

To the memory of Dr. Elkan R. Blout (1919–2007), our inspirational mentor. His passion for scientific rigor and international health will be forever cherished.

Foreword

The number of people who live in Asia is greater than the total number of people who live in the rest of the world. More than 160 cities in Asia have a population of at least one million people. Thus, when new infectious diseases threaten populations in Asia, huge segments of the global population are at risk. At the same time, Asians are thoroughly integrated with the rest of the world, providing skilled expertise and becoming trading partners in all continents.

Infectious diseases ordinarily show no preference for infection or disease according to race or ethnic background. A few exceptions exist, due to the host–pathogen evolution that happened before the recent era of rapid travel. Such exceptions occur usually because the infectious agent was newly introduced to one population only after having existed and evolved for hundreds or thousands of years in a different population. As air travel became popular in the last few generations of people, it became increasingly difficult for populations to remain in isolation. Thus, in 2003, SARS in China rapidly became SARS in Canada.

Throughout history, a major source of new infections of people has been old infections of animals. For some, such as Ebola or Lassa, transmission to people is rare and self-limiting, though frighteningly lethal for the few unfortunate individuals who get infected. And Ebola and Lassa are indigenous for Africa, not Asia. A more common example of a lethal infection that originates in animals and may cause repeated problems anywhere in the world is rabies. These viruses kill all the people they infect; transmission from person to person to cause new epidemics does not occur. To cause new epidemics in people, a virus must be readily transmitted by people before they are in the final stages of disease. This happens with SARS, flu, and AIDS.

Because dangerous viruses are usually transmitted before they cause severe clinical symptoms, a fundamental principle of public health is surveillance. Such surveillance must be done to track the spread of the infectious agent itself, not just the associated disease. Monitoring clinical AIDS disease rather than the spread of HIV allows a massive expansion of the epidemic before realizing that large segments of the population may be incubating a lethal disease. And for many infectious agents, such as avian flu, SARS, and rabies, it is important to do surveillance on the carrier animals, as well as people.

Fortunately, modern biotechnology provided us with new ways to design vaccines and other interventions to respond to such disease agents, when new opportunities for rapid movement of people began to flourish. But the challenges are often great and the time is limited. Our best chance for success is through collaboration and the sharing of information, ideas, results, and solutions. This book, entitled *Emerging Infections in Asia*, helps define the problems, and challenges us to work together for solutions. Successful responses could save many lives in this generation and future generations.

Bangkok, Thailand   Pornchai Matangkasombut

Preface

In the 1997 annual Harvard AIDS Institute think-tank meeting at the Endicott House in a suburb of Boston, Dr. Natth Bhamarapravati of Thailand reported an interesting observation: emerging infections in Asia seemed to have become a regular event. Not only had we seen new pathogens such as Nipah virus appear in the region, but infectious diseases originating elsewhere in the world also seemed to be spreading more rapidly in Asia. By then, many of us were convinced that Asia would soon surpass Africa in the number of people living with HIV/AIDS because the total population of Asia is much larger than the population of sub-Saharan Africa.

Then came the 2003 SARS epidemic. Soon after the so-called "atypical pneumonia" appeared in southern China, Dr. Ruan Li of China CDC started frequent telephone discussions about the disease with us at the Harvard School of Public Health, where he had previously spent a sabbatical leave as a Fogarty scholar. Our communication continued even when he himself was quarantined. During those difficult times, we often recalled the previous discussions about the increasing vulnerability of Asia to becoming an epicenter for new infectious diseases. It was also at that time that we decided to put together a book about SARS in Asia after the outbreak was under control and we had collected more facts.

The plan to publish this book was finally formulated in 2004, following the editing process of the book *AIDS in Asia*. The first section of that book is a "snapshot" of the HIV/AIDS epidemic in each of the Asian countries or regions. We asked our contributors to include a historic review of the AIDS epidemic in the context of the infectious diseases in their respective home countries. After all the chapters were submitted, we began to face some interesting questions. Why has Asia become a hotbed for new infectious diseases? Is it really a recent phenomenon or just periodic renewal of our attention?

We asked our contributors to consider these questions when they wrote their chapters, and we hope that our book can help readers make their own conclusions and ask more questions. This volume focuses on SARS, AIDS, avian influenza, and several other emerging infectious diseases that originated in Asia. It does not include "old" infectious diseases like Dengue fever, Japanese Encephalitis, and rabies, all of which seem to have gained new strength in recent years.

This volume also does not include recent events that have occurred since 2006, such as the Chikungunya outbreak in India. This disease is not new and did not originate in Asia. The Chikungunya virus was first identified in Tanzania in the 1950s and was shown to cause limited outbreaks in Africa and southeast Asia transmitted by the *Aedes aegypti* and *A. albopictus* (Asian Tiger mosquito).

There are also other emerging animal infectious diseases in Asia that should be closely monitored. For instance, serious regional outbreaks of foot and mouth diseases have frequently been reported since the 1990s. In 2007, the spread of Porcine Respiratory and Reproductive Syndrome Virus (PRRSV) in China reached a crisis level in the pork industry.

Infectious disease outbreaks limited to animals such as these were not a focus for this book. However, outbreaks of diseases in animals should serve to remind us that some animal infections move to people, as did SARS and flu. This reminds us that we must mobilize our vigilance. This may then raise our awareness to ask the right questions.

Boston, MA   Yichen Lu
Boston, MA   M. Essex
Cambridge, MA   Bryan Roberts

Acknowledgments

The editors thank Bill Tucker and his team at Springer Publishing for providing critical support and encouragement to this project. The editors thank Molly Pretorius Holme, Lendsey Melton, and Alexandra Lu for their enormous help with the editing process. Thanks also are due to Elizabeth Liao and Robert Brier for departmental support; Yang Wang and Song Xin for translation; Zhang Yin of Hong Kong Polytechnic University, James Song of Toronto University, and Ms. Jin Zhe of Beijing for providing the photographs for the book cover. The editors would like to thank the collaborative authors for their dedication of time and effort to this publication.

Contents

Part 3   HIV/AIDS

Part 4   Other Infections

Contributors

Tanvir Ahmed
International Centre for Diarrhoeal Disease Research, Bangladesh: Centre for
Health and Population Research, Dhaka, Bangladesh

Prasert Auewarakul
Department of Microbiology, Faculty of Medicine Siriraj Hospital, Mahidol
University, Bangkok 10700, Thailand, sipaw@mahidol.ac.th

Remi N. Charrel
Unité des Virus Emergents, UMR190 (Universite - IRD) Faculte de Medecine, 27
Blvd Jean Moulin 13005 Marseille, France, Remi.Charrel@medecine.univ-mrs.fr

Yi-Ming Arthur Chen
Institute of Microbiology and Immunology, AIDS Prevention and Research Center,
National Yang-Ming University, Taipei 112, Taiwan, ROC, Arthur@ym.edu.tw

Bryan T. Eaton
CSIRO Livestock Industries, Australian Animal Health Laboratory, Geelong, VIC,
Australia, Bryan.eaton@csiro.au

M. Essex
Department of Immunology and Infectious Diseases, Harvard School of Public
Health, FXB Building, 665 Huntington Avenue, Boston, MA 02115, USA,
messex@hsph.harvard.edu

Kee Tai Goh
College of Medicine Building, 16, College Road, Singapore, Singapore 169854,
goh_kee-tai@moh.gov.sg

Zhihong Hu
State Key Laboratory of Virology, Wuhan Institute of Virology, Chinese Academy
of Sciences, Wuhan 430071, P.R. China, huzh@wh.iov.cn

Yoshihiro Kawaoka
Division of Virology, Department of Microbiology and Immunology, and
International Research Center for Infectious Diseases, Institute of Medical
Science, University of Tokyo, Shirokanedai, Minato-ku, Tokyo 108-8639, Japan

Core Research for Evolutional Science and Technology, Japan Science and Technology Agency, Saitama 332-0012, Japan

Department of Pathological Sciences, School of Veterinary Medicine, University of Wisconsin-Madison, Madison, WI, USA, kawaokay@svm.vetmed.wisc.edu

Zhuang Ke
Modern Virology Research Center, College of Life Science, Wuhan University, Wuhan, Hubei, P.R. China, zhuangky@hotmail.com

Xavier de Lamballerie
Unité des Virus Emergents, UMR190 (Universite - IRD) Faculte de Medecine, 27 Blvd Jean Moulin 13005 Marseille, France, Xavier.de-lamballerie@medecine. univ-mrs.fr

Li Ruan
Department of Biotech Center for Viral Disease Emergency, National Institute for Viral Disease Control and Prevention, Chinese Center for Disease Control and Prevention, Beijing 100052, China, ruanl@public3.bta.net.cn

Yichen Lu
Department of Immunology and Infectious Diseases, Harvard School of Public Health, FXB Building, 665 Huntington Avenue, Boston, MA 02115, USA, yichenlu@hsph.harvard.edu

John S. Mackenzie
Australian Biosecurity Cooperative Research Centre for Emerging Infectious Disease; Curtin University of Technology, Perth, WA, Australia, j.mackenzie@curtin.edu.au

Firdausi Qadri
International Centre for Diarrhoeal Disease Research, Bangladesh: Centre for Health and Population Research, Dhaka, Bangladesh

Bryan Roberts
Apex Consulting Group, 35 Lawrence Street, Cambridge, MA 02139, USA, bryanr1@comcast.net

Zhengli Shi
State Key Laboratory of Virology, Wuhan Institute of Virology, Chinese Academy of Sciences, Wuhan 430071, P.R. China, zlshi@wh.iov.cn

Kyoko Shinya
The International Center for Medical Research and Treatment, Kobe University, n-5-1, Kusunoki-Cho, Chuo-Ku, Kobe, 650-0017, Japan, shinya@med.kobe-u.ac.jp

Jae-Hoon Song
Samsung Medical Center, Sungkyunkwan University School of Medicine, Asian-Pacific Research Foundation for Infectious Diseases, Seoul, Korea, jhsong@smc.samsung.co.kr

Srikanth Prasad Tripathy
National AIDS Research Institute, Bhosari, Pune 411026, India,
stripathy@nariindia.org

Sriram Prasad Tripathy
Indian Council of Medical Research, Pune, India, sriramtripathy@hotmail.com

Lin-Fa Wang
CSIRO Livestock Industries, Australian Animal Health Laboratory, Geelong,
VIC, Australia, Linfa.Wang@csiro.au

Annelies Wilder-Smith
Department of Community, Occupational and Family
Medicine, National University Singapore, (MD3), Yong Loo Lin School
of Medicine, 16 Medical Drive, Singapore, Singapore 117597

Gui Xien
Zhongnan Hospital of Wuhan University, 169 Donghu Road, Wuhan, Hubei,
P.R. China, znact@126.com

Ali Mohamed Zaki
Dr. Fakeeh Hospital, Jeddah 21461, Saudi Arabia

Guang Zeng
Chinese Center for Disease Control and Prevention, 27 Nan Wai Lu,
Xuan Wu Qu, Beijing 100050, China, zeng4605@vip.sina.com.

Part 1
Avian Flu

Influenza: Biology, Infection, and Control

Bryan Roberts

I had a little bird
Its name was Enza
I opened the window
And in-flew-Enza

Jump rope song (USA, 1918)

Overview

The growth of the human population has profoundly affected the global ecosystem, influencing the animal population balance, the availability of fresh water, arable land, biotic production, and atmospheric gases. The human ecological impact has significantly accelerated the evolutionary change of numerous organisms. For example, the production of human medicine and food has resulted in the rapid evolution of drug-resistant pathogenic organisms as well as plants and insects resistant to pesticides (Palumbi, 2001). Recently, the nutritional support of the human population has relied on the vast monoculture of domestic mammals and birds, which has facilitated the emergence of pathogenic enzootic organisms that infect both animals and humans. This chapter will focus on the global threat to human health represented by the highly contagious enzootic virus influenza. It will also discuss current efforts and future improvements to protect humans from global influenza epidemics and pandemics.

Human Population Growth and the Evolution of Infectious Disease

The evolution and global dispersal of human populations over many millennia have profoundly influenced the pattern and development of infectious human pathogens. McMichael and Weiss have outlined five major transitions in human ecology that have profoundly influenced the profile and properties of organisms that infect humans (McMichael, 2004; Weiss & McMichael, 2004).

Y. Lu et al. (eds.), *Emerging Infections in Asia.*
© Springer Science+Business Media, LLC 2008

1. The primary ecological transition of the human population occurred several million years ago with the emergence of our early ancestors in Africa from arboreal habitats into the open savannah. Contact with animals in the savannah resulted in infection with new enzootic agents. This trend continued during the emergence of *Homo sapiens* and the subsequent migration of Neolithic hunter-gatherers out of Africa approximately 100,000 years ago.

2. The second transition originated about 10,000 years ago with the development of agriculture, following the domestication of animals and plants. This practice resulted in the establishment of stable settlements, in which the number and density of humans and animals increased, facilitating the transmission of pathogens between species. Ultimately, this enzootic exchange of pathogens led to the development of infectious organisms that were exclusively propagated and maintained within the expanding human population. This mechanism of evolution over the last 10,000 years has been suggested for measles, mumps, rubella, and smallpox. Recently, the emergence of HIV and Hepatitis C from animal sources, and their establishment and global transmission within human populations, have been observed.

3. The third transition was the continental expansion of human populations, which resulted in the geographic isolation of populations that evolved different types of enzootic and human pathogens. When these distinct human populations throughout the Eurasian continent made contact through trade or warfare, catastrophic epidemics ensued. These occurred during the period 1000 BCE and 1500 CE, culminating in the Black Death in 1347 CE, which killed approximately one-third of the European population.

4. The fourth transition was initiated in 1500 CE when Europeans undertook global exploration followed by widespread colonization of countries in Africa, Asia, and the New World. This resulted in the global distribution of infectious diseases and the eradication of naive native populations by the introduction of new diseases such as measles and smallpox.

5. The fifth transition started during the eighteenth century and is characterized by the uncontrolled upward spiral of the human population despite wars, famine, and disease. The growth rate of the human population rose significantly in the eighteenth century, coincident with the European Industrial Revolution, when agricultural practice was rendered more efficient, and manufacturing was facilitated by the application of power-driven machinery.

This trend intensified into the twentieth century when the global population grew from 1.6 billion in 1900 to 6.1 billion by 2000. The bulk of the global population growth occurred after the Second World War, predominantly in the developing world, namely, Asia, Africa, and South America (United Nations, 2004). In 2005, the global population was about 6.5 billion, with 5.3 billion living in the developing world. The economic and health disparities between the developed and the developing are constantly expanding, with the latter sustaining a tenfold higher infant mortality rate, more than two-thirds of the 13 million deaths due to infectious diseases, and 50% of the population living on less than $2 per day (Roberts &

Lu, 2004). During this period, urban settlements have become the predominant human habitat with estimates of 7% of the world's population living in megacities (United Nations, 2004). The UN 2000 forecasts that the world's population will increase 30% by 2030 and of these additional 2 billion people, 1.9 billion will live in the cities and towns of South America, Asia, and Africa. Toward the end of this century the majority of the world's population will be living in cities and large towns (United Nations, 2004). This trend toward urban living and the redistribution of the human population will profoundly impact the profile and spread of infectious diseases. Moreover, during the second half of the twentieth century, the development of global communication and economic interactions has led to an enormous increase in global travel both by air and sea. The redistribution and urbanization of large portions of the human population, together with the vast increase in global air travel, have already dramatically altered the pattern and kinetics of disease dissemination. During the twentieth century, this was clearly demonstrated by the global spread of the chronic diseases AIDS and Hepatitis C, caused by HIV1 and HCV, respectively. In 1999, the coronavirus that originally caused severe acute respiratory syndrome in southern China was globally distributed within 3 months (Vijayanand et al., 2004), and the flavivirus West Nile Virus introduced into the eastern USA from the Middle East was efficiently disseminated across the continent within 3 years (Petersen & Roehrig, 2001).

Biology of Influenza Virus

Current databases indicate that 1,415 pathogens cause diseases in humans, of which 61.6% are enzootic; that is, they infect humans and other animal species (Cleaveland et al., 2001). Pathogens that infect multiple hosts evolve independently in different populations, resulting in changes in their pathogenicity, host range, and transmission characteristics. Influenza virus is a major enzootic pathogen that is transmitted among humans, domestic animals, and wild animals and profoundly impacts human health and economics.

Influenza Virus Reservoirs

Influenza viruses are negative-strand RNA viruses belonging to the Orthomyxoviridae family. Based on antigenic differences in the nucleoprotein and matrix proteins, influenza viruses are divided into three distinct types, A, B, and C (Murphy, 1996). The viral genome is divided into eight negative-sense single-stranded linear segments in the type A and B subtypes, and seven segments in the type C virus.

Influenza C viruses have been isolated only from humans and swine, where they cause mild upper respiratory tract infections (Baigent & McCauley, 2003). The influenza B subtype has been isolated only from humans and seals and causes severe disease in humans, including lower respiratory tract infections, pneumonia, and encephalitis (Baigent & McCauley, 2003). During the first 2 years of the twenty-first century, the influenza B strain variant B/Victoria/2/87 reemerged from Asia and spread globally, causing widespread human epidemic outbreaks (Shaw et al., 2002). The influenza A type viruses maintain an extensive subtype reservoir in wild aquatic birds and infect a range of mammals, avian species, and humans. Inducing significant morbidity and mortality worldwide, these influenza A type viruses are one of the major causes of human infection and are the focus of this chapter.

Influenza Type A Virus Biology

The influenza type A virus comprises eight genomic segments named according to the proteins they encode, namely HA, NA, M, PB1, PB2, NS, PA, and NP. These eight RNA segments encode 11 structural and nonstructural proteins that facilitate cellular uptake, protein synthesis, RNA replication, and the assembly and release of progeny virions. Viral subtypes are defined by the possession of 1 of 15 antigenically distinct hemagglutinins (HA) and 1 of 9 neuraminidase (NA) antigens. The 15 hemagglutinins (H1–H15) and 9 neuraminidases (N1–N9) are perpetuated in nature in shorebirds, waterfowl, and gulls (Alexander, 2000>; Hinshaw et al., 1980). In these aquatic wild bird populations, influenza viruses normally replicate without disease symptoms. This genetically diverse reservoir of influenza A subtypes in wild birds is well adapted to its natural hosts and exhibits an evolutionary stasis with minimal variation in its surface protein sequence, suggestive of a long-established and balanced host and pathogen interactions (Webster et al., 1992).

Molecular evidence suggests that specific viral subtypes from this avian reservoir have been transmitted to domestic birds, ocean-dwelling mammals, seals and whales, and land-dwelling mammals including horses, pigs, and humans (Webster et al., 1992). A broad spectrum of influenza A subtypes infects domestic poultry, the majority causing mild respiratory disease; yet subtypes H5N1, H5N2, H7N1, and H7N3 have mutated and become highly pathogenic and cause lethal infections (Capua & Alexander, 2004). In land-dwelling mammals, the influenza A subtypes H7N7 and H3N8 cause epidemic disease in horses, H1N1, H1N2, and H3N2 in pigs, and H3N2, H2N2, and H1N1 in humans (Webster et al., 1992).

The transmission and replication of influenza subtypes in new host animals or birds depend on the interaction of the virus and its encoded proteins with cells and tissues of the host that support virus propagation and spread within the population. The two viral surface proteins HA and NA interact cooperatively to define this host specificity, by determining the efficiency of viral attachment to, entry into, fusion with, and release from, host cells. The cell surface receptor recognized by HA is sialic acid attached to galactose by either alpha-2,3 Gal or alpha-2,6 Gal linkages (Gambaryan et al., 1995). The HA of influenza viruses isolated from the avian reservoir bind to sialic acid linked to galactose by an alpha-2,3 linkage and those that infect mammals recognize sialic acid linked to galactose by an alpha-2,6 linkage. The release of viral progeny relies on the NA cleavage of cell surface sialic acid that is linked to galactose in the same structural conformation recognized by the HA. This clearance of sialic acid residues from the cell surface obviates virus–cell interactions and facilitates the release of virions from infected cells.

The infection of cells by influenza virus relies on the cleavage of the precursor HA into proteins HA1 and HA2 by host cell trypsin-like proteases. The tissue distribution of trypsin-like proteases within the host organism restricts virus replication to distinct sites, generally the mucosal surfaces of the respiratory and gastrointestinal tracts. The efficiency of HA cleavage is influenced by the structure of its protease cleavage site, and the presence of multiple basic amino acids flanking this site facilitates cleavage by ubiquitous proteases such as furin. The cleavage of HA by ubiquitous proteases that are widely distributed in the host organism permits viral replication at sites throughout the body, resulting in a lethal disease causing major organ and tissue damage. The mutational introduction of basic amino acids flanking the protease cleavage site that enhance and broaden protease recognition has been clearly demonstrated as a major factor in the evolution of nonvirulent avian viruses into highly pathogenic avian influenza viruses in domestic poultry (Capua & Alexander, 2004).

The replication of viral genetic information within infected cells requires compatible interactions between viral proteins and cellular components to facilitate the unraveling of viral ribonucleic acid complexes, the replication of viral RNA segments, and virion assembly and release.

The specificity of the infection of animals by influenza virus subtypes illustrates the subtlety of interactions that define the host range. This is elegantly illustrated in the antibody profile of workers exposed to poultry infected by different avian influenza subtypes. The presence of antibodies in human serum samples demonstrated that they were infected productively by the avian virus subtypes, H7N7, H7N3, and H5N1, but not H7N1 or H5N2 (Hayden & Croisier, 2005; Puzelli et al., 2005).

The lethality of an influenza strain is a function of its transmission efficiency in the population and its pathogenicity, replication, and tissue tropism within the infected host. Viral pathogenesis is complex and contributed by a number of different determinants including the efficiency of HA cleavage by proteases (Steinhauer, 1999), viral polymerase activity (Almond, 1977), the viral gene products NP (Bean & Webster, 1978; Oxford et al., 1978; Scholtissek & Murphy, 1978) and NS (Treanor et al., 1989) that interact to facilitate the growth, dissemination, and transmission within the host species.

In new host organisms, the influenza viral genomes are unstable and accumulate sequence alterations that evolve into new variants. Sequence changes in influenza A virus occur by two mechanisms, the continuous accumulation of mutations within genomic segments called "genetic drift" and the exchange of entire genomic segments between different viruses referred to as "genetic shift."

The continuous accumulation of sequence alterations by genetic drift facilitates the rapid development of resistance of influenza to small-molecule drugs. This phenomenon is illustrated by the widespread resistance to amantidine in circulating human influenza viruses and the rapid appearance of cases of resistance to oseltamivir in humans infected with H5N1 (Bright et al., 2006; Le et al., 2005). This questions the wisdom of investing in the development of small-molecule drugs whose effective treatment of highly mutable RNA viruses, such as influenza, is short lived.

During the coinfection of a host permitting the multiplication of mammalian and avian influenza viruses, "genetic shift" occurs, when the exchange of complete genomic segments results in the formation of new reassortants. Those reassortants that exhibit a new surface HA and/or NA are new subtypes that can propagate widely in susceptible avian and mammalian populations. The emergence of a new influenza subtype that infects naive humans causes the establishment of global pandemic disease. Following pandemic disease in humans, the new subtype continues to circulate in the population and accumulates genomic mutations by genetic drift that is disseminated in the viral population by replication and recombination. This process results in the establishment of subtype variants that cause annual epidemics in humans. In a similar fashion, genetic variation occurs in influenza strains that circulate in other mammals and birds, and cause periodic epidemic outbreaks.

The extraordinary genetic malleability of this segmented RNA virus has resulted in the evolution of an extensive reservoir of subtypes in wild aquatic birds, which spread selectively and mutate in domestic poultry and mammals, causing significant disease outbreaks.

Influenza Type A Infections of Horses and Swine

In horses, epidemic disease is caused by infection with genetic variants of the subtypes H7N7 and H3N8 (Webster et al., 1992). Equine influenza was first recognized in 1956 in a widespread epidemic in Eastern Europe caused by subtype H7N7 (Daly et al., 2004). This influenza virus continued in circulation, and its last confirmed outbreak occurred in 1979. In 1963, a new subtype, H3N8, was identified in a disease outbreak in the USA, which spread globally, and its genetic variants remain the major cause of equine influenza (Daly et al., 2004).

Influenza was first recorded in pigs during the pandemic outbreak of 1918 (Koen, 1919), and the virus was isolated in 1930 (Shope, 1931). During most of the twentieth century, swine influenza was caused by the genetic drift of the predominant circulating subtype H1N1. However, in 1998, a severe influenza outbreak in swine in the USA was caused by a new pathogenic subtype H3N2. This subtype was shown to be a triple reassortant H3N2, containing the HA, NA, and PB1 segments from humans, the M, NS, and NP segments from swine, and the PA and PB2 segments from birds (Webby et al., 2000). This subtype became endemic in swine and, by coinfection with the H1N1 subtype, created a further reassortant H1N2 (Karasin et al., 2000). Currently, the three subtypes H1N1, H1N2, and H3N2 circulate worldwide in swine and their variants cause epidemic outbreaks. The evolution of subtypes and their variants in swine illustrates the extensive genetic change that can occur rapidly in the segmented RNA genome of the influenza virus.

Influenza Type A Infections of Domestic Poultry

A highly pathogenic disease of domestic birds called fowl plague was identified in Italy in 1878 (Perroncito, 1878), which led to the isolation of the first influenza virus type A in 1902 (Horimoto & Kawaoka, 2001). Domestic fowl are infected by a wide range of influenza A subtypes, the majority of which exhibit infections of low virulence characterized by mild respiratory disease and lowered egg production. Highly pathogenic avian influenzas are generally confined to subtypes bearing the surface HA H5 or H7 that cause highly lethal disease with flock mortalities up to 100% (Capua & Alexander, 2004). Highly pathogenic subtypes display HA H5 or H7 on their surface, which contains multiple basic amino acids proximal to the protease cleavage site. The efficient cleavage of the HA facilitates widespread infection of the avian tissues and the rapid onset of lethal disease. Recent scientific results support the conclusion that wild bird populations propagate influenza strains that exhibit no disease symptoms or those that cause only mild infections (Rohm et al., 1995; Banks et al., 2000, 2001). However, highly pathogenic H5 and H7 influenza strains arise in domestic poultry as a result of mutations in nonlethal viruses introduced from wild birds (Garcia et al., 1996; Perdue et al., 1998).

Records kept since 1959 identified 19 highly pathogenic primary influenza isolates in domestic fowl, which were either self-limiting or controlled by culling flocks (Fouchier et al., 2003). Diagnostic assays recently identified the mutation of low pathogenic subtypes into highly pathogenic variants, which caused widespread outbreaks in domestic fowl and severely impacted animal health and regional economies. These disease outbreaks occurred in Pennsylvania, USA, in 1983 (Webster & Kawaoka, 1988), Mexico in 1993 (Villarreal & Flores, 1997), Pakistan in 1994 (Naeem, 1998), Italy in 1999 (Capua & Marangon, 2000), and Chile in 2002 (Rojas et al., 2002), and demonstrate the global distribution of highly pathogenic influenza infections in domestic poultry stocks. In the period from 1997 to 2004, the incidence of worldwide infections with highly pathogenic strains of H5 and H7 has exceeded 28 lethal outbreaks in domestic poultry (Capua & Alexander, 2004).

In 1996, a highly pathogenic H5N1 virus was isolated from an infected goose in southern China, which reassorted with the other seven genes from the avian influenza H6N1. This virus caused disease in chickens in Hong Kong and was controlled by the culling of millions of chickens in southern China. Despite these containment efforts, this H5N1 strain spread widely in Southeast Asian countries including Japan, Vietnam, Laos, Cambodia, Thailand, and Indonesia, causing widespread lethal infections of domestic poultry (Writing Committee of the World Health Organization Consultation on Human Influenza A/H5, 2005). Wild ducks were shown to propagate and transmit the highly pathogenic H5N1 virus without manifesting disease symptoms, implying their potential role in the dissemination of this lethal subtype throughout Southeast Asia (Sturm-Ramirez et al., 2005). During mid-2005, it was reported that the H5N1 pathogenic virus caused a lethal epidemic in migratory waterfowl that led to the death of thousands of waterfowl in northwestern China, over 3,000 miles away from its epicenter of origin in southern China (Chen et al., 2005). In this case, the avian vector of the pathogenic H5N1 viruses was not clearly established. However, the ongoing global dissemination of pathogenic H5N1 virus is due to its transmission from domestic poultry to wild migratory aquatic birds. Currently, the spread of H5N1 from northwestern China has resulted in the lethal infection of wild birds and domestic poultry in Siberia, the Urals, Turkey, Romania, Iraq, Greece, Italy, and Africa and is threatening the vast domestic poultry stocks in Europe and the Americas.

The reason for the recent escalation of highly pathogenic avian influenza virus infections in domestic poultry is not known. It could be due to their population size, genetic composition, conditions of containment, or other factors associated with the monoculture of poultry. However, this increase in highly pathogenic strains of influenza in poultry in the second half of the twentieth century parallels the 244% increase in poultry meat production during this period. Currently, 65% of this meat is generated by four poultry producers, the USA, China, EU, and Brazil, with production in the developing world exceeding that in the developed world in both enclosed and free-range facilities (Tilman, 1999). This domestication of poultry has established ideal conditions for the growth and rapid evolution of enzootic pathogens such as influenza virus. This has resulted in two unprecedented occurrences: highly pathogenic H5N1 influenza virus evolved in domestic poultry in 1996 and established global transmission in wild migratory aquatic birds; this pathogenic H5N1 virus grows, directly infects, , and produces lethal disease in humans.

Characteristics of Influenza Infections in Humans

The history of influenza infections in humans during the twentieth century is well recorded, and this information is reviewed in order to understand the issues and obstacles that confront efforts to control outbreaks in the future. The majority of the information is derived from documentation in the developed countries, as information from the developing regions is more difficult to assemble and consequently less complete. Even the information from countries with well-established public health systems is not completely reliable, especially during pandemic outbreaks. The compiling of clinical and lethality records was difficult during pandemic outbreaks due to the social disruption caused by the rapid onset of acute disease and its impact on the general population. In addition, it appears that in some instances clinical and lethality records were distorted because of the implementation of inappropriate social and political pressures (Barry, 2004). Despite the shortcomings of this historical database, it is an important record of the timing and impact of influenza disease within society and highlights the tasks implicit in the control of this disease. However, it would be imprudent to rely on this information as being predictive of the nature and characteristics of future influenza outbreaks, especially because there are dramatic changes in the size, distribution, and disease susceptibility of the human population and its ongoing activities that are driving major evolutionary changes in the biology and pathology of influenza viruses.

Influenza Infections in Humans

Influenza is a highly contagious acute respiratory infection that is efficiently transmitted between humans by the inhalation of contaminated droplets or by direct contact. Records show it to be one of the most significant infectious diseases of humans. The causative agent of influenza disease was finally established in 1933 by the isolation of a filterable agent, characterized as influenza type A virus, from human patients (Smith et al., 1933). In the 1940s, influenza virus grown in embryonated eggs was purified and formulated into an inactivated vaccine that was shown to produce protective immunity in human clinical studies. Influenza immunity in humans is principally related to protective antibodies that inactivate the surface protein HA.

However, a variation of influenza HA was shown in 1947 to undermine this variant-specific immunity, requiring the preparation of new vaccines to protect against these variants (Francis et al., 1947). This observation led to an initiative from participants at the International Congress of Microbiology in 1947 to recommend that WHO organize an international effort to survey and collate the global spread of influenza viruses. As a consequence, a program was established by WHO to monitor the global epidemiology of influenza and to isolate new strains and make them available to vaccine manufacturers (Payne, 1953). Currently, the program is coordinated by five Collaborating Centers in Atlanta, Memphis, London, Melbourne, and Tokyo, collating information from over 110 national laboratories in 82 countries. Sensitive and rapid methods of nucleic acid and protein sequencing and immune-based assays for antibody identification have been harnessed to identify influenza subtypes and variants that infect humans. The WHO Global Influenza Surveillance System coordinates this information on the antigenic variation and the epidemiology of influenza viruses, and this database is used to select new strains and variants for influenza vaccines.

Pandemic Disease in Humans

The emergence of new viral subtypes originating from the avian reservoir that transmits lethal infections in humans undermines the strain-specific immunity in the population and can instigate global pandemic disease. Potter estimated that during the last three centuries there were ten pandemic outbreaks that occurred on average once every 33 years (Potter, 2001). During the twentieth century, three pandemic strains emerged, H1N1 in 1918, H2N2 in 1957, and H3N2 in 1968; each viral subtype contained a novel HA. Retrospective molecular analyses indicate an avian origin for the HAs in the pandemic strains of 1957 and 1968 (Webster & Laver, 1972; Kawaoka et al., 1989). The origin of the 1918 HA is unclear. Its sequence is partially related to the avian HA but it may have emerged from a mammalian source and not directly from the avian reservoir (Reid et al., 2004). It is assumed that these pandemic strains derive by the reassortment of strains of avian origin with strains that propagate in humans. These reassortants most likely deriveupon the coinfection of a mammal, possibly swine, which permit the growth of both avian and human influenza strains.

In 1918, pandemic disease appeared at about the same time in North America, Europe, and Asia, its severity increasing with time in the human population. This is the most lethal recorded pandemic with estimates of global deaths ranging from 20 to 100,000 million (Barry, 2004). During the 1918 pandemic, the number of deaths in accordance to age demonstrated a W-shaped distribution with peaks of mortality in infants, young adults, and the elderly, whereas the 1957 and 1968 pandemics data conformed to a U-shaped distribution with peaks in the deaths of infants and the elderly (Luk et al., 2001).

In 1957, the pandemic started in southern China and spread to Hong Kong by April 1957. The new subtype H2N2 responsible for the pandemic was identified after the vaccinologist Maurice Hilleman read in the *New York Times* that 250,000 people in Hong Kong had a respiratory infection (Hilleman, 1999). The first wave of disease in the USA and Europe started in August and peaked in October, followed by a second wave at the beginning of 1958. Approximately 2 million deaths were recorded worldwide with greater than 50% attack rates in children aged 5–19 years (Glezen, 1996).

The last pandemic in 1968 was initiated by the novel subtype H3N2 in Hong Kong in July and followed by infections in the USA during the winter of 1968–1969 and outbreaks in Europe during the winter of 1969–1970. This outbreak was relatively benign and it has been suggested that this was possibly due to immunity in the population supplied by the NA antigen, which was present in the new subtype H2N2 that started the previous pandemic in 1957 and remained in circulation up until 1968 (Cox & Subbarao, 2000). The global deaths exceeded 1 million, and in the USA two-thirds of all deaths occurred in persons of age 45–64 years (Simonsen et al., 1998).

Estimates from these pandemics in the twentieth century suggest that up to 30% of the total human population became infected. In susceptible populations such as schoolchildren and nursing home occupants, infection rates were as high as 40–50% (Cox & Subbarao, 2000). These records show that each pandemic exhibits a different level of lethality and that the age-related death statistics exhibited different profiles, indicating that influenza is a complex clinical syndrome in humans.

Epidemic Disease in Humans

Following pandemic disease, the new viral subtype remains in circulation in the human population for 10–40 years, and it progressively mutates to produce genetic variants that cause annual epidemics. The severity of epidemics is a reflection of the mutational changes in epitopes of the surface antigens HA and NA, and the degree of their mismatch with the protective antibodies resident in the human population. In temperate regions, annual epidemics occur in the winter season, between November and March in the Northern Hemisphere, and April and September in the Southern Hemisphere, whereas in subtropical and tropical areas, influenza is present throughout the year (Cox & Subbarao, 2000). The CDC estimates that these epidemics are responsible for 20,000–30,000 annual deaths in the USA and the WHO estimated that 250,000–500,000 deaths occur every year around the world (World Health Organization, 2003).

Surveillance data indicate that in recent times the majority of new antigenic influenza variants originate in China from where they spread globally (Cox & Subbarao, 2000). Due to the introduction of a new viral subtype into the human population, its genetic variants form epidemic strains that progressively decline in virulence and ultimately disappear from circulation in the human population, as shown in Fig. 1 (Simonsen et al., 1998). The cause of this clearance is not known. It is assumed that strains are disadvantaged by the establishment of widespread immunity in the human population and that ultimately they reach a biological limit in the formation of viable antigenically distinct variants. The pandemic/epidemic cycle is restarted by the transmission of a new influenza subtype into the human population, which initiates the spread of pandemic disease.

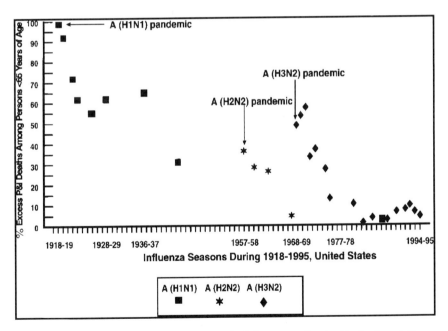

Fig. 1 The age distribution of deaths in the United States associated with the three influenza pandemics of the twentieth century and the interpandemic seasons that followed each pandemic (Reproduced with permission from Simonsen et al., 1998.)

Avian Influenza Pandemic Alert, 1997

Since the last influenza pandemic in 1968, the human population during the current interpandemic period has experienced rapid growth and redistribution to large urban areas. At the same time, global poverty and infectious diseases have increased dramatically. The support of this burgeoning human population requires enormous dedication of land resources to agriculture and energy generation that results in significant global ecological disruptions. The most dramatic impact on the ecology and evolution of influenza viruses has been caused by the vast increase in the production of domestic poultry during the last half of the twentieth century.

Coincident with the growth of the commercial monoculture of poultry, there has been an emergence of highly pathogenic avian influenza viruses that cause sporadic lethal outbreaks in poultry flocks. Intensive surveillance studies have catalogued the mutational changes in genomic and protein sequences of avian influenza viruses and their relationship to transmission, circulation, and pathogenesis among domestic poultry, wild birds, and humans. The data indicate that avian subtypes containing HAs H5 and H7 are highly pathogenic in domestic fowl. This correlates with the substitution of multiple basic amino acids proximal to the protease cleavage site, which facilitates the efficient cleavage of the HA precursor HA0 resulting in widespread infection of the avian tissues and the rapid onset of lethal disease. Avian influenza subtypes bearing HAs H5 and H7 demonstrate direct transfer and replication in humans, yet currently are limited in secondary spread within the human population. Workers exposed to infected poultry were shown to have antibodies against the avian strains H7N7, H7N3, and H5N1 but not H7N1 or H5N2 (Hayden & Croisier, 2005; Puzelli et al., 2005). These studies indicate that only specific viral subtypes are able to infect humans, implying the subtlety of interactions between viral and cellular proteins that define host range.

To date, the only subtype that demonstrates significant lethality in humans is H5N1. In 1996, a highly pathogenic H5N1 virus was isolated from an infected goose in southern China, which reassorted with the other seven genes from the avian influenza H6N1. In 1997, this strain caused disease in domestic chickens in Hong Kong and was transmitted to humans, killing 6 of 18 infected people (Writing Committee of the World Health Organization Consultation on Human Influenza A/H5, 2005). This event resulted in the declaration of a Phase 3 Pandemic Alert in accordance with the WHO Pandemic Preparedness Plan (World Health Organization, 1999). Thereafter, the virus was controlled by the culling of millions of chickens in southern China; yet in 2003 H5N1 infections occurred in two people in Fujian Province, China, resulting in the death of one person. This H5N1 strain spread widely in the southeast Asian countries including Japan, Vietnam, Laos, Cambodia, Thailand, and Indonesia, causing 112 infections and 57 deaths between December 2003 and August 2005 (Writing Committee of the World Health Organization Consultation on Human Influenza A/H5, 2005). The cumulative H5N1 infections in these countries amounted to 132 people with severe clinical symptoms of whom 64 died, indicating a lethality of 48% for this new strain in humans. The lethality of H5N1 infections is derived from a small database, which reflects the lethality in individuals that demonstrate clinical symptoms and does not include infections with mild symptoms that were not reported. The transmission of H5N1 strains to humans was correlated in numerous countries by contact with infected domestic birds on farms and in wet markets; convincing evidence of transmission between humans has not been established.

Lectin-binding studies of cells along the human airway demonstrated that sialic acid bound by human HAs occurred mainly in nasal mucosal cells, whereas those recognized by the avian HAs were found in the lower airway on epithelial cells in the paranasal sinuses, pharynx, trachea, bronchi, and alveoli (Shinya et al., 2006; Van Riel et al., 2006). These observations are consistent with autopsy data on a patient who died from avian influenza in Thailand (Uiprasertkul et al., 2005). The attachment of H5N1 virus to the lower respiratory tract may explain the requirement for close contact with diseased birds for the infection in humans. Moreover, the inability of the virus to propagate in the upper respiratory airways may limit viral transmission in the human population in water droplets generated by coughing and sneezing.

An H5N1 virus isolated in 2004 from a Vietnamese who died from avian influenza demonstrated the standard trimeric HA structure at a resolution of 2.95Å. It displayed the characteristic receptor-binding domain embedded in a globular head and a membrane proximal domain containing the signature alpha helical stalk and HA1/HA2 cleavage site, which is a major contributor to its pathogenesis. Superimposition studies of HA domains from this Vietnamese isolate with those of human, swine, and avian viruses demonstrated that its was most closely related to the H1 HA, reconstructed from the virus responsible for the 1918 pandemic (Stevens et al., 2006).

Molecular studies demonstrate that influenza viruses switch from avian to mammalian receptor specificity, by the substitution of one or two amino acids in the receptor-binding region of the HA. This was established for the conversion of avian HAs into the H1, H2, and H3 that caused the twentieth-century human pandemics, and H1 in swine and H3 in horses and seals responsible for recent epizootic disease (Rogers et al., 1983; Connor et al., 1994; Matrosovitch et al., 2000; Nobusawa et al., 2000). Mutational analysis of the Vietnamese H5N1 isolate indicates that the replacement of individual amino acids in the receptor-binding domain modulates the avian alpha 2,3 sialic acid receptor selectivity (Stevens et al., 2006). However, the introduction of two amino acid substitutions into the receptor-binding region of the progenitor duck avian influenza virus reduced binding to 2,3 sialic acid but retained binding of 2,6 sialic acid equivalent to the human virus control (Harvey et al., 2004). These studies imply that in the future the substitution of a small number of appropriate amino acids in the receptor-binding domain of HA could alter the avian/human receptor selectivity of the H5N1 virus and facilitate its efficient human transmission.

The rapid global dissemination of H5N1 virus by aquatic wild birds has significantly increased its replication in domestic poultry, and their human contact facilitates its progressive accumulation of genetic alterations and enhances the probability of the emergence of lethal pandemic disease.

Influenza Surveillance: Implications and Applications

Surveillance studies illustrate a complex picture of the ecology, evolution, and transmission of pathogenic avian influenza viruses in domestic poultry, wild birds, and humans. To date, our understanding of the molecular determinants of host range, transmission between species, and pathogenesis is rudimentary, and consequently, sequence alterations are not predictive. There are trends in this data that have implications for the health of both domestic animals and humans.

1. The growth in the domestic poultry industry fosters the evolution of the contagious enzootic pathogen influenza, threatening the health of domestic poultry and humans. During the twentieth century, virulent influenza infections in domestic poultry have gravitated from local self-limiting outbreaks to worldwide dissemination of pathogenic strains that persist and are not controlled by large-scale culling of stocks. This trend threatens the domestic poultry industry and the nutritional welfare of humans dependant on this abundant and affordable meat source. It would appear logical for authorities regulating animal and human health to develop methods of controlling influenza infections of domestic poultry.

2. Pathogenic influenza strains that evolve in domestic poultry have recently shown large-scale transmission into wild waterfowl populations (Chen et al., 2005). The ecology of this phenomenon is complex. It appears that some species, such as ducks, transmit highly pathogenic H5N1 strains without disease symptoms. This indicates that migratory aquatic birds could be responsible for the distribution of H5N1 throughout south-east Asia and its ongoing global spread. Furthermore, the lethal infection of wild waterfowl could result in selective pressures within these populations that destabilize their reservoirs of influenza strains. The 15 subtypes of HA (H1–H15) and 9 subtypes of NA (N1–N9) identified in shorebirds, waterfowl, and gulls (Hinshaw et al., 1980) could diversify their sequences and hasten the establishment of new strains that infect domestic poultry and humans.

3. Highly pathogenic avian influenza virus strains from domestic fowl have shown direct transmission to and lethal infection of humans. However, to date, they are unable to affect secondary transmission between humans. The coinfection of humans or swine with both avian and human influenza viruses could result in a reassortant virus that transmits efficiently between humans. The pandemic reassortant virus will display the avian HA and transmit between humans, and its lethality in humans will depend on the final composition of its avian and human genomic segments. Alternatively, the direct adaptation of a pathogenic avian strain during the infection of humans could result in a variant comprising exclusively avian genomic segments, which efficiently transmits between humans. If this variant is derived by minimal sequence alterations, it may retain its high lethality in humans. Moreover, the adaptation of an avian virus comprising exclusively avian genomic segments that transmits efficiently in humans raises the possibility that this strain may cocirculate between and within the human and bird populations. Such a variant would dramatically enhance the transmission

characteristics of infection in both the bird and human populations and make the task of local containment and control of the global spread of pandemic disease more difficult. The probability of the adaptation in humans of an avian strain with these lethality and transmission characteristics is not known but should not be discounted. Our knowledge of the ecology and epidemiologic development of influenza is rudimentary. Few influenza authorities would have anticipated the unprecedented emergence and global spread of a highly pathogenic avian influenza strain from domestic poultry that induced lethal disease by the direct infection of humans and wild waterfowl in 1996.

Control of Influenza Infections in Humans

Vaccines prevent many infectious diseases in humans and are regarded as the most successful medical intervention to date. Despite the value they represent to society, vaccines only comprise 2% of the total global pharmaceutical market (Rappuoli et al., 2002). The main reason for this paradox is financial in that successful vaccines provide a low return on investment because they progressively eliminate disease and ultimately erode their own market. Influenza is an exception in that vaccines against epidemic disease induce protective immunity against the surface HA of circulating variants. New genetic influenza variants are not recognized by the protective antibodies in the human population and require the annual develop-ment of new vaccines to control epidemic disease. Pandemics are initiated in humans by the introduction of an influenza subtype that displays a novel HA, which transmits infection to naive members of the population. The control of pandemics is difficult because disease outbreak in the population must occur before the causative strain can be identified and the isolate made available for manufacturers to initiate vaccine development. Thereafter, it is a race to produce sufficient vaccine to protect the population before the highly contagious acute disease spreads globally and achieves peak infection rates. In contrast, genetic variants of the pandemic strain circulate in the human population causing annual epidemics. These strains are identified by surveillance and the candidates selected early in the spring, allowing time for vaccine production for the coming winter influenza season.

Control of Influenza Epidemic Infections

Annual influenza epidemics are caused by genetic variants of the influenza type A and B viruses circulating in the human population. The predominant A type virus variants currently circulating are derived from subtype H3N2 which initiated the 1968 pandemic and the 1918 pandemic strain H1N1 which reemerged in Tianjin, China, in 1977 (Cox & Subbarao, 2000). The influenza B strain variants currently circulating are derived predominantly from B/Victoria/2/87 which reemerged in

Asia in 2000–2001 and spread globally, causing widespread human epidemic outbreaks (Shaw et al., 2002). The control of epidemics caused by these variants is achieved by the use of two vaccine types: an inactivated viral vaccine and a cold-adapted attenuated live vaccine. New vaccines are developed annually because of genetic variants that circumvent the HA-specific protective immunity in the human population.

The current inactivated vaccine contains antigen from the three viral strains, two influenza A strains and one influenza B strain, selected annually by the Vaccine and Related Biological Products Advisory Committee (VRBPAC) of the FDA using the WHO Influenza Surveillance Data. The selection of strains occurs in spring and the vaccine is available for distribution in late fall. The annual trivalent vaccine is prepared by a process developed in the 1940s in which vaccine virus grown in germ-free embryonated chicken eggs is inactivated chemically, purified, disrupted, and formulated for delivery by injection. This process requires specialized facilities for handling large quantities of eggs and is limited by the availability of germ-free eggs, the generation of egg-adapted viruses, and the retention of sterility during egg inoculation and viral harvest. Following the selection of variant viruses, the preparation of the annual vaccine and its safety and potency testing takes 7–8 months. The estimated total global production of epidemic influenza vaccine in 2003 was approximately 300 million doses, 65% of which was produced in Europe by Sanofi Aventis, Glaxo Smith Kline, and Novartis/Chiron (PAHO Meeting, 2005).

Improvements in Inactivated Influenza Vaccines

The growth of virus for vaccines in cell culture is the subject of research and development to improve the quantity and quality of the antigen (Brown et al., 1999). This is important because the supply of germ-free eggs is limited and difficult to manipulate and retain sterility. Moreover, a significant portion of the human population has acquired allergies to egg proteins, which obviate their use in current influenza vaccines. The clinical evaluation and marketing of a cell-based influenza vaccine is anticipated within the next decade. The use of adjuvants that enhance immune responses and reduce the amount of antigen in inactivated vaccines is under evaluation by US and European agencies. These advances will improve the production process and the yield of inactivated influenza vaccines.

Live Attenuated Cold-Adapted Influenza Vaccine

Recently, attenuated live vaccines have been developed using cold-adapted virus as an alternative annual vaccine for prevention of epidemic influenza (Maassab & Bryant, 1999). The HA and NA of the three variants selected for the annual vaccine are expressed in cold-adapted viruses that are delivered to recipients by nasal spray.

The manufacturer of this vaccine, Medimmune, estimated in 2006 a production capacity of 15 million doses per month. These vaccines are effective and currently represent a small fraction of the influenza vaccine sales, limited by novelty and cost. There is also a concern that the circulation of live influenza vaccines in the human population could facilitate the formation of pathogenic reassortants with a coinfecting influenza virus in recipients.

Both of these vaccines are primarily marketed in the developed world and segments of the developing world population. Despite the annual distribution of new vaccines, epidemics cause approximately 20,000–30,000 deaths annually in the USA. In a survey in the USA from 1972 to 1992, the cumulative epidemic influenza deaths were 426,000 individuals (Simonsen et al., 1997). The reason for this was problems with distribution methods and complacency among recipients. In the USA, annual direct costs due to influenza hospitalizations in 1981 were $1–3 billion and the socio-economic burden was $10–15 billion (Szucs, 1999). It is difficult to determine the annual global deaths due to epidemics, but WHO estimates are between 250,000 and 500,000 individuals worldwide each year (World Health Organization, 2003). The major cause of mortality is the lack of vaccine availability and its distribution throughout the developing world. The cumulative deaths due to epidemic influenza indicate its equivalent importance to the pandemic disease and the need for improved vaccines and their distribution.

Control of Pandemic Influenza Outbreaks

Pandemic disease is initiated when a new viral subtype spreads within the human population due to a lack of immunity against its novel HA. Once the pandemic strain is identified and made available to vaccine manufacturers it takes 6–8 months to prepare the vaccine for distribution. The key issue for the protection of the human population is that the vaccine be available before the global spread of pandemic disease and the establishment of major infections within the population. The records from previous pandemic outbreaks during the twentieth century indicate that major pandemic diseases were prevalent or at peak level before adequate stocks of vaccine were produced.

In 1957, the disease started in southern China and Hong Kong in April. By August, within 3 months of the availability of the vaccine strain for manufacture, production was at maximum capacity in the USA.. However, the first pandemic disease wave started in the USA in August and peaked in November, and only 48 million doses of vaccine were produced. So within 6 months, insufficient vaccine had been prepared to control the first disease wave (Wood, 2001).

In 1968, the strain was available in September and vaccine production started within 2 months, in November. However within 4 months of starting vaccine production, the disease was at peak within the USA with only 20 million doses of vaccine available (Murray, 1969).

In 1976, a pandemic alert was initiated by an outbreak of "swine flu" in Fort Dix and vaccine manufacturers prepared 150 million doses of vaccine within 3 months, sufficient to protect the entire US population. This outstanding yield of vaccine was achieved using a new reassortant virus that showed high growth in eggs and the assurance by the government of a market for all the vaccine produced (Wood, 2001). The process was extended by 2 months because of the passing of indemnification legislation for the assurance of vaccine sales and new vaccine safety and standardization procedures and independent vaccine testing by the FDA. Despite improved production capacity, the overall period for vaccine distribution was still 7–8 months (Barry et al., 1977).

In 1997, the occurrence of 18 human infections by the avian influenza virus H5N1 in Hong Kong resulted in the declaration of a pandemic alert, consistent with the new WHO Pandemic Preparedness Plan (World Health Organization, 1999). Due to the lack of human-to-human transmission of H5N1, large-scale vaccine production was postponed and only the early stages of vaccine development were undertaken. Yet, to produce the first samples of vaccine for small-scale clinical evaluation it took 7 months, much longer than in alerts in 1957, 1968, and 1976. A reason for this delay was that the pathogenicity of the H5N1 isolate in humans required the stringent use of biological containment facilities (BSL 3+) to manipulate the viral isolates. In addition, the lethality of H5N1 virus in embryonated eggs required the application of reverse genetics to produce an attenuated surrogate to produce vaccine virus in eggs (Wood, 2001).

An important issue with pandemic vaccines is that, because the protective HA antigen is new, many recipients in the population are immunologically naive. During the pandemics of 1957 and 1968, the infants and young adults were naive, whereas the older members of the population had been primed by previous infection with related strains. In contrast, in the current H5N1 pandemic alert, the entire global population is immunologically naive to the HA H5 in the new subtype. Immunity against the NA N1 may reduce disease severity and exhibit a biphasic distribution in the human population represented by two distinct age groups. These populations include individuals over 50 years of age who were infected by H1N1 before its disappearance from circulation in humans in 1957 and young adults under 29 years of age infected by H1N1 which inexplicably resumed circulation in 1977.

Clinical studies in the last quarter of the twentieth century using three subtypes H1N1, H2N2, and H5N3 in naive recipients demonstrated a need for high antigen concentration in single-dose vaccines or two inoculations of vaccine with a lower antigen dose (Wood, 2001). This indicates that much more antigen will be required to be produced to generate vaccines for unprimed recipients. Moreover, time must be allocated to evaluate clinically the antigen dose required to induce protective immunity in a naive population.

So despite the early vaccine development efforts already accomplished for a H5N1 vaccine, it will require tremendous coordination to produce and distribute vaccine to control an H5N1pandemic outbreak. First, the viral strain must be isolated in containment facilities and the surface antigens manipulated and attenuated for safe and effective growth of vaccine virus in secured stocks of germ-free eggs.

Following the coordinated production of vaccine by different manufacturers, the safety and efficacy of the final product must be evaluated in animal and human studies. Finally, when vaccine is produced, it must be distributed and administered to the population in an orderly sequence to protect individuals at high risk, infants and the elderly, and those who fulfill essential social functions, followed by general distribution. Vaccine distribution and administration rely on the public health infrastructure within each country. Even in developed countries, there has been a progressive erosion of public health services, which is evidenced by the difficulties many countries, including the USA, have in administering the annual epidemic influenza vaccine. The situation in many developing countries is dire because the deficiencies in their public health personnel and infrastructure make the distribution of vaccine to their populations extremely difficult (Brugha et al., 2002).

It is clear that during pandemic alerts it is very difficult to prepare sufficient vaccine before the disease peaks in the population. This problem is more pronounced now than in 1957 and 1968 because the population has grown significantly, requiring more vaccine and the disease will spread more rapidly because of the vast increase in global travel (Garrett, 1994).

Containment of Pandemic Outbreaks at Site of Origin

Recently, two independent groups investigated the concept of attempting to contain and eliminate emerging pandemic disease at the source from which the viral variant originated by computer modeling (Ferguson et al., 2005; Longini et al., 2005). Both groups advocate a combination of quarantine (social distancing) and antiviral therapy using oseltamivir to treat infected individuals and as a prophylactic for healthy contacts and the local population. Longini et al. also suggest using a poorly matched H5N1 vaccine if it is available. The modeling data suggest that if the exercise is started within weeks of the first transmissible infection and the disease spread is relatively slow, it would be possible within their programming parameters to contain the spread of the pandemic variant. This computer-based outcome relies on the early identification of a single outbreak epicenter in rural Thailand, the rapid and coordinated delivery of antivirals and vaccine, the staff to implement medical treatment and enforce quarantine, and the cooperation of the local indigenous population. It also assumes the efficacy of antiviral treatment of infections caused by the highly genetically variable influenza viruses and does not take into account that resistance to this antiviral has been detected in certain H5N1 infections of humans in southeast Asia (Le et al., 2005). These modeling data are encouraging and suggest that under ideal circumstances this approach may contain an emerging pandemic or at least delay its spread, and thus increase the time available for the production of an effective vaccine. Yet from a practical point of view, a disease spreading with predetermined characteristics and constraints within the confines of a computer program is far removed from the reality of its dissemination in the tropical rural communities of an impoverished southeast Asian country.

Pandemic Preparedness Plans

The procedures that define the stages of pandemic disease outbreak and international and national responses are outlined in the WHO Pandemic Preparedness Plan (World Health Organization, 1999) and reports prepared by a number of national health agencies. The WHO defines six phases in the establishment of a pandemic: two phases are interpandemic, during which old and new viral strains that pose a risk to humans are confined to animal populations; three phases of pandemic alert, during which a new virus from animals infects humans and gradually evolves the capacity to transmit between humans; and one phase of pandemic, which is declared following increased and sustained transmission of disease within the general population. The current situation (in 2006) is a pandemic alert phase 3, declared in 1997, in which the H5N1 from domestic birds infects humans without significant transmission between humans and is spreading around the globe because of the infection of wild migratory aquatic birds.

During a pandemic outbreak, the Preparedness Plan requires the coordination of rapid and disciplined responses by international and national agencies, pharmaceutical companies, healthcare workers, and essential government and service employees. This outcome may be difficult to achieve, given the history of poor interactions and territorial disputes among many agencies and the complex chain of command that would impede prompt and focused actions by essential civilian and military personnel. Responses to natural disasters on the national and international levels are replete with examples of these problems.

In an upcoming pandemic, it is not possible to predict either the number of infections in the population that will need medical treatment or the timing and extent of lethal infections. Most preparedness plans do not articulate a clear organizational response to outbreaks with either different levels of infections in the population that require medical treatment or hospitalization, or the coordination of social and essential services required to handle various levels of lethality of disease in the population. The majority of preparedness plans anticipate a disease profile of low-lethality infections in humans. This seems peculiar when confronted by the global spread of an avian strain H5N1 which exhibits unprecedented lethal infections of humans (Writing Committee of the World Health Organization Consultation on Human Influenza A/H5, 2005). Assuming the upcoming pandemic would exhibit transmission and lethality characteristics similar to the pandemic of 1918, with the present-day population six times larger, the lethality estimates would range from 120 to 600 million.

Despite advances in medical treatments, the health system would be soon overwhelmed by the number of acute infections that would occur over a short time span. In addition, the social and essential services dealing with the large number of deaths over a short timeframe would face enormous logistical difficulties. These are clearly complex and sensitive issues, but failure to adequately address them undermines the concept of preparedness and fails to inform the general population of the constructive roles they could undertake to minimize the disruption of essential social services and unrest within the population.

Development of Cross-Protective Influenza Vaccines

Since the last influenza pandemic in 1968, there have been great advances in the technologies that identify and sequence new influenza variants, define their transmission within bird and mammalian populations, and unravel their infection and growth characteristics in cells. However, little progress has occurred in the generation of new influenza vaccines for the prevention of epidemic and pandemic outbreaks. The derivation of an influenza vaccine that induces cross-protective immunity against all viral subtypes that infect humans would yield a universal vaccine impervious to variations in the surface glycoproteins HA and NA. The ideal cross-protective vaccine would induce long-lived immunity against all subtypes of human influenza virus and avian subtypes that infect humans, and thereby eliminate epidemic and pandemic diseases. This concept was first established by researchers at CDC in 1995 (Slepushkin et al., 1995) and has been subsequently confirmed and extended by academic and pharmaceutical groups reviewed later.

The influenza virus displays three membrane proteins, the HA and NA which demonstrate continuous sequence variation and the M2 protein whose sequence is highly conserved. The 97 amino acids of the M2 protein comprise three domains: 24 extracellular residues, 19 transmembrane residues, and 54 intracellular residues (Lamb et al., 1985). The M2 protein is a homotetramer composed of two disulfide-linked dimers that assemble across the cell membrane to form a proton-selective ion channel (Sugrue & Hay, 1991). Sequencing studies show that M2 protein is highly conserved and that the extracellular domain shows very little change in all human viruses sequenced since the first human virus was isolated in 1933 (Ito et al., 1991; Fiers et al., 2004). The M2 protein is present in low concentration on the virion surface but is abundantly represented on the surface of influenza-infected cells (Lamb et al., 1985; Zebedee & Lamb, 1988). M2 mediates proton influx into endosomes which results in the dissociation of the viral ribonucleoprotein from the matrix protein facilitating the replication of viral RNA (Helenius, 1992). Consistent with this role in viral multiplication, a monoclonal antibody that attaches to the M2 extracellular domain inhibits viral replication in cell culture and in infected mice (Zebedee & Lamb, 1988; Treanor et al., 1990).

The analysis of convalescent sera from humans infected with the influenza A virus H3N2 demonstrated the presence of antibodies to the M2 protein (Black et al., 1993). Studies at CDC demonstrated that an M2/insect fusion protein induced heterosubtypic antibodies in mice that conferred protection against a lethal heterologous viral challenge (Slepushkin et al., 1995). These data were confirmed and it was demonstrated that cross-protective immunity could be induced by the 24 highly conserved amino acids of the extracellular domain of M2 when presented in soluble fusion proteins and virus-like particles (Nierynck et al., 1999; Mozdzanowska et al., 2003; Fan et al., 2004; Liu et al., 2004; Ionescu et al., 2006). These studies demonstrated that the cross-protective immune response based on antibodies was long lasting and could be significantly enhanced by the presentation of multiple copies of the M2 sequence in soluble recombinant proteins or virus-like particles and when formulated with appropriate adjuvants. It was shown that these M2 recombinant proteins induced cross-protective antibodies in rodents, ferrets and rhesus monkeys. Moreover, conserved sequences have been identified from other influenza proteins including HA, nucleoprotein, and matrix proteins that induce cross-protective immunity in rodents (Levi & Arnon, 1996; Epstein et al., 2002).

The databanks of the influenza genome sequences of human and avian subtypes and variants (Ghedin et al., 2005; Obenauer et al., 2006) can be utilized to collate the entire repertoire of conserved sequences and define their subtype distribution. Those sequences shown individually to induce immunity would be assembled into a multivalent recombinant protein. The arrangement and number of individual epitopes within the recombinant protein can be adjusted to assure the optimal induction of robust cross-protective immunity against all human viral subtypes and those avian subtypes that infect humans. These recombinant proteins can be prepared as stable soluble products or virus-like particles in bacterial or insect expression systems and formulated with appropriate adjuvants for clinical evaluation in humans. A successful clinical outcome would lead to an affordable subunit vaccine for administration to children within the pediatric schedule, which, with appropriate boosting, would confer lifelong immunity against influenza infection. Ideally, a successful universal influenza vaccine would eliminate both epidemic and pandemic diseases and the associated mortality and socioeconomic burdens.

The same approach could be used to define the equivalent conserved sequences in avian, swine, and equine influenzas, and develop universal vaccines that protect these domestic animals and limit the enzootic spread of influenza viruses.

The successful development of universal influenza vaccines would ideally confine influenza strains to the wild aquatic bird population and obviate disease in domestic animals and humans. The investment to develop such vaccines would be minimal compared to funds currently dedicated to global surveillance, annual epidemic vaccine development, and the effort of preparing for upcoming pandemics, not to mention the direct costs and the socioeconomic burden of annual epidemic and periodic pandemic disease.

The achievement of this goal will require the formation of an international organization with an unwavering dedication to the development of vaccines for the global control of infectious diseases including influenza. This new organization would need adequate funding, with a mandate to oversee the global control of infectious disease without national, regional, or a for-profit bias. This concept of a Global Infectious Disease Authority has been previously described (Roberts & Lu, 2004).

Conclusion

The control of influenza infections in humans is in serious need of modernization and improvement. The control of annual epidemics relies on antiquated vaccine production methodologies that generate insufficient quantities of vaccine for the effective protection of the human population. The control of pandemic outbreaks by vaccination is improbable because experience from the pandemics of 1957 and

1968 clearly demonstrates that the global spread and the peak of infection in the population preceded the manufacture of significant quantities of vaccine. The growth of the human population and its global mobility will assure rapid pandemic spread and will require more vaccine in a shorter time period than in previous outbreaks.

The large-scale monoculture of domestic birds has facilitated the unprecedented evolution and widespread dissemination of highly pathogenic avian viruses that cause not only lethal infections of poultry but also directly transmit disease to wild birds and humans. The infection of humans by the avian subtype H5N1 causes severe disease that is highly lethal but it is currently limited by the lack of transmission between humans. A variant of this highly pathogenic strain that transmits efficiently between humans would result in the global spread of this highly contagious infection that could rapidly overwhelm medical and societal infrastructures and lead to widespread deaths and political and social unrest. The threat posed by influenza infections to human society transcends that of most infectious diseases and dwarfs natural disasters and terrorist threats. The recent changes in influenza evolution and transmission calls for a global initiative to develop more effective vaccines that produce broad cross-protective immunity and eliminate epidemic and pandemic diseases in humans.

References

Almond, J. W. (1977). A single gene determines the host range of influenza. *Nature*, 270, 617–618.

Alexander, D.J. (2000). A Review of avian influenza in different bird species. Veterinary Microbiology 74, 3–13.

Baigent, S. J., & McCauley, J. W. (2003). Influenza type A in humans, mammals and birds: Determinants of virus host-range and interspecies transmission. *BioEssays*, 25, 657–671.

Banks, J., Speidel, E. C., McCauley, J. W., & Alexander, D. J. (2000). Phylogenetic analysis of H7 hemagglutinin subtype influenza A viruses. *Archives of Virology*, 145, 1047–1058.

Banks, J., Speidel, E. C., Moore, E., Plowright, L., Piccirillo, A., Capua, I., Cordioli, P., Fioretti, A., & Alexander, D. J. (2001). Changes in the hemagglutinin and the neuraminidase genes prior to the emergence of highly pathogenic H7N1 avian influenza viruses in Italy. *Archives of Virology*, 146, 963–973.

Barry, J. M. (2004). *The Great Influenza*. Penguin, Harmondsworth.

Barry, D. W., Mayner, R. E., Meisler, J. M., & Seligmann Jr., E. B. (1977). Evaluation and control of vaccines for the National Influenza Immunization Program. *Journal of Infectious Diseases*, 136, S407–S414.

Bean, W. J., & Webster, R. G. (1978). Phenotypic properties associated with influenza genome segments. In *Negative Strand Viruses and the Host Cell* (Mahy, B. W. J., & Barry, R. D., Eds), pp. 685–692. Academic, London.

Black, R. A., Rota, P. A., Gorodkova, N., Klenk, H. D., & Kendal, A. P. (1993). Antibody response of the M2 protein of influenza A virus expressed in insect cells. *Journal of General Virology*, 74, 143–146.

Bright, R. A., Shay, D. K., Shu, B., Cox, N. J., & Klimov, A. I. (2006). Adamatane resistance among Influenza A viruses isolated early during the 2005–2006 influenza season in the United States. *JAMA*, 295(8), 891–894.

Brown, F., Robertson, J. S., Schild, G. C., & Wood, J. M. (1999). Inactivated influenza vaccines prepared in cell culture. *Developments in Biological Standardization*, 98.

Brugha, R., Sterling, M., & Walt, G. (2002). GAVI, the first steps: Lessons for the Global Fund. *Lancet*, 359, 435–438.

Capua, I., & Alexander, D. J. (2004). Avian influenza: Recent developments. *Avian Pathology*, 33, 393–404.

Capua, I., & Marangon, S. (2000). The avian influenza epidemic in Italy, 1999–2000: a review. *Avian Pathology*, 29, 289–294.

Chen, H., Smith, G. J. D., Zhang, S. Y., Qin, K., Wang, J., Li, K. S., Webster, R. G., Peiris, J. S. M., & Guan, Y. (2005). H5N1 virus outbreak in migratory waterfowl. *Nature*, 436, 191–192.

Cleaveland, S., Laurenson, M. K., & Taylor, L. H. (2001). Diseases of humans and their domestic mammals: Pathogen characteristics, host range and the risk of emergence. *Philosophical Transactions of the Royal Society of London. Series B*, 356, 991–999.

Connor, R. J., Kawaoka, Y., Webster, R. G., & Paulson, J. C. (1994). Receptor specificity in human, avian and equine H2 and H3 influenza isolates. *Virology*, 205, 17–23.

Cox, N. J., & Subbarao, K. (2000). Global epidemiology of influenza: Past and present. *Annual Reviews of Medicine*, 51, 407–421.

Daly, J. M., Newton, J. R., & Mumford, J. A. (2004). Current perspectives on control of equine influenza. *Veterinary Research*, 35, 411–423.

Epstein, S. L., Tumpey, T. M., Misplon, J. A., Lo, C-Y., Cooper, L. A., Subbarao, K., Renshaw, M., Sambhara, S., & Katz, J. M. (2002). DNA vaccine expressing conserved influenza virus proteins protective against H5N1 challenge infection in mice. *Emerging Infectious Diseases*, 8, 796–801.

Fan, J., Liang, X., Horton, M. S., Perry, H. C., Citron, M. P., Heidecker, G. J., Fu, T-M., Joyce, J., Przysiecki, C. T., Keller, P. M., Garsky, V. M., Ionescu, R., Rippeon, Y., Shi, L., Chastain, M. A., Condra, J. H., Davies, M-E., Liao, J., Emini, E. A., & Shiver, J. W. (2004). Preclinical study of influenza virus A M2 peptide conjugate vaccines in mice, ferrets and rhesus monkeys. *Vaccine*, 22, 2993–3003.

Ferguson, N. M., Cummings, D. A. T., Cauchemez, S., Fraser, C., Riley, S., Meeyai, A., Iamsirithaworn, S., & Burke, D. S. (2005). Strategies for containing an emerging influenza pandemic in Southeast Asia. *Nature*, 437, 209–214.

Fiers, W., De Filette, M., Birkett, A., Nierynck, S., & Min Jou, W. (2004). A universal influenza A vaccine. *Virus Research*, 103, 173–176.

Fouchier, R. A. M., Osterhaus, A. D. M. E., & Brown, I. H. (2003). Animal influenza virus surveillance. *Vaccine*, 21, 1754–1757.

Francis Jr., T., Salk, J. E., & Quilligan, J. J. J. (1947). Experience with vaccination against influenza in the spring of 1947. *American Journal of Public Health*, 37, 1013–1016.

Gambaryan, A. S., Piskarev, V. E., Yamskov, I. A., Sakharov, A. M., Tuzikov, A. B., Bovin, N. V., Nifant'ev, N. E., & Matrosovich, M. N. (1995). Human influenza virus recognition of oligosaccharides. *FEBS Letters*, 366, 57–60.

Garcia, M., Crawford, J. M., Latimer, J. W., RiveraCruz, E., & Perdue, M. L. (1996). Heterogeneity in the hemagglutinin gene and emergence of the highly pathogenic phenotype among recent H5N2 avian influenza strains in Mexico. *Journal of General Virology*, 77, 1493–1504.

Garrett, L. (1994). *The Coming Plague: Newly Emerging Diseases in a World Out of Balance*. Farrar, Strauss and Giroux, New York.

Ghedin, E., Sengamalay, N. A., Shumway, M., Zaborsky, J., Feldblyum, T., Subbu, V., Spiro, D. J., Sitz, J., Koo, H., Bolotov, P., Dernovoy, D., Tatusova, T., Bao, Y., St George, K., Taylor, J. U., Lipman, D. J., Fraser, C. M., Taubenberger, J. K., & Salzberg, S. L. (2005). Large-scale sequencing of human influenza reveals the dynamic nature of viral genome evolution. *Nature*, 437, 1162–1166.

Glezen, W.P. (1996) Emerging Infections: Pandemic Influenza. Epidemiologic Reviews 18(1), 64–76.

Harvey, R., Martin, A. C. R., Zambon, M., & Barclay, W. S. (2004). Restrictions to the adaptation of influenza A virus H5 hemagglutinin to the human host. *Journal of Virology*, 78, 502–507.

Hayden, F., & Croisier, A. (2005). Transmission of avian influenza viruses to and between humans. *Journal of Infectious Diseases*, 192, 1311–1314.

Helenius, A. (1992). Unpacking the incoming influenza virus. *Cell*, 69, 577–578.

Hilleman, M. R. (1999). Personal historical chronicle of six decades of basic and applied research in virology, immunology and vaccinology. *Immunological Reviews*, 170, 7–27.

Hinshaw, V. S., Webster, R. G., & Turner, B. (1980). The perpetuation of orthomyxoviruses and paramyxoviruses in Canadian waterfowl, *Journal of Microbiology*, 26, 622–629.

Horimoto, T., & Kawaoka, Y. (2001). Pandemic threat posed by avian influenza A viruses. *Clinical Microbiology Reviews*, 14, 129–149.

Ionescu, R. M., Przysiecki, C. T., Liang, X., Garsky, V. M., Fan, J., Wang, B., Troutman, R., Pippeon, Y, Flanagan, E., Shiver, J., & Shi, L. (2006). Pharmaceutical and immunological evaluation of human papillomavirus viruslike particle as an antigen carrier. *Journal of Pharmaceutical Science*, 95, 70–79.

Ito, T., Gorman, O. T., Kawaoka, Y., Bean, W. J., & Webster, R. G. (1991). Evolutionary analysis of the influenza A virus M gene with comparison of the M1 and M2 proteins. *Journal of Virology*, 65, 5491–5498.

Karasin, A. I., Olsen, C. W., & Anderson, G. A. (2000). Genetic characterization of an H1N2 influenza isolated from a pig in Indiana. *Journal of Clinical Microbiology*, 38, 2453–2456.

Kawaoka, Y., Krauss, S., & Webster, R. G. (1989). Avian to human transmission of the PB1 gene of influenza A viruses in the 1957 and 1968 pandemics. *Journal of Virology*, 63, 4603–4608.

Koen, J. S. (1919). A practical method for field diagnosis of swine diseases. *American Journal of Veterinary Medicine*, 14, 468–470.

Lamb, R. A., Zebedee, S. L., & Richardson, C. D. (1985). Influenza virus M2 protein is an integral membrane protein expressed on the infected-cell surface. *Cell*, 40, 627–633.

Le, Q. M., Kiso, M., Someya, K., Sakai, Y., Nguyen, T, H., Nguyen, K. H. L., Dinh Pham, N., Nguyen, H. N., Yamada, S., Muramoto, Y. Horimoto, T., Takada, A., Goto, H. Suzuki, T., Suzuki, Y., & Kawaoka, Y. (2005). Isolation of drug resistant H5N1 virus. *Nature*, 437, 1108.

Levi, R., & Arnon, R. (1996). Synthetic recombinant influenza vaccine induces efficient long-term immunity and cross strain protection. *Vaccine*, 14, 85–92.

Liu, W., Peng, Z., Liu, Z., Lu, Y., Ding, J., & Chen, Y-H. (2004). High epitope density in a single recombinant protein molecule of the extracellular domain of influenza A virus M2 protein significantly enhances protective immunity. *Vaccine*, 23, 366–371.

Longini, I. M., Nizam, A., Xu, S., Ungchusak, K., Hanshaoworakul, W., Cummings, D. A. T., & Halloran, M. E. (2005). Containing pandemic influenza at the source. *Science*, 309, 1083–1087.

Luk, J., Gross, P., & Thompson, W. W. (2001). Observations on mortality during the 1918 influenza pandemic. *Clinical Infectious Diseases*, 33, 1375–1378.

Maassab, H. F., & Bryant, M. L. (1999). The development of live attenuated cold adapted influenza virus vaccine for humans. *Reviews in Medical Virology*, 9, 237–244.

Matrosovitch, M., Tuzikov, A., Bovin, N., Gambaryan, A., Klimov, A., Castrucci, M. R., Donatelli, I., & Kawaoka, Y. (2000). Early alterations of the receptor-binding properties of H1, H2 and H3 avian influenza virus hemagglutinins after their introduction into mammals. *Journal of Virology*, 74, 8502–8512.

McMichael, A. J. (2004). Environmental and social influences on emerging infectious diseases: Past, present and future. *Philosophical Transactions of the Royal Society of London. Series B*, 359, 1049–1058.

Mozdzanowska, K., Feng, J. Q., Eid, M., Kragol, G., Cudic, M., Otvos, L., & Gerhard, W. (2003). Induction of Influenza type A virus specific resistance by immunization of mice with a synthetic multiple antigenic peptide vaccine that contains ectodomains of matrix protein 2. *Vaccine*, 21, 2616–2626.

Murphy, F. A. (1996). Virus taxonomy. In *Virology* (Fields, B. N., Knipe, D. M. & Howley, P. M., Eds.), pp. 15–57, Lippincott-Raven, Philadelphia.

Murray, R. (1969). Production and testing in the USA of influenza virus vaccine made from the Hong Kong variant in 1868–69. *Bulletin of the World Health Organization*, 41, 495–496.

Naeem, K. (1998). The avian influenza outbreak in South Central Asia. In Proceedings of the International Symposium on Avian Influenza American Association of Avian Pathologists. Pennsylvania, Athens, Georgia, USA, pp. 31–35.

Nierynck, S., Deroo, T., Saelens, X., Vanlandschoot, P., Min Lou, W., & Fiers, W. (1999). A universal influenza A vaccine based on the extracellular domain of the M2 protein. *Nature Medicine*, 5, 1157–1163.

Nobusawa, E., Ishihara, H., Morishita, T., Sato, K., & Nakajima, K. (2000). Change in receptor-binding specificity of recent human influenza A viruses (H3N2): A single amino acid change in hemagglutinin altered its recognition of sialyloligosaccharides. *Virology*, 278, 587–596.

Obenauer, J. C., Denson, J., Mehta, P. K., Su, X., Mukatira, S., Finkelstein, D. B., Xu, X., Wang, J., Ma, J., Fan, Y., Rakestraw, K. M., Webster, R. G., Hoffman, E., Krauss, S., Zheng, J., Zhang, Z., & Naeve, C. W. (2006). Large-scale sequence analysis of avian influenza isolates. *Science*, 311, 1576–1580.

Oxford, J. S., McGeoch, D. J., Schild, G. C., & Beare, A. S. (1978). Analysis of virion RNA segments and polypeptides of influenza A virus recombinants of defined virulence. *Nature*, 273, 778–779.

PAHO Meeting. (2005). *Avian Influenza and Pandemic Preparedness: The Vaccine Industry Perspective*. Washington, DC, 21 November 2005.

Palumbi, S.R. (2001). Humans as the world's greatest evolutionary force. Science. 293,5536,1786–1790.

Payne, A. M. (1953). The influenza programme of WHO. *Bulletin of the World Health Organization*, 8, 755–774.

Perdue, M., Crawford, J., Garcia, M., Latimer, J., & Swayne, D. (1998). Occurrence and possible mechanisms of cleavage site insertions in the avian influenza hemagglutinin gene. In Proceedings of the 4th International Symposium on Avian Influenza. Athens, Georgia, USA, pp. 182–193.

Perroncito, E. (1878). Epizoozia tifoide nei gallinacei. *Annals of the Academy of Agriculture*, 21, 87–93.

Petersen, L. R., & Roehrig, J. T. (2001). West Nile Virus: A reemerging global pathogen. *Emerging Infectious Disease*, 7(4), 611–614.

Potter, C. W. (2001). A history of influenza. *Journal of Applied Microbiology*, 91, 572–579.

Puzelli, S., Di Trani, L., Fabiani, C., Campitelli, L., De Marco, M. A., Capua, I, Aguilera, J. F., Zambom, M., & Donatelli, I. (2005). Serological analysis of serum samples from humans exposed to avian H7 influenza viruses in Italy between 1999 and 2003. *Journal of Infectious Diseases*, 192, 1318–1322.

Rappuoli, R., Miller, H. I., & Falkow, S. (2002). The intangible value of vaccines. *Science*, 297, 937–939.

Reid, A. H., Fanning, T. G., Janczewski, T. A., Lourens, R. M., & Tanbenberger, J. K. (2004). Novel origin of the 1918 pandemic influenza virus nucleoprotein gene. *Journal of Virology*, 78, 12462–12470.

Roberts, B. E., & Lu, Y. (2004). *Infectious Diseases in Asia: Implications for Global Health in Aids in Asia* (Lu, Y. & Essex, M., Eds), Kluwer/Plenum, New York.

Rogers, G. N., Paulson, J. C., Daniels, R. S., Skehel, J. J., Wilson, I. A., & Wiley, D. C. (1983). Single amino acid substitutions in influenza haemagglutinin change receptor specificity. *Nature*, 304, 76–78.

Rohm, C., Horimoto, T., Kawaoka, Y., Suss, J., & Webster, R. G. (1995). Do hemagglutinin genes of highly pathogenic avian influenza viruses constitute unique phylogenetic lineages? *Virology*, 209, 664–670.

Rojas, H., Moreira, R., Avalos, P., & Marangon, S. (2002). Avian influenza in poultry in Chile. *Veterinary Record*, 151, 188.

Scholtissek, C., & Murphy, B. R. (1978). Host range mutants of an influenza A virus. *Archives of Virology*, 58, 323–333.

Shaw, M. W., Xu, X., Normand, S., Ueki, R. T., Kumimoto, G. Y., Hall, H, Kimov, A., Cox, N. J., & Subbarao, K. (2002). Reappearance and global spread of variants of influenza B/ Victoria/2/87 lineage viruses in the 2000–2001 and 2001–2002 seasons. *Virology*, 303, 1–8.

Shinya, K., Ebinall, M., Shinya, Y., Ono, M., Kasai, N., & Kawaoka, Y. (2006). Influenza virus receptors in the human airway. *Nature*, 440, 435–436.

Shope, R. E. (1931). Swine influenza filtration experiments and etiology. *Journal of Experimental Medicine*, 54, 373–385.

Simonsen, L., Clarke, M. J., Williamson, G. D., Stroup, D. F., Arden, N. H., & Schonberger, L. B. (1997). The impact of influenza epidemics on mortality: Introducing a severity index. *American Journal of Public Health*, 87, 1944–1950.

Simonsen, L., Clarke, M. J., Schonberger, L. B., et al. (1998). Pandemic versus epidemic influenza mortality: A pattern of changing age distribution. *Journal of Infectious Diseases*, 178, 53–60.

Slepushkin, V.A., Katz, J.M., Black R.A., Gamble, W.A., Rota, P.A., & Cox, N.J. (1995). Protection of mice against influenza A virus challenge by vaccination with baculovirus-expressed M2 protein. Vaccine 13(15) 1399–1402.

Smith, W., Andrews, C. H., & Laidlaw, P. P. (1933). A virus obtained from influenza patients. *Lancet*, 2, 66–68.

Steinhauer, D. A. (1999). Minireview role of hemagglutinin cleavage for the pathogenicity of influenza virus. *Virology*, 258, 1–20.

Stevens, J., Blixt, O, Tumpey, T. M., Taubenberger, J. K., Paulson, J. C., & Wilson, I. A. (2006). Structure and receptor specificity of the hemagglutinin from an H5N1 influenza virus. *Sciencexpress Research article*, http://www.sciencexpress.org, 20 March 2006.

Sturm-Ramirez, K. M., Hulse-Post, D. J., Govorkova, E. A., Humberd, J., Seiler, P., Puthavathana, P., Buranathai, C., Nguyen, T. D. Chaisingh, A., Long, H. T., Naipospos, T. S. P., Chen, H., Ellis, T. M., Guan, Y., Peiris, J. S. M., & Webster, R. G. (2005). Are ducks contributing to the endemicity of highly pathogenic H5N1 influenza virus in Asia? *Journal of Virology*, 79, 11269–11279.

Sugrue, R. J., & Hay, A. J. (1991). Structural characteristics of the M2 protein of influenza A viruses: Evidence that it forms a tetrameric channel. *Virology*, 180, 617–624.

Szucs, T. (1999). The socio-economic burden of influenza. *The Journal of Antimicrobial Chemotherapy*, 44, Topic B, 11–15.

Tilman, D. (1999). Global environmental impacts of agricultural expansion: The need for sustainable and efficient practices. *Proceedings of the National Academy of Sciences of the United States of America*, 96, 5995–6000.

Treanor, J. J., Snyder, M. H., London, W. T., & Murphy, B. R. (1989). The B allele of the NS gene of avian influenza viruses but not the A allele attenuates a human influenza A virus for squirrel monkeys. *Virology*, 171, 1–9.

Treanor, J. J., Tierney, E. L., Zebedee, S. L., Lamb, R. A., & Murphy, B. R. (1990). Passively transferred monoclonal antibody to the M2 protein inhibits influenza A virus replication in mice. *Journal of Virology*, 64, 1375–1377.

Uiprasertkul, M., Puthavathana, P., Sangsiriwut, K., Pooruk, P., Srisook, K., Peiris, M., Nicholls, J. M., Chokephaibulkit, K., Vanprapar, N., & Auewarakul, P. (2005). Influenza A H5N1 replication sites in humans. *Emerging Infectious Diseases*, 11, 1036–1041.

United Nations. (2004). *World Population Prospects: The 2004 Revision*. United Nations, New York.

Van Riel, D., Munster, V. J. deWit, E. Rimmelzwaan, G. F., Fouchier, R. A. M., Osterhaus, A. D. M. E., & Kuiken, T. (2006). H5N1 virus attachment to lower respiratory tract. *Sciencexpress Brevia*, http://www.sciencexpress.org, 23 March 2006.

Vijayanand, P., Wilkins, E., & Woodhead, M. (2004). Severe acute respiratory syndrome (SARS): A review. *Clinical Medicine*, 4, 152–160.

Villarreal, C. L., & Flores, A. O. (1997). The Mexican avian influenza H5N2 outbreak. In Proceedings of the International Symposium on Avian Influenza American Association of Avian Pathologists, Pennsylvania, Athens, Georgia, USA, pp. 18–22.

Webby, R. J., Swenson, S. L., Krauss, S. L., Gerrish, P. J., Goyal, S. M., & Webster, R. G. (2000). Evolution of swine H3N2 influenza viruses in the United States. *Journal of Virology* 74, 8243–8251.

Webster, R. G., & Kawaoka, Y. (1988). Avian influenza. *Critical Reviews in Poultry Biology*, 1, 211–246.

Webster, R. G., & Laver W. G. (1972). The origin of pandemic influenza. *Bulletin of the World Health Organization*, 47, 449–452.

Webster, R. G., Bean, W. J., Gorman, O. T., Chambers, T. M., & Kawaoka, Y. (1992). Evolution and ecology of influenza A viruses. *Microbiological Reviews*, 56, 152–179.

Weiss, R. A., & McMichael, A. J. (2004). Social and environmental risk factors in the emergence of infectious diseases. *Nature Medicine*, 10(Suppl. 12), S70–S76.

Wood, J. M. (2001). Developing vaccines against pandemic influenza. *Philosophical Transactions of the Royal Society of London. Series B*, 356, 1953–1960.

World Health Organization. (1999). *Influenza Pandemic Preparedness Plan. The Role of WHO and Guidelines for National and Regional Planning*. WHO, Geneva.

World Health Organization. (2003). *Influenza Fact Sheet #211*, revised March 2003 WHO, Geneva.

Writing Committee of the World Health Organization Consultation on Human Influenza A/H5. (2005). Avian influenza A (H5N1) infections in humans. *New England Journal of Medicine*, 353, 1374–1385.

Zebedee, S. L., & Lamb, R. A. (1988). Influenza A virus M2 protein: Monoclonal antibody restriction of virus growth and detection of M2 in virions. *Journal of Virology*, 62, 2762–2772.

The Past and Present Threat of Avian Influenza in Thailand

Prasert Auewarakul

Abstract Avian influenza H5N1 infection was first identified in Thailand in January 2004. Since then, there have been three major outbreaks in the cold season of 2003–2004 and in the rainy and cold seasons of 2004–2005 and 2005–2006. More than 62 million birds died or were culled. The burden shifted from large industrial farming in the first outbreak to small farms, backyard chickens, and free-grazing ducks. Up to November 2005, there were 20 confirmed cases of human H5N1 infection. Thirteen of these died. Most of the confirmed cases were solitary ones except for three persons in a single family, and epidemiological evidence indicated that person-to-person transmission may have been involved in this cluster. However, sequence analysis of the virus in the cluster did not suggest any changes that might enhance the viral ability to get transmitted among humans. H5N1 viruses in Thailand and Vietnam belong to a single lineage genetically and are antigenically distinguishable from the viruses of the same genotype Z from southern China and Indonesia. Despite the seemingly subsiding epidemic in Thailand, the problem is far from resolved. H5N1 viruses are still sporadically isolated from domestic poultry as well as from wildlife. More important, isolates were also found in asymptomatic animals. Natural selection may have adapted the virus to a less aggressive form. This would make the virus more elusive and difficult to control. A threat of a pandemic strain emerging from the H5N1 virus is still imminent.

A national strategic plan for avian influenza control and influenza pandemic preparedness has been implemented. The plan aims at effective control of avian influenza spread in animals as well as in humans for a three-year period and at efficient pandemic preparedness within one year. Nevertheless, more regional and international collaboration is needed. With proper collective preparedness, there is a hope that the threatening influenza pandemic can be prevented by confining and eliminating a potential pandemic strain at its origin.

In December 2003, poultry farms in the eastern, central, and northern regions of Thailand experienced large-scale die-offs. The outbreak started from the eastern region of the country. The disease caused rapid death, with a very high attack rate. At that time, H5N1 outbreaks had been reported in South Korea, Vietnam, and Japan (OIE, 2005). A few humans with pneumonia were suspected to originate from contact with sick or dead poultry. Final diagnosis in these patients was not

Y. Lu et al. (eds.), *Emerging Infections in Asia.*
© Springer Science+Business Media, LLC 2008

done as clinical samples were not available at the time when proper diagnostic testing became available.

On 23 January 2004, the first case of human H5N1 infection in Thailand was reported. It was a boy from Kanchanaburi, a province about 100 km west of Bangkok. He was admitted to Siriraj Hospital in Bangkok and was diagnosed to have severe progressive pneumonia. The patient was initially treated with broad spectrum antibiotics, and respiratory samples were tested for influenza virus. The laboratory result showed that the patient harbored influenza virus, and sequencing of the viral RNA indicated that the virus belonged to the H5 subtype (Chokephaibulkit et al., 2005; Puthavathana et al., 2005). When this result was reported to the Ministry of Public Health, the government announced that there was a highly pathogenic avian influenza (AI) outbreak in Thailand. The Department of Livestock Development (DLD) confirmed the presence of H5N1 viruses in poultry on the same day. Subsequent analysis of the virus from patients and animals confirmed that it was H5N1 AI virus of genotype Z and was closely related to the virus from Vietnam (Viseshakul et al., 2004; Puthavathana et al., 2005).

The Course of Outbreaks in Humans and Poultry

Figure 1 shows the time distribution of the outbreak in humans and poultry in Thailand (DLD, 2005a). The outbreak activity has a clear seasonal variation. The disease activity starts at the beginning of the rainy season (July), peaks in October at the transition from the rainy season to winter, and subsides in March when summer starts. The first round of outbreaks in early 2004 was widely spread.

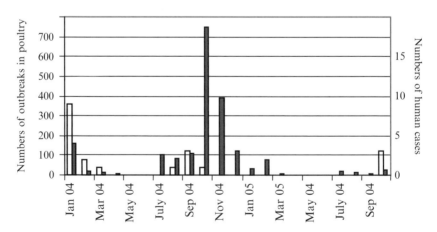

Fig. 1 Time distribution of avian influenza outbreaks in poultry (*solid bars*) and humans (*open bars*) in Thailand (DLD, 2005a)

Subsequent outbreaks in 2004 and 2005 had a more restricted geographical distribution. Most of the outbreaks were in the central and lower northern regions of the country, along the major river basin, where poultry density is the highest, especially free-grazing ducks (Fig. 2). Outbreaks in humans and poultry had similar time and geographical distributions, indicating poultry as the source of infection in humans. Repetitive outbreaks in same areas suggested that even though there was no apparent disease between the outbreaks, the virus remained resident either in domestic animals or wildlife in that area. The similarity of the viruses between the outbreaks further proved that latter outbreaks were caused by the remnant viruses from previous outbreaks and not by a reintroduced virus (Amonsin et al., 2005).

Up to the end of October 2005, there have been a total of 20 confirmed cases in humans, of which 13 died. Of the 20 cases, 12 were in the first round of the outbreak in the winter of 2003–2004, 5 were in the rainy season and winter of 2004, and 3 were in 2005 (Centers for Disease Control and Prevention, 2004; Beigel et al., 2005; Chotpitayasunondh et al., 2005). Besides these 20 cases, there were 23 suspected cases with comparable clinical and epidemiological features but lack laboratory confirmation. Most of the suspected cases were in the early part of the first outbreak when the laboratory test was not readily available and surveillance and specimen referral system had not been well established. They also had direct contact with dying poultry except for one cluster that probably resulted from person-to-person transmission (Ungchusak et al., 2005).

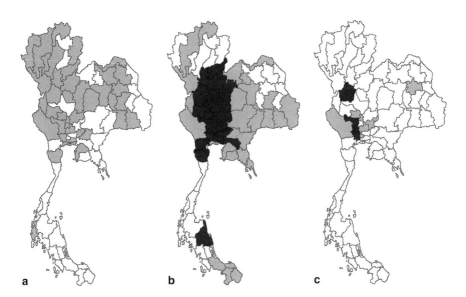

a   b   c

Fig. 2 Geographical distribution of the (**a**) first (January 2004 to April 2004), (**b**) second (July 2004 to March 2005), and (**c**) third rounds of avian influenza outbreaks (July 2005 to September 2005) in poultry. In (**b**) and (**c**), black and gray shades represent provinces with outbreaks involving more and less than 5,000 birds, respectively (DLD, 2005a)

Origin and Evolution of the Virus

All H5N1 AI viruses since the first outbreak in 1997 carry H5 and N1 genes that originated from a common ancestor closely related to a goose virus isolated from Guangdong in 1996 (A/Goose/Gaungdong/1/96) (Li et al., 2004). Although the virus responsible for the 1997 outbreak in Hong Kong was completely eliminated by a total depopulation of poultry on the island, the ancestral virus still circulated in southern China and gave rise to several genotypes by reassortment with other AI viruses. Since 1997, many of these genotypes have emerged, disappeared, and been replaced by other genotypes (Guan et al., 2002, 2004). The genotype Z emerged in 2002 and became the dominant phenotype that caused the explosive outbreak in Southeast Asia in 2003–2004. The genotype Z viruses have multiple sublineages that can categorize Thailand and Vietnam isolates into one cluster and viruses from Indonesia and China into other clusters (Li et al., 2004). All the viruses in the outbreaks since 2004 belong to the genotype Z. This suggested that the genotype Z has the optimal genetic makeup for efficient spread among poultry.

All Thailand isolates contain multiple basic amino acid substitutions at the protease cleavage site in the HA protein, a 20-codon deletion in the NA gene, and a 5-codon deletion in the NS gene, which are characteristics of the genotype Z viruses. Amino acid residues at the receptor-binding site of HA of human viruses were similar to those of chicken viruses. The presence of amantadine resistance in the Thailand viruses was indicated by a mutation in the M2 transmembrane protein and was phenotypically confirmed. The Thailand viruses contained more avian-specific residues than did the 1997 Hong Kong H5N1 viruses, suggesting that the virus may have adapted to allow a more efficient spread in avian species (Viseshakul et al., 2004; Puthavathana et al., 2005).

It was initially hypothesized that the Thailand–Vietnam clade might be more efficient in causing disease in humans, because there was no human infection in Indonesia earlier in the outbreak, despite extensive spread of the disease in poultry. However, the more recent outbreak of human infection in Indonesia indicated that the Indonesian clade is also pathogenic in man (Kandun et al., 2006). Whether this is a result of viral adaptation or a property of the original virus is unclear.

Influenza is a rapidly evolving virus. Experiments in ducks demonstrated that only a single round of nonlethal infection in one host could exert enough selection pressure to cause an antigenic drift and reduce virulence (Hulse-Post et al., 2005). It is therefore likely that the endemic virus will gradually become less pathogenic in ducks, which is a natural host of influenza virus. Observation of the outbreak pattern in the third round (rainy season 2005) suggested that pathogenicity in other avian species may not be similar to what had been observed in the first round of outbreaks. In the latest outbreak, a smaller fraction of sick and dying animals was observed and more viruses were isolated from apparently healthy animals. Experimental data have shown that the viruses in 2005 were indeed less pathogenic in ducks (Hulse-Post et al., 2005; Sturm-Ramirez et al., 2005). Interestingly, the H5N1 viruses of 1997 were also nonpathogenic in ducks. The virus became pathogenic in ducks in 2002–2003 and reverted to a nonpathogenic strain in 2005 (Chen et al., 2004; Sturm-Ramirez et al., 2005). This probably indicated a temporary loss of the equilibrium between the virus and its natural host by the adaptation into a new host, that is, domestic poultry. The reduction of pathogenicity in 2005 suggested that the virus is setting a new equilibrium with its natural host.

Effect on Poultry Industry

The impact on the poultry industry during the first outbreak was devastating. Because Thailand is a major poultry meat exporting country, direct loss in production caused by the outbreak and culling, the trade ban imposed by importing countries, and reduced domestic consumption caused severe economic loss in the industry. More than 62 million birds were either killed by the disease or culled for outbreak control (Tiensin et al., 2005). The government compensated farmers for their losses. Farmers were entitled to compensation of 75% of the value of animals that were destroyed. Different sectors of the poultry industry vary in their practice of biosecurity and outbreak prevention. After the first outbreak, most large-scale industries improved biosecurity measures. Consequently, little problem remained in the large-scale industry sector in the second and third outbreaks. The major concern remains in the small-scale backyard farms of chickens and ducks, where it is very difficult to employ proper biosecurity. Another area of concern is the farms in the central part of Thailand, where paddy fields are plentiful. It is a common practice of free-grazing duck raising in Thailand to move flocks of ducks from field to field by trucks to let them feed on the dropped grains after the harvest. Flocks can move over a very long distance in search of a suitable feeding area. Because ducks can be infected and can shed virus without clinical sign, migrating flocks are ideal for spreading the disease (Chen et al., 2004; Sturm-Ramirez et al., 2005). The geographical distribution of the outbreaks coincided with the area with the highest density of free-grazing duck raising (Gilbert et al., 2006). This further supports the belief that free-grazing ducks may have been a major source of the spread of disease.

Another activity that the government has been trying to control is cock fighting. It involves not only the movement of fighting cocks from place to place for fighting, but also close contact between cocks and people, which can increase the chance of transmission to humans. The control measures now in place are registration and the obligatory screening of fighting cocks and temporary prohibition of cock fighting during the peak of influenza outbreaks (DLD, 2005b).

Impact on Wildlife

Open-bill storks are probably the most affected species in Thailand (Keawcharoen et al., 2005). They are migratory birds that migrate to central Thailand in winter. Some of the birds remain in Thailand all year round. Open-bill storks are vulnerable to infection, probably because they live in big flocks in the wetlands of central Thailand. Continuous surveillance confirmed the presence of virus in these birds. Evidence of H5N1 infection was also found in other birds, such as sparrows and pigeons, which share natural habitats with humans and domestic poultry. Although free-living birds are not likely to play a major role in the introduction of new outbreaks, it is possible that these birds may spread the infection locally between farms and maintain the viral reservoir locally between outbreaks.

Disease Manifestation in Humans

Of the 20 confirmed cases, 11 were children under the age of 14 years and 13 died, leading to a mortality of 65% (Chotpitayasunondh et al., 2005). In most of the confirmed cases, the source of infection was backyard chickens. Most of the patients had a fever as the starting symptom followed by coughing, dyspnea, and pneumonia in a median time of 4 days. About half of the patients (53%) had rhinorrhea, 71% had sore throat, 53% had myalgia, and 41% had diarrhea (Chotpitayasunondh et al., 2005). Abnormal chest radiographs in these patients included interstitial infiltration and patchy lobar infiltrates in a variety of patterns (single lobe, multiple lobes, unilateral, or bilateral distributions). In patients who developed ARDS (acute respiratory distress syndrome), the radiographic pattern progressed to a diffuse bilateral ground-glass appearance (Beigel et al., 2005; Chotpitayasunondh et al., 2005). An autopsy study showed that the lung, but not upper airway epithelium, was the site of viral replication, and the cellular target of the virus was the alveolar epithelial cell (Uiprasertkul et al., 2005). The most remarkable laboratory findings in these patients were lymphopenia, leucopenia, and thrombocytopenia. More importantly, the lymphocyte counts were significantly different between fatal cases and survivors and between patients with and without ARDS (Chotpitayasunondh et al., 2005). This suggested that a simple blood count can not only help in the preliminary diagnosis of bird flu, but can also be used as a prognostic marker. Most of these patients were treated with Oseltamivir, but it is not clear whether the treatment changed the course of the illness.

Unusual Disease Manifestation

Although most confirmed AI infections in humans caused respiratory infection and pneumonia, there were some cases with other manifestations. A case presenting with acute diarrhea and later developing fatal respiratory failure was reported (Apisarnthanarak et al., 2004). Viral replication could be detected in an autopsy sample from the intestine of a patient even in the absence of diarrhea (Uiprasertkul et al., 2005). This suggested that the virus may have a tropism for the intestinal tract similar to the infection in avian species. Reports from Vietnam also showed other unusual manifestations of H5N1 infection in humans, such as encephalitis (de Jong et al., 2005). This will make the disease surveillance more difficult, and monitoring of only pneumonia and respiratory failure may not be adequate to cover all cases of human H5N1 infection.

Human-to-Human Transmission and the Risk of Pandemic Disease

Avian and human influenza viruses were thought to be separated by the receptor preference: avian viruses use $2,3$-α-linked sialic acid while human viruses use $2,6$-α-linked sialic acid (Suzuki, 2005). H5N1 AI viruses showed avian-type receptor specificity (Matrosovich et al., 1999; Gambaryan et al., 2004). Nevertheless, they can infect humans. Infection by the H5N1 virus in humans is not efficient, and person-to-person transmission cannot readily occur. The inability of the virus to transmit from person to person is the only barrier preventing the virus from becoming a pandemic strain. Experimental data showed that only two substitutions in the receptor-binding site of the hemagglutinin gene are needed to change the receptor-binding preference of H5N1 virus from $2,3$- to $2,6$-α-linked sialic acid (Harvey et al., 2004). It is not known whether this receptor preference is the only barrier the virus needs to cross to infect humans efficiently.

Although several clusters of H5N1 infections have been observed in Thailand, Vietnam, and Indonesia, it is difficult to prove human-to-human transmission, as most of these patients had exposure to poultry and it is not possible to prove whether they contracted the disease from animals or humans. The very low sequence variability among the viruses in the outbreak made it impossible to infer chain of transmission from sequence data.

It was a unique incidence in Thailand that allowed an inference of probable person-to-person transmission (Ungchusak et al., 2005). It was a cluster of three patients: a young girl, her mother, and her aunt. The girl and her aunt lived in Kamphaengphet where there was an AI outbreak in poultry. The mother lived in Nonthaburi, a province near Bangkok where there was no AI outbreak and did not have any contact with poultry. She went to take care of her sick daughter 1 day before the girl died. The mother had an onset of fever 4 days later, went back to Nonthaburi, had pneumonia, and died 14 days later. The aunt who also took care of the sick girl also developed pneumonia 8 days after the girl's death. Although she had contact with a dead chicken, the last exposure was 17 days before the onset of fever, which was too long for an incubation period of influenza. Because the mother and the aunt had no contact with poultry within a time interval compatible with an incubation period of influenza and the time of onset after exposure to the index case was compatible with the incubation period of AI, it was concluded that the two cases were likely to contract the disease from the index case (Ungchusak et al., 2005). As soon as this cluster was recognized, effort was made to contain possible further person-to-person transmission. All household members, other family contacts, exposed neighbors, and exposed health care workers were placed under active surveillance for fever and respiratory symptoms for 14 days. Fortunately, there was no further transmission or evidence that the virus in this cluster facilitated more efficient human-to-human transmission. However, if the virus is allowed to transmit from humans to humans without interruption, it is likely that it will eventually evolve to become more transmissible in humans. It is therefore crucial that every effort has to be made to prevent human-to-human transmission.

Disease in Mammals

AI virus H5N1 infection was observed in several mammalian species, including cat, tiger, leopard, and dog (Keawcharoen et al., 2004; Thanawongnuwech et al., 2005; Songsermn et al., 2006; Butler, 2006). The exposure that led to the infection was mostly from feeding on the carcasses of infected poultry. The infection caused severe disease, with high mortality in these animals. Experimental infections were also reported in cats, mice, ferrets, monkey, and pigs (Rimmelzwaan et al., 2001, 2003; Kuiken et al., 2003, 2004; Govorkova et al., 2005; Maines et al., 2005). Most of these animals presented severely fatal disease manifestations except for pigs, in which the infection caused only mild disease (Choi et al., 2005). Nevertheless, the virulence of H5N1 virus in mammals is probably heterogeneous among strains and is continuously evolving. Experimental data suggested that the virus is evolving to become more pathogenic in mammals and that the genetic determinants of virulence lie in the polymerase genes, resulting in a high-replication phenotype (Govorkova et al., 2005; Li et al., 2005). This further emphasized the danger of this virus and suggested that it may also become more pathogenic and transmissible in humans.

Control Measure

Active surveillance of suspected cases is continuously employed by the public health authority in Thailand. Cases of pneumonia in those who have history of exposure to poultry are reported to the Department of Disease Control and investigated for the presence of H5N1 virus by viral culture and RT-PCR. Clusters of pneumonia and pneumonia in hospital personnel are also the targets of surveillance and disease control in order to detect human-to-human transmission of severe influenza of pandemic potential. Emphasis has been made to detect any potential pandemic strain as early as possible. Recent studies using computer simulation predicted that early detection and proper outbreak control by social distancing measures and antiviral drugs may be effective in containing the outbreak and eliminating the potential pandemic virus provided the virus does not have a greater ability to get transmitted than does the previous pandemic strains, that is, it has a basic reproductive number below 1.6–1.8 (Ferguson et al., 2005; Longini et al., 2005). The amount of the antiviral drug Oseltamivir that should be enough for the elimination of a potential pandemic virus has been predicted differently between the two studies: 100,000 to 1 million and 3 million courses (Ferguson et al., 2005; Longini et al., 2005). Having that in mind, the Ministry of Public Health has started to stockpile Oseltamivir, and as of October 2005, the amount stockpiled is 72,500 courses (725,000 tablets).

Outbreaks in poultry are monitored and controlled by the DLD. Specifically, if the poultry death rate in any facility was greater than 10% within a single day, all birds, their products, and other potentially contaminated materials have to be destroyed without delay. Cloacal swabs of affected flocks would then be collected for laboratory confirmation. Subsequently, neighboring flocks would be destroyed immediately or quarantined and destroyed when H5N1 laboratory diagnosis was confirmed. Movement of poultry and their products would be restricted to a 1–5-km radius.

In the first round of outbreaks, neighboring flocks within a 5-km radius were preemptively culled as quickly as possible. After July 2004, preemptive culling was implemented only within a village, within an area of 1 km around an outbreak, or on suspected farms. DLD has launched a nationwide surveillance program (known as "x-ray survey") in January 2004, October 2004, and July 2005. The program was conducted in close collaboration with the Ministry of Agriculture and Cooperatives, Ministry of Public Health, provincial governors, volunteer public health workers, and DLD livestock workers (DLD, 2005b). The program is planned to be launched biannually, in the winter before Chinese New Year and in the rainy season. These two periods are considered the riskiest times of the year because there is an unusually high volume of movement of poultry for the Chinese New Year festivities, which can promote the spreading of the virus. Furthermore, the high humidity and low temperature in the rainy season may be optimal for the viral spread.

Other specific measures include the control of free-grazing ducks and fighting cocks. There have been serious debates over the continuation of raising free-grazing ducks. The practice is favored by environmentalists because it makes efficient use of the paddy field after harvesting and provides biological pest control, as they prey on the golden apple snail, a major pest for rice cultivation. Although the debates are not yet totally resolved, long distance moving of flocks by trucks is temporarily prohibited, especially moving from or into the central region of the country where the disease is not yet fully eliminated. The flocks are registered and allowed to migrate only in a limited zone. The limitation of grazing area by zoning was designed so that there will be no extensive movement, so as to limit the area of potential contamination. The zoning strategy is also implemented to other poultry, dividing the country into five zones: central, north, northeast, east, and south, in order to limit movement of poultry from the central plan to the other regions that are disease-free, especially the eastern region where most exporting poultry industry farms are located.

In contrast to other countries in the region, Thailand does not use the AI vaccine in poultry. Although the illegal vaccine may have been used to some extent, the official policy is still against the vaccine (FAO Newsroom, 2006).

Although the decision was probably influenced mainly by the international trade barrier, the major scientific concern against vaccination in poultry is the risk of having undetectable asymptomatic infection that may shed the virus and spread the infection (Swayne et al., 2001; Liu et al., 2003). With the changing phenotype of the virus towards lower virulence in ducks, the vaccination policy may need to be reconsidered, because without vaccination the ducks will be asymptomatically infected as well and vaccination is effective in reducing the level of viral shedding (Tian et al., 2005). A previous report showing the ability of vaccination to abort an outbreak in a chicken farm strongly supports the use of the vaccine in adjunction to biosecurity measures (Ellis et al., 2004).

Sufficient facility for viral testing is crucial for the success of outbreak control and surveillance. Both the National Institute of Health and the National Institute of Animal Health have strengthened their diagnostic capability and extended the service to their regional laboratories.

National Influenza Plan

Two national plans, National Strategic Plan for Avian Influenza Control and National Strategic Plan for Influenza Pandemic Preparedness for a 3-year period (2005–2007), have been set and endorsed by the cabinet since January 2005 (Wibulpolprasert et al., 2005).

The National Strategic Plan for Avian Influenza Control has targets within the 3-year period as follows:

1. No outbreak of AI in economic poultry in 2 years.
2. Reduce outbreak in domestic poultry, fighting cocks, exotic birds, and migratory birds to a level that is not considered a problem in 3 years.
3. No outbreak in other animals in 3 years.
4. No disease contract from animals to humans in 2 years.
5. Thailand is efficiently prepared to handle an influenza pandemic in 1 year.

The National Strategic Plan for Influenza Pandemic Preparedness has targets within the 3-year period as follows:

1. To strengthen an effective influenza surveillance system, including clinical surveillance in the communities, work places, educational institutions, and every public health facilities, as well as establishing 12 centers for laboratory surveillance of the viruses throughout the country within 3 years.
2. To enable Thailand to be ready for efficient management of the emergency situations during the influenza pandemic within 2 years.
3. To stockpile antiviral drugs (Oseltamivir) so as to treat 325,000 patients (3,250,000 tablets) and to stockpile the raw materials for manufacturing antiviral drugs (Oseltamivir) so as to treat 1,625,000 patients within 5 years.
4. To develop the capacity to manufacture or stockpile influenza vaccines within 5 years.

5. In case of an influenza pandemic, hospitals throughout the country have the capacity of up to 100,000 beds for taking care of influenza patients in critical conditions. In case of outbreaks in specific areas, field hospitals with a capacity of 5,000 beds will be ready for services.

The threat of influenza pandemic is eminent. While any AI virus has a potential to evolve and eventually become a pandemic strain, the present danger is the H5N1 virus, which has already crossed the interspecies barrier from avian to human. Without proper intervening measures, it is just a matter of time before the virus adapts to transmit efficiently from person to person and become the next pandemic virus. Effective control of the outbreak in animals, prevention of exposure in humans, and early detection of a potential pandemic strain are essential to the success of preventing the pandemic. Preparedness in case of a pandemic is also crucial to minimize the loss of human life. Strong international collective effort is essential for the success.

References

Amonsin, A., Payungporn, S., Theamboonlers, A., Thanawongnuwech, R., Suradhat, S., Pariyothorn, N., Tantilertcharoen, R., Damrongwantanapokin, S., Buranathai, C., Chaisingh, A., Songserm, T., & Poovorawan, Y. (2005). Genetic characterization of H5N1 influenza A viruses isolated from zoo tigers in Thailand. *Virology*, 26 Sep [Epub ahead of print].

Apisarnthanarak, A., Kitphati, R., Thongphubeth, K., Patoomanunt, P., Anthanont, P., Auwanit, W., Thawatsupha, P., Chittaganpitch, M., Saeng-Aroon, S., Waicharoen, S., Apisarnthanarak, P., Storch, G. A., Mundy, L. M., & Fraser, V. J. (2004). Atypical avian influenza (H5N1). *Emerg Infect Dis*, 10, 1321–4.

Beigel, J. H., Farrar, J., Han, A. M., Hayden, F. G., Hyer, R., de Jong, M. D., Lochindarat, S., Nguyen, T. K., Nguyen, T. H., Tran, T. H., Nicoll, A., Touch, S., & Yuen, K. Y. (2005). Avian influenza A (H5N1) infection in humans. *N Engl J Med*, 353, 1374–85.

Butler, D. (2006). Thai dogs carry bird-flu virus, but will they spread it? *Nature*, 439, 773.

Centers for Disease Control and Prevention. (2004). Cases of influenza A (H5N1) – Thailand, 2004. *MMWR Morb Mortal Wkly Rep*, 53, 100–3.

Chen, H., Deng, G., Li, Z., Tian, G., Li, Y., Jiao, P., Zhang, L., Liu, Z., Webster, R. G., & Yu, K. (2004). The evolution of H5N1 influenza viruses in ducks in southern China. *Proc Natl Acad Sci U S A*, 101, 10452–7.

Choi, Y. K., Nguyen, T. D., Ozaki, H., Webby, R. J., Puthavathana, P., Buranathal, C., Chaisingh, A., Auewarakul, P., Hanh, N. T., Ma, S. K., Hui, P. Y., Guan, Y., Peiris, J. S., & Webster, R. G. (2005). Studies of H5N1 influenza virus infection of pigs by using viruses isolated in Vietnam and Thailand in 2004. *J Virol*, 79, 10821–5.

Chokephaibulkit, K., Uiprasertkul, M., Puthavathana, P., Chearskul, P., Auewarakul, P., Dowell, S. F., & Vanprapar, N. (2005). A child with avian influenza A (H5N1) infection. *Pediatr Infect Dis J*, 24, 162–6.

Chotpitayasunondh, T., Ungchusak, K., Hanshaoworakul, W., Chunsuthiwat, S., Sawanpanyalert, P., Kijphati, R., Lochindarat, S., Srisan, P., Suwan, P., Osotthanakorn, Y., Anantasetagoon, T., Kanjanawasri, S., Tanupattarachai, S., Weerakul, J., Chaiwirattana, R., Maneerattanaporn, M., Poolsavathitikool, R., Chokephaibulkit, K., Apisarnthanarak, A., & Dowell, S. F. (2005). Human disease from influenza A (H5N1), Thailand, 2004. *Emerg Infect Dis*, 11, 201–9.

de Jong, M. D., Bach, V. C., Phan, T. Q., Vo, M. H., Tran, T. T., Nguyen, B. H., Beld, M., Le, T. P., Truong, H. K., Nguyen, V. V., Tran, T. H., Do, Q. H., & Farrar, J. (2005). Fatal avian influenza A (H5N1) in a child presenting with diarrhea followed by coma. *N Engl J Med*, 352, 686–91.

DLD. (2005a). Date of updating: 31 October 2005. Department of Livestock Development. Date of access: 31 October 2005, http://www.dld.go.th/home/bird_flu/history.html

DLD. (2005b). Date of posting: 20 July 2005. Department of Livestock Development. Date of access: 31 October 2005, http://www.dld.go.th/home/duck/chick&duck.pdf

Ellis, T. M., Leung, C. Y., Chow, M. K., Bissett, L. A., Wong, W., Guan, Y., & Malik Peiris, J. S. (2004). Vaccination of chickens against H5N1 avian influenza in the face of an outbreak interrupts virus transmission. *Avian Pathol*, 33, 405–12.

FAO Newsroom. (2006). Thailand shares secrets of success. Date of posting: 21 July 2006. FAO. Date of access: 1 January 2007, http://www.fao.org/newsroom/en/focus/2006/1000348/article_1000352en.html

Ferguson, N. M., Cummings, D. A., Cauchemez, S., Fraser, C., Riley, S., Meeyai, A., Iamsirithaworn, S., & Burke, D. S. (2005). Strategies for containing an emerging influenza pandemic in Southeast Asia. *Nature*, 437, 209–14.

Gambaryan, A. S., Tuzikov, A. B., Pazynina, G. V., Webster, R. G., Matrosovich, M. N., & Bovin, N. V. (2004). H5N1 chicken influenza viruses display a high binding affinity for Neu5Acalpha2–3Galbeta1-4(6-HSO(3))GlcNAc-containing receptors. *Virology*, 326, 310–6.

Gilbert, M., Chaitaweesub, P., Parakamawongsa, T., Premashthira, S., Tiensin, T., Kalpravidh, W., Wagner, H.,& Slingenbergh, J. (2006). Free-grazing ducks and highly pathogenic avian influenza, Thailand. *Emerg Infect Dis*, 12, 227–34.

Govorkova, E. A., Rehg, J. E., Krauss, S., Yen, H. L., Guan, Y., Peiris, M., Nguyen, T. D., Hanh, T. H., Puthavathana, P., Long, H. T., Buranathai, C., Lim, W., Webster, R. G., & Hoffmann, E. (2005). Lethality to ferrets of H5N1 influenza viruses isolated from humans and poultry in 2004. *J Virol*, 79, 2191–8.

Guan, Y., Peiris, J. S., Lipatov, A. S., Ellis, T. M., Dyrting, K. C., Krauss, S., Zhang, L. J., Webster, R. G., & Shortridge, K. F. (2002). Emergence of multiple genotypes of H5N1 avian influenza viruses in Hong Kong SAR. *Proc Natl Acad Sci U S A*, 99, 8950–5.

Guan, Y., Poon, L. L., Cheung, C. Y., Ellis, T. M., Lim, W., Lipatov, A. S., Chan, K. H., Sturm-Ramirez, K. M., Cheung, C. L., Leung, Y. H., Yuen, K. Y., Webster, R. G., & Peiris, J. S. (2004). H5N1 influenza: A protean pandemic threat. *Proc Natl Acad Sci U S A*, 101, 8156–61.

Harvey, R., Martin, A. C., Zambon, M., & Barclay, W. S. (2004). Restrictions to the adaptation of influenza a virus h5 hemagglutinin to the human host. *J Virol*, 78, 502–7.

Hulse-Post, D. J., Sturm-Ramirez, K. M., Humberd, J., Seiler, P., Govorkova, E. A., Krauss, S., Scholtissek, C., Puthavathana, P., Buranathai, C., Nguyen, T. D., Long, H. T., Naipospos, T. S., Chen, H., Ellis, T. M., Guan, Y., Peiris, J. S., & Webster, R. G. (2005). Role of domestic ducks in the propagation and biological evolution of highly pathogenic H5N1 influenza viruses in Asia. *Proc Natl Acad Sci U S A*, 102, 10682–7.

Kandun, I. N., Wibisono, H., Sedyaningsih, E. R., Yusharmen, Hadisoedarsuno, W., Purba, W., Santoso, H., Septiawati, C., Tresnaningsih, E., Heriyanto, B., Yuwono, D., Harun, S., Soeroso, S., Giriputra, S., Blair, P. J., Jeremijenko, A., Kosasih, H., Putnam, S. D., Samaan, G., Silitonga, M., Chan, K. H., Poon, L. L., Lim, W., Klimov, A., Lindstrom, S., Guan, Y., Donis, R., Katz, J., Cox, N., Peiris, M., & Uyeki, T. M. (2006). Three Indonesian clusters of H5N1 virus infection in 2005. *N Engl J Med*, 355, 2186–94.

Keawcharoen, J., Oraveerakul, K., Kuiken, T., Fouchier, R. A., Amonsin, A., Payungporn, S., Noppornpanth, S., Wattanodorn, S., Theambooniers, A., Tantilertcharoen, R., Pattanarangsan, R., Arya, N., Ratanakorn, P., Osterhaus, D. M., & Poovorawan, Y. (2004). Avian influenza H5N1 in tigers and leopards. *Emerg Infect Dis*, 10, 2189–91.

Keawcharoen, J., Amonsin, A., Oraveerakul, K., Wattanodorn, S., Papravasit, T., Karnda, S., Lekakul, K., Pattanarangsan, R., Noppornpanth, S., Fouchier, R. A., Osterhaus, A. D., Payungporn, S., Theamboonlers, A., & Poovorawan, Y. (2005) Characterization of the hemagglutinin and neuraminidase genes of recent influenza virus isolates from different avian species in Thailand. *Acta Virol*, 49, 277–80.

Kuiken, T., Rimmelzwaan, G. F., Van Amerongen, G., & Osterhaus, A. D. (2003). Pathology of human influenza A (H5N1) virus infection in cynomolgus macaques (Macaca fascicularis). *Vet Pathol*, 40, 304–10.

Kuiken, T., Rimmelzwaan, G., van Riel, D., van Amerongen, G., Baars, M., Fouchier, R., & Osterhaus, A. (2004). Avian H5N1 influenza in cats. *Science*, 306, 241.

Li, K. S., Guan, Y., Wang, J., Smith, G. J., Xu, K. M., Duan, L., Rahardjo, A. P., Puthavathana, P., Buranathai, C., Nguyen, T. D., Estoepangestie, A. T., Chaisingh, A., Auewarakul, P., Long, H. T., Hanh, N. T., Webby, R. J., Poon, L. L., Chen, H., Shortridge, K. F., Yuen, K. Y., Webster, R. G., & Peiris, J. S. (2004). Genesis of a highly pathogenic and potentially pandemic H5N1 influenza virus in eastern Asia. *Nature*, 430, 209–13.

Li, Z., Chen, H., Jiao, P., Deng, G., Tian, G., Li, Y., Hoffmann, E., Webster, R. G., Matsuoka, Y., & Yu, K. (2005). Molecular basis of replication of duck H5N1 influenza viruses in a mammalian mouse model. *J Virol*, 79, 12058–64.

Liu, M., Wood, J. M., Ellis, T., Krauss, S., Seiler, P., Johnson, C., Hoffmann, E., Humberd, J., Hulse, D., Zhang, Y., Webster, R. G., & Perez, D. R. (2003). Preparation of a standardized, efficacious agricultural H5N3 vaccine by reverse genetics. *Virology*, 314, 580–90.

Longini, I. M., Jr., Nizam, A., Xu, S., Ungchusak, K., Hanshaoworakul, W., Cummings, D. A., & Halloran, M. E. (2005). Containing pandemic influenza at the source. *Science*, 309, 1083–7.

Maines, T. R., Lu, X. H., Erb, S. M., Edwards, L., Guarner, J., Greer, P. W., Nguyen, D. C., Szretter, K. J., Chen, L. M., Thawatsupha, P., Chittaganpitch, M., Waicharoen, S., Nguyen, D. T., Nguyen, T., Nguyen, H. H., Kim, J. H., Hoang, L. T., Kang, C., Phuong, L. S., Lim, W., Zaki, S., Donis, R. O., Cox, N. J., Katz, J. M., & Tumpey, T. M. (2005). Avian influenza (H5N1) viruses isolated from humans in Asia in 2004 exhibit increased virulence in mammals. *J Virol*, 79, 11788–800.

Matrosovich, M., Zhou, N., Kawaoka, Y., & Webster, R. (1999). The surface glycoproteins of H5 influenza viruses isolated from humans, chickens, and wild aquatic birds have distinguishable properties. *J Virol*, 73, 1146–55.

OIE. (2005). Update on avian influenza in animals (type H5). Date of updating: 10 October 2005. World Organization for Animal Health. Date of access: 11 November 2005, http://www.oie.int/downld/AVIAN%20INFLUENZA/A_AI-Asia.htm

Puthavathana, P., Auewarakul, P., Charoenying, P. C., Sangsiriwut, K., Pooruk, P., Boonnak, K., Khanyok, R., Thawachsupa, P., Kijphati, R., & Sawanpanyalert, P. (2005). Molecular characterization of the complete genome of human influenza H5N1 virus isolates from Thailand. *J Gen Virol*, 86, 423–33.

Rimmelzwaan, G. F., Kuiken, T., van Amerongen, G., Bestebroer, T. M., Fouchier, R. A., & Osterhaus, A. D. (2001). Pathogenesis of influenza A (H5N1) virus infection in a primate model. *J Virol*, 75, 6687–91.

Rimmelzwaan, G. F., Kuiken, T., van Amerongen, G., Bestebroer, T. M., Fouchier, R. A., & Osterhaus, A. D. (2003). A primate model to study the pathogenesis of influenza A (H5N1) virus infection. *Avian Dis*, 47, 931–3.

Songsermn, T., Amonsin, A., Jam-on, R., Sae-Heng, N., Meemak, N., Pariyothorn, N., Payungporn, S., Theamboonlers, A., & Poovorawan, Y. (2006). Avian influenza H5N1 in naturally infected domestic cat. *Emerg Infect Dis*, 12, 681–3.

Sturm-Ramirez, K. M., Hulse-Post, D. J., Govorkova, E. A., Humberd, J., Seiler, P., Puthavathana, P., Buranathai, C., Nguyen, T. D., Chaisingh, A., Long, H. T., Naipospos, T. S., Chen, H., Ellis, T. M., Guan, Y., Peiris, J. S., & Webster, R. G. (2005). Are ducks contributing to the endemicity of highly pathogenic H5N1 influenza virus in Asia? *J Virol*, 79, 11269–79.

Suzuki, Y. (2005). Sialobiology of influenza: Molecular mechanism of host range variation of influenza viruses. *Biol Pharm Bull*, 28, 399–408.

Swayne, D. E., Beck, J. R., Perdue, M. L., & Beard, C. W. (2001). Efficacy of vaccines in chickens against highly pathogenic Hong Kong H5N1 avian influenza. *Avian Dis*, 45, 355–65.

Thanawongnuwech, R., Amonsin, A., Tantilertcharoen, R., Damrongwatanapokin, S., Theamboonlers, A., Payungporn, S., Nanthapornphiphat, K., Ratanamungklanon, S., Tunak, E., Songserm, T.,

Vivatthanavanich, V., Lekdumrongsak, T., Kesdangsakonwut, S., Tunhikorn, S., & Poovorawan, Y. (2005). Probable tiger-to-tiger transmission of avian influenza H5N1. *Emerg Infect Dis*, 11, 699–701.

Tian, G., Zhang, S., Li, Y., Bu, Z., Liu, P., Zhou, J., Li, C., Shi, J., Yu, K., & Chen, H. (2005). Protective efficacy in chickens, geese and ducks of an H5N1-inactivated vaccine developed by reverse genetics. *Virology*, 341, 153–62.

Tiensin, T., Chaitaweesub, P., Songserm, T., Chaisingh, A., Hoonsuwan, W., Buranathai, C., Parakamawongsa, T., Premashthira, S., Amonsin, A., Gilbert, M., Nielen, M., & Stegeman, A. (2005). Highly pathogenic avian influenza H5N1, Thailand, *Emerg Infect Dis*, 11, 1664–72.

Uiprasertkul, M., Puthavathana, P., Sangsiriwut, K., Pooruk, P., Srisook, K., Peiris, M., Nicholls, J. M., Chokephaibulkit, K., Vanprapar, N., & Auewarakul, P. (2005). Influenza A H5N1 replication sites in humans. *Emerg Infect Dis*, 11, 1036–41.

Ungchusak, K., Auewarakul, P., Dowell, S. F., Kitphati, R., Auwanit, W., Puthavathana, P., Uiprasertkul, M., Boonnak, K., Pittayawonganon, C., Cox, N. J., Zaki, S. R., Thawatsupha, P., Chittaganpitch, M., Khontong, R., Simmerman, J. M., & Chunsutthiwat, S. (2005). Probable person-to-person transmission of avian influenza A (H5N1). *N Engl J Med*, 352, 333–40.

Viseshakul, N., Thanawongnuwech, R., Amonsin, A., Suradhat, S., Payungporn, S., Keawchareon, J., Oraveerakul, K., Wongyanin, P., Plitkul, S., Theamboonlers, A., & Poovorawan, Y. (2004). The genome sequence analysis of H5N1 avian influenza A virus isolated from the outbreak among poultry populations in Thailand. *Virology*, 328, 169–76.

Wibulpolprasert, S., Chunsuttiwat, S., Ungchusak, K., Kanchanachitra, C., Teokul, W., & Prempree, P. (Eds). (2005). *National strategic plan for avian influenza control and influenza pandemic preparedness in Thailand, 2005–2007.* The Ministry of Public Health and the Thai Health Promotion Foundation, Thailand.

Transmission of Avian Influenza Viruses to Humans: Viral Receptor Specificity and Distribution in Human Airways

Yoshihiro Kawaoka and Kyoko Shinya

Direct transmission of highly pathogenic avian influenza (HPAI) viruses to humans was not considered a major risk prior to 1997. In 1997, however, H5N1 HPAI viruses were transmitted to humans in Hong Kong. Six of 18 infected individuals died, marking the first fatal infection of humans with wholly avian influenza viruses (Claas et al., 1998a,b; Subbarao & Shaw, 2000). Since then, H5N1 HPAI viruses have spread throughout southeast Asia and recently into Europe and Africa. To date, more than 200 individuals have been infected and about half have succumbed to the infection (World Health Organization, 2006). Despite the continued transmission of H5N1 HPAI viruses to humans, these viruses have not yet acquired the ability to spread efficiently among humans. Here, we discuss the factors that lead to human infections with H5N1 HPAI viruses as they relate to the binding of the virus to its cellular receptor.

Influenza Virus and Its Cellular Receptors

Sialic Acids on the Surface of Cells

The receptors of influenza viruses are oligosaccharides with sialic acid (SA) as their terminal components (sialyloligosaccharides; Fig. 1). Oligosaccharides exist as side chains of glycoproteins and glycolipids, and are involved in various cell functions, including protection of the cell surface, intermolecular recognition, and the regulation of cellular interactions (Duksin & Bornstein, 1977; Gu and Taniguchi, 2004; Reed et al., 1981; Rougon et al., 1982).

SA is a generic term for nine-carbon acidic amino sugars. So far, more than 40 natural variants have been described (Schauer, 2000). The amino group is always substituted with either an N-acetyl or N-glycolyl group, yielding N-acetylneuraminic (NeuAc) or N-glycolylneuraminic (NeuGc) acid, respectively. NeuAc is the precursor of several SA species and is widely distributed in animal cells, including human cells (Irie et al., 1998). By contrast, NeuGc has only been detected on nonhuman animal cells (Irie et al., 1998). SAs link to their neighboring galactose moiety by an $\alpha2,3$-(SA$\alpha2,3$Gal) or an $\alpha2,6$-linkage (SA$\alpha2,6$Gal).

Y. Lu et al. (eds.), *Emerging Infections in Asia.*
© Springer Science+Business Media, LLC 2008

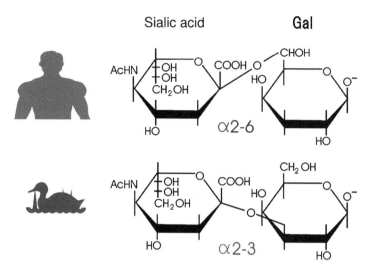

Fig. 1 The difference in receptor-binding specificity between human and avian influenza A viruses. Avian influenza viruses bind more efficiently to SAα2,3Gal sialyoligosaccharides, whereas human influenza viruses have evolved to bind efficiently to SAα2,6Gal sialyoligosaccharides

Receptor Distribution

The distribution of sialyloligosaccharides differs among animal species and cell types. Epithelial cells in the intestinal tract of ducks (the preferential site of avian influenza virus replication) are characterized by SAα2,3Gal sialyloligosaccharides (Ito et al., 2000; Suzuki, 2005; Suzuki et al., 2000), whereas epithelial cells in human airways (the preferential site of human influenza virus replication) primarily express sialyloligosaccharides with an α2,6-linked SA (Baum & Paulson, 1990) (see also section Receptor-Binding Specificity of H5N1 HPAI Viruses). These differences in receptor distribution are mirrored by the preferential binding of avian and human influenza viruses to SAα2,3Gal (Hinshaw et al., 1983; Ito et al., 2000) and SAα2,6Gal (Rogers & Paulson, 1983; Suzuki, 2005) sialyloligosaccharides, respectively. Pigs, often considered as "mixing vessels" for the creation of avian–human reassortant viruses, contain both SAα2,6Gal and SAα2,6Gal sialyloligosaccharides on the epithelial cells of their trachea.

Receptor-Binding Specificity of the Hemagglutinin Protein

The receptor-binding specificity of influenza viruses is a critical factor in influenza virus host-range restriction. When a virus with an avian-derived hemagglutinin (HA) gene is introduced into the human population, it may need to change its receptor-binding specificity from avian to human type for efficient human-to-human transmission. This assumption is based on the finding that the earliest isolates of the

1918, 1957, and 1968 pandemic influenza viruses – all of which contained HA genes of avian origin – acquired the ability to preferentially recognize SAα2,6Gal rather than SAα2,3Gal sialyloligosaccharides (Matrosovich et al., 2000; Stevens et al., 2004).

The receptor-binding specificity of influenza viruses is determined by the viral surface glycoprotein HA, which mediates viral binding to cellular receptors and the fusion of the viral and endosomal membranes. Experimental (Matrosovich et al., 1993; Rogers et al., 1983) and crystallographic (Lin & Cannon, 2002) data have shown that the receptor-binding specificity is determined by the amino acids that form the receptor-binding pocket. For example, for H2 and H3 HAs, the specificity for SAα2,3Gal sialyloligosaccharides is primarily determined by glutamine and glycine at positions 226 and 228, respectively, whereas leucine and serine at these positions result in preferential binding to SAα2,3Gal sialyloligosaccharides (Connor et al., 1994; Rogers et al., 1983). Consequently, HAs of avian origin contain Gln266 and Gly228, whereas human virus isolates are characterized by Leu226 and Ser228. For viruses of the H1 subtype, the nature of the amino acid at position 190 of HA is critical: aspartate, which is found in human and swine virus isolates, determines preferential binding to α2,6-linked SA, whereas glutamate (found in avian virus isolates) results in preferential binding to α2,3-linked SA (Kobasa et al., 2004; Matrosovich et al., 2000; Stevens et al., 2006). The amino acids at positions 136, 190, and 225 of HA also affect receptor-binding affinity and specificity (Stevens et al., 2006). For viruses of the H3 subtype, changes in receptor specificity after their introduction into humans have also been described (Ryan-Poirier et al., 1998), further emphasizing that mutations in HA are critical for human adaptation of influenza viruses. Moreover, analysis of H5 viruses demonstrated that amino acids at positions 182 or 192 independently changed the preferential receptor-binding specificity from "avian" to "human type" (Yamada et al., 2006).

Transmission of H5N1 HPAI Viruses to Humans

The direct transmission of wholly avian viruses to humans was considered a rare event, due to the earlier-described differences in receptor-binding specificity between human and avian influenza viruses. The continued transmission of H5N1 HPAI viruses to humans since 1997 has challenged this assumption and revitalized the question of how avian influenza viruses infect humans.

H5N1 HPAI Infections in Humans

Typically, human influenza virus infections are characterized by upper respiratory symptoms, such as coughing and sneezing with generalized fatigue and high fever. By contrast, while human infections with H5N1 HPAI viruses do cause these upper respiratory symptoms, they also result in lower respiratory and digestive symptoms. H5N1 virus isolation from infected individuals often requires tracheobronchial washes

(Uiprasertkul et al., 2005), whereas "typical" human influenza viruses can be isolated from nasopharyngeal swabs. H5N1 HPAI viruses thus grow efficiently in the lower airways of infected individuals, but to only a limited extent in the upper airways.

The Distribution of Virus Receptors in Human Airways

The continued transmission of H5N1 HPAI viruses to humans and the finding of lower respiratory symptoms in infected individuals (Uiprasertkul et al., 2005) have prompted scientists to reassess the distribution of virus receptors in human airways.

Studies with in vitro differentiated human epithelial cells from tracheal/bronchial tissues have shown that human cells not only express SAα2,6Gal, but also SAα2,3Gal sialyloligosaccharides (Matrosovich et al., 2004). Nonciliated epithelial cells (which account for most epithelial cells) were shown to express SAα2,6Gal sialyloligosaccharides, whereas ciliated cells (the minor population of epithelial cells) expressed those with 2,3-linkages (Matrosovich et al., 2004). Consequently, nonciliated cells were predominantly infected by human virus isolates, whereas ciliated cells were preferentially infected by avian influenza viruses, again highlighting the importance of sialyloligosaccharide distribution for host range. More importantly, the finding of avian-type influenza virus receptors on human cells offers an explanation for the recent human infections with H5N1 HPAI viruses.

Other studies of human respiratory tissue have also revealed differences in the sialyloligosaccharide distribution between the upper and the lower airways (Shinya et al., 2006): Epithelial cells in nasal mucosa, paranasal sinuses, pharynx, and trachea contain predominantly sialyloligosaccharides with α2,6-linkage, whereas nonciliated cuboidal bronchiolar cells at the junction between the respiratory bronchiole and alveolus, and type II cells, which line the alveolar wall, express predominantly SAα2,3Gal sialyloligosaccharides (Fig. 2). The lower respiratory symptoms associated with human H5N1 HPAI infections may therefore be explained by the presence of SAα2,3Gal sialyloligosaccharides in the lower human airway. The finding that H5N1 HPAI viruses attach to and infect primarily type II pneumocytes, alveolar macrophages, and nonciliated cuboidal epithelial cells in the terminal bronchioles of the lower respiratory tract of humans also supports this conclusion (Shinya et al., 2006; van Riel et al., 2006). The low frequency of avian-type receptors in the upper human airway may restrict efficient H5N1 virus replication at this site and, consequently, limit human-to-human virus transmission via droplets generated by coughing and sneezing.

Receptor-Binding Specificity of H5N1 HPAI Viruses

The 1997 H5N1 HPAI viruses have been shown to bind to SAα2,3Gal but not SAα2,6Gal sialyloligosaccharides (Matrosovich et al., 1999). However, we now

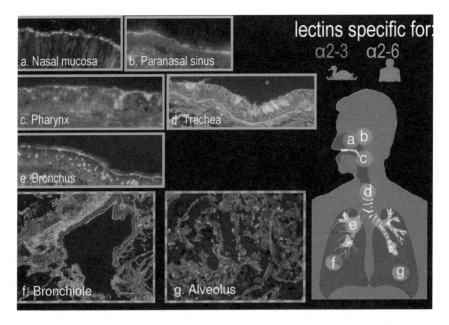

Fig. 2 Influenza virus receptor distribution in human airways. Staining with lectins that specifically recognize α2,3- or α2,6-linked sialyloligosaccharides reveals human-type receptors in the
upper human airway (green), but avian-type receptors in the lower respiratory organs (red). From
Nature, 440, 435–436. 2006 (See figure insert for color reproduction)

know that the receptor-binding specificity of influenza viruses is not an insur-
mountable host-range barrier, given the earlier-described detection of SAα2,3Gal
sialyloligosaccharides on human cells. A comparison of the receptor specificity of
the 1997 H5N1 human index virus with that of an avian H5N9 virus (A/turkey/
Ontario/7732/66) revealed differences between the human and avian H5 viruses in
their recognition of sialyloligosaccharides (Iwatsuki-Horimoto et al., 2004). These
differences in receptor binding could be traced to differences in both the oligosac-
charide side chains and the nature of the amino acids surrounding the receptor-
binding pocket.

The receptor-binding specificities of more recent H5N1 HPAI viruses have also
been assessed (Gambaryan et al., 2006; Shinya et al., 2005). Although most of these
viruses preferentially bind to SAα2,3Gal sialyloligosaccharides, two human isolates
(A/Hong Kong/212/2003, A/Hong Kong/213/2003) had acquired an increased
affinity for human-type receptors that were accompanied by a reduced affinity for
the avian-type receptor. In addition, some recent human H5N1 virus isolates have
been shown to bind to both SAα2,3Gal and SAα2,6Gal sialyloligosaccharides
(Le et al., 2005).

Further insight into how H5N1 HPAI viruses infect humans has come from
the x-ray crystallographic structure of the A/Vietnam/1203/2004 (VN1204)

H5N1 virus, which, in mammalian models, is one the most pathogenic H5N1 HPAI viruses. Although it primarily recognizes SAα2,3Gal sialyloligosaccharides, the HA of VN1204 more closely resembles the HA of the 1918 human pandemic virus than that of an avian H5 virus (A/duck/Singapore/3/1997) (Stevens et al., 2006). Replacement of glutamine at position 226 and glycine at position 228 with leucine and serine, respectively, reduces the affinity of VN1204 HA for SAα2,3Gal sialyloligosaccharides while increasing that for 2,6-linked sugars.

Do H5N1 HPAI Viruses Adapt to Humans?

The HA proteins of two human H5N1 virus isolates that could bind to human-like receptors (A/Hong Kong/212/2003, A/Hong Kong/213/2003) have been characterized by a serine-to-alanine change at position 227 (H3 numbering)(Gambaryan et al., 2006). The same mutation was detected in human H5N1 viruses isolated from fatal cases in Vietnam in 2005 and in Turkey in 2006 (Butler, 2006a; Le et al., 2005). Given that several human H5N1 virus isolates have acquired this mutation, it may be that this amino acid replacement is critical for virus adaptation to humans. Recently, human H5N1 influenza viruses have also been isolated that contain amino acid changes in their HAs, which allow more efficient binding to SAα2,6Gal sialyloligosaccharides (Yamada et al., 2006). The adaptation of HPAI viruses to humans is of great concern since it may yield a pandemic influenza virus. No efficient human-to-human transmission has yet been reported for any of these viruses.

Why Have H5N1 HPAI Viruses Not Yet Caused a Pandemic?

Although it is known for nearly a decade now that H5N1 HPAI viruses are transmitted to humans, these viruses have not yet adapted to transmit efficiently among humans (Ungchusak et al., 2005). Limited human-to-human transmission may have occurred recently among members of a family in Indonesia (with seven of eight infected family members succumbing to the infection) (Butler, 2006b); however, virus spread beyond this family cluster has not been documented.

Multiple factors determine the ability of a virus to efficiently infect and replicate within a cell, and transmit its progeny to other cells. As discussed earlier, the difference in the receptor-binding specificity of influenza viruses may not prevent human infection with avian influenza viruses. The ability to recognize human-type receptors and infect cells of the upper human airway is likely necessary for the generation of a pandemic H5N1 virus. However, a change in receptor-binding specificity alone is not sufficient to cause a human pandemic virus, because none of the human H5N1 viruses with altered receptor-binding specificity were transmitted efficiently among humans.

In addition to human-type receptor-binding specificity, other mutations are likely required for the efficient replication of avian influenza viruses in humans. A prime candidate is the glutamic acid-to-lysine change at position 627 of the PB2 protein (a subunit of the viral polymerase complex). This amino acid replacement is a critical determinant of H5N1 virus pathogenicity in mice and most likely in other mammals. Several studies have demonstrated that this replacement affects efficient viral growth in mammalian cells, with lysine at this position providing a replicative advantage (Hatta et al., 2001; Naffakh et al., 2000; Subbarao et al., 1998). Lysine was found at position 627 of the PB2 of an H7N7 virus isolated from a veterinarian who died during an influenza virus outbreak in the Netherlands in 2003 (Fouchier et al., 2004), and in half of H5N1 viruses isolated from humans in Vietnam and Thailand. Similarly, several H5N1 viruses isolated from tigers in Thailand had lysine at position 627 of their PB2 proteins (Amonsin et al., 2006). Collectively, these data suggest that this lysine residue is critical for efficient virus replication in mammals. A human H5N1 virus (isolated in Turkey in early 2006) contained mutations at position 227 of the HA protein and 627 of the PB2 protein, which allowed recognition of human-type receptors and efficient replication in human cells. The finding of a human H5N1 virus isolate containing these two key features raised great concern of an imminent pandemic. However, this virus was also not transmitted efficiently among humans, indicating that further adaptive changes are necessary for efficient human-to-human spread.

Prospect

The ongoing transmission of H5N1 HPAI viruses to humans increases the risk of one of these viruses ultimately acquiring the requisite combination of mutations to allow efficient replication in humans as well as efficient human-to-human transmission. In order to avoid an H5N1 virus pandemic, it is critical that we limit, if we are unable to prevent, avian-to-human transmission of H5N1 HPAI viruses.

Acknowledgments We thank Susan Watson and Gabriele Neumann for editing the manuscript. Our original work described in this review was supported by Core Research for Evolutional Science and Technology (CREST) grants from the Japan Science and Technology Corporation Agency (JST), Japan, by grants-in-aid from the Ministry of Education, Culture, Sports, Science and Technology and the Ministry of Health, Labor and Welfare, Japan, and by grants from the National Institutes of Health, NIAID.

References

Amonsin, A., Payungporn, S., Theamboonlers, A., Thanawongnuwech, R., Suradhat, S., Pariyothorn, N., Tantilertcharoen, R., Damrongwantanapokin, S., Buranathai, C., Chaisingh, A., Songserm, T., & Poovorawan, Y. (2006). Genetic characterization of H5N1 influenza A viruses isolated from zoo tigers in Thailand. *Virology, 344*, 480–491.

Baum, L.G., & Paulson, J.C. (1990). Sialyloligosaccharides of the respiratory epithelium in the selection of human influenza virus receptor specificity. *Acta Histochem.*, *40*, 35–38.

Butler, D. (2006a). Alarms ring over bird flu mutations. *Nature, 439,* 248–249.

Butler, D. (2006b). Family tragedy spotlights flu mutations. *Nature, 442,* 114–115.

Claas, E.C., de Jong, D.C., van Reek, B.R., Rimmelzwaan, G.F., & Osterhaus, A.D. (1998a). Human influenza virus A/HongKong/156/97 (H5N1) infection. *Vaccine, 16,* 977–978.

Claas, E.C., Osterhaus, A.D., van Reek, B.R., De Jong, J.C., Rimmelzwaan, G.F., Senne, D.A., Krauss, S., Shortridge, K.F., & Webster, R.G. (1998b). Human influenza A H5N1 virus related to a highly pathogenic avian influenza virus. *Lancet, 351,* 472–477.

Connor, R.J., Kawaoka, Y., Webster, R.G., & Paulson, J.C. (1994). Receptor specificity in human, avian, and equine H2 and H3 influenza virus isolates. *Virology, 205,* 17–23.

Duksin, D., & Bornstein, P. (1977). Changes in surface properties of normal and transformed cells caused by tunicamycin, an inhibitor of protein glycosylation. *Proc. Natl Acad. Sci. U. S. A., 74,* 3433–3437.

Fouchier, R.A., Schneeberger, P.M., Rozendaal, F.W., Broekman, J.M., Kemink, S.A., Munster, V., Kuiken, T., Rimmelzwaan, G.F., Schutten, M., Van Doornum, G.J., Koch, G., Bosman, A., Koopmans, M., & Osterhaus, A.D. (2004). Avian influenza A virus (H7N7) associated with human conjunctivitis and a fatal case of acute respiratory distress syndrome. *Proc. Natl Acad. Sci. U. S. A., 101,* 1356–1361.

Gambaryan, A., Tuzikov, A., Pazynina, G., Bovin, N., Balish, A., & Klimov, A. (2006). Evolution of the receptor binding phenotype of influenza A (H5) viruses. *Virology, 344,* 432–438.

Gu, J., & Taniguchi, N. (2004). Regulation of integrin functions by N-glycans. *Glycoconj. J., 21,* 9–15.

Hatta, M., Gao, P., Halfmann, P., & Kawaoka, Y. (2001). Molecular basis for high virulence of Hong Kong H5N1 influenza A viruses. *Science, 293,* 1840–1842.

Hinshaw, V.S., Webster, R.G., Naeve, C.W., & Murphy, B.R. (1983). Altered tissue tropism of human-avian reassortant influenza viruses. *Virology, 128,* 260–263.

Irie, A., Koyama, S., Kozutsumi, Y., Kawasaki, T., & Suzuki, A. (1998). The molecular basis for the absence of N-glycolylneuraminic acid in humans. *J. Biol. Chem., 273,* 15866–15871.

Ito, T., Suzuki, Y., Suzuki, T., Takada, A., Horimoto, T., Wells, K., Kida, H., Otsuki, K., Kiso, M., Ishida, H., & Kawaoka, Y. (2000). Recognition of N-glycolylneuraminic acid linked to galactose by the alpha2,3 linkage is associated with intestinal replication of influenza A virus in ducks. *J. Virol., 74,* 9300–9305.

Iwatsuki-Horimoto, K., Kanazawa, R., Sugii, S., Kawaoka, Y., & Horimoto, T. (2004). The index influenza A virus subtype H5N1 isolated from a human in 1997 differs in its receptor-binding properties from a virulent avian influenza virus. *J. Gen. Virol., 85,* 1001–1005.

Kobasa, D., Takada, A., Shinya, K., Hatta, M., Halfmann, P., Theriault, S., Suzuki, H., Nishimura, H., Mitamura, K., Sugaya, N., Usui, T., Murata, T., Maeda, Y., Watanabe, S., Suresh, M., Suzuki, T., Suzuki, Y., Feldmann, H., & Kawaoka, Y. (2004). Enhanced virulence of influenza A viruses with the haemagglutinin of the 1918 pandemic virus. *Nature, 431,* 703–707.

Le, Q.M., Kiso, M., Someya, K., Sakai, Y.T., Nguyen, T.H., Nguyen, K.H., Pham, N.D., Ngyen, H.H., Yamada, S., Muramoto, Y., Horimoto, T., Takada, A., Goto, H., Suzuki, T., Suzuki, Y., & Kawaoka, Y. (2005). Avian flu: Isolation of drug-resistant H5N1 virus. *Nature, 437,* 1108.

Lin, A.H., & Cannon, P.M. (2002). Use of pseudotyped retroviral vectors to analyze the receptor-binding pocket of hemagglutinin from a pathogenic avian influenza A virus (H7 subtype). *Virus Res., 83,* 43–56.

Matrosovich, M.N., Gambaryan, A.S., Tuzikov, A.B., Byramova, N.E., Mochalova, L.V., Golbraikh, A.A., Shenderovich, M.D., Finne, J., & Bovin, N.V. (1993). Probing of the receptor-binding sites of the H1 and H3 influenza A and influenza B virus hemagglutinins by synthetic and natural sialosides. *Virology, 196,* 111–121.

Matrosovich, M., Zhou, N., Kawaoka, Y., & Webster, R. (1999). The surface glycoproteins of H5 influenza viruses isolated from humans, chickens, and wild aquatic birds have distinguishable properties. *J. Virol., 73,* 1146–1155.

Matrosovich, M., Tuzikov, A., Bovin, N., Gambaryan, A., Klimov, A., Castrucci, M.R., Donatelli, I., & Kawaoka, Y. (2000). Early alterations of the receptor-binding properties of H1, H2, and H3 avian influenza virus hemagglutinins after their introduction into mammals. *J. Virol., 74,* 8502–8512.

Matrosovich, M.N., Matrosovich, T.Y., Gray, T., Roberts, N.A., & Klenk, H.D. (2004). Human and avian influenza viruses target different cell types in cultures of human airway epithelium. *Proc. Natl Acad. Sci. U. S. A., 101,* 4620–4624.

Naffakh, N., Massin, P., Escriou, N., Crescenzo-Chaigne, B., & van der Werf, S. (2000). Genetic analysis of the compatibility between polymerase proteins from human and avian strains of influenza A viruses. *J. Gen. Virol., 81,* 1283–1291.

Reed, B.C., Ronnett, G.V., & Lane, M.D. (1981). Role of glycosylation and protein synthesis in insulin receptor metabolism by 3T3-L1 mouse adipocytes. *Proc. Natl Acad. Sci. U. S. A., 78,* 2908–2912.

Rogers, G.N., & Paulson, J.C. (1983). Receptor determinants of human and animal influenza virus isolates: Differences in receptor specificity of the H3 hemagglutinin based on species of origin. *Virology, 127,* 361–373.

Rogers, G.N., Paulson, J.C., Daniels, R.S., Skehel, J.J., Wilson, I.A., & Wiley, D.C. (1983). Single amino acid substitutions in influenza haemagglutinin change receptor binding specificity. *Nature, 304,* 76–78.

Rougon, G., Deagostini-Bazin, H., Hirn, M., & Goridis, C. (1982). Tissue- and developmental stage-specific forms of a neural cell surface antigen linked to differences in glycosylation of a common polypeptide. *EMBO J., 1,* 1239–1244.

Ryan-Poirier, K., Suzuki, Y., Bean, W.J., Kobasa, D., Takada, A., Ito, T., & Kawaoka, Y. (1998). Changes in H3 influenza A virus receptor specificity during replication in humans. *Virus Res., 56,* 169–176.

Schauer, R. (2000). Achievements and challenges of sialic acid research. *Glycoconj. J., 17,* 485–499.

Shinya, K., Hatta, M., Yamada, S., Takada, A., Watanabe, S., Halfmann, P., Horimoto, T., Neumann, G., Kim, J.H., Lim, W., Guan, Y., Peiris, M., Kiso, M., Suzuki, T., Suzuki, Y., & Kawaoka, Y. (2005). Characterization of a human H5N1 influenza A virus isolated in 2003. *J. Virol., 79,* 9926–9932.

Shinya, K., Ebina, M., Yamada, S., Ono, M., Kasai, N., & Kawaoka, Y. (2006). Avian flu: Influenza virus receptors in the human airway. *Nature, 440,* 435–436.

Stevens, J., Corper, A.L., Basler, C.F., Taubenberger, J.K., Palese, P., & Wilson, I.A. (2004). Structure of the uncleaved human H1 hemagglutinin from the extinct 1918 influenza virus. *Science, 303,* 1866–1870.

Stevens, J., Blixt, O., Tumpey, T.M., Taubenberger, J.K., Paulson, J.C., & Wilson, I.A. (2006). Structure and receptor specificity of the hemagglutinin from an H5N1 influenza virus. *Science, 312,* 404–410.

Subbarao, K., & Shaw, M.W. (2000). Molecular aspects of avian influenza (H5N1) viruses isolated from humans. *Rev. Med. Virol., 10,* 337–348.

Subbarao, K., Klimov, A., Katz, J., Regnery, H., Lim, W., Hall, H., Perdue, M., Swayne, D., Bender, C., Huang, J., Hemphill, M., Rowe, T., Shaw, M., Xu, X., Fukuda, K., & Cox, N. (1998). Characterization of an avian influenza A (H5N1) virus isolated from a child with a fatal respiratory illness. *Science, 279,* 393–396.

Suzuki, Y. (2005). Sialobiology of influenza: Molecular mechanism of host range variation of influenza viruses. *Biol. Pharm. Bull., 28,* 399–408.

Suzuki, Y., Ito, T., Suzuki, T., Holland Jr., R.E., Chambers, T.M., Kiso, M., Ishida, H., & Kawaoka, Y. (2000). Sialic acid species as a determinant of the host range of influenza A viruses. *J. Virol., 74,* 11825–11831.

Uiprasertkul, M., Puthavathana, P., Sangsiriwut, K., Pooruk, P., Srisook, K., Peiris, M., Nicholls, J.M., Chokephaibulkit, K., Vanprapar, N., & Auewarakul, P. (2005). Influenza A H5N1 replication sites in humans. *Emerg. Infect. Dis., 11,* 1036–1041.

Ungchusak, K., Auewarakul, P., Dowell, S.F., Kitphati, R., Auwanit, W., Puthavathana, P., Uiprasertkul, M., Boonnak, K., Pittayawonganon, C., Cox, N.J., Zaki, S.R., Thawatsupha, P., Chittaganpitch, M., Khontong, R., Simmerman, J.M., & Chunsutthiwat, S. (2005).

Probable person-to-person transmission of avian influenza A (H5N1). *N. Engl. J. Med., 352,* 333–340.

van Riel, D., Munster, V.J., de Wit, E., Rimmelzwaan, G.F., Fouchier, R.A., Osterhaus, A.D., & Kuiken, T. (2006). H5N1 virus attachment to lower respiratory tract. *Science, 312,* 399.

World Health Organization. (2006). Epidemiology of WHO-confirmed human cases of avian influenza A(H5N1) infection. *Wkly. Epidemiol. Rec., 81,* 249–257.

Yamada, S., Suzuki, Y., Suzuki, T., Le, M.Q., Nidom, C.A., Sakai-Tagawa, Y., Muramoto, Y., Ito, M., Kiso, M., Horimoto, T., Shinya, K., Sawada, T., Kiso, M., Usui, T., Murata, T., Lin, Y., Hay, A., Haire, L.F., Stevens, D.J., Russell, R.J., Gamblin, S.J., Skehel, J.J., & Kawaoka, Y. (2006). Haemagglutinin mutations responsible for the binding of H5N1 influenza A viruses to human-type receptors. *Nature, 444,* 378–382.

Part 2
SARS

Investigation of Animal Reservoir(s) of SARS-CoV

Zhihong Hu and Zhengli Shi

Introduction

Severe acute respiratory syndrome (SARS) is a novel infectious disease in the new millennium. It has been ascertained that a new coronavirus, SARS-CoV, is the etiological agent of SARS. While the extraordinarily rapid isolation and full genome sequencing of SARS-CoV constituted a remarkable scientific achievement, identification of the actual animal reservoir(s) of SARS-CoV is more difficult. Initial evidences indicated that the masked palm civet (*Paguma larvata*) was the primary suspect of the animal origin of SARS (Guan et al., 2003; Song et al., 2005). Recent studies suggested that horseshoe bat is one of the real reservoirs (Lau et al., 2005; Li et al., 2005) and masked palm civet may have only served as an intermediate amplification host for SARS-CoV and fulfilled efficient interspecies transmission (Lau et al., 2005). This chapter will summarize the studies on the animal reservoir(s) of SARS-CoV.

Investigation of Animals and Animal Traders in Markets in 2003

Search for the animal host of SARS-CoV started early during the SARS outbreak. In May 2003, a breakthrough occurred with the identification of a SARS-CoV-like virus in animals in a live-animal market in Shenzhen, Guangdong Province, China. Guan et al. (2003) investigated 25 animals from eight different species in the market. SARS-CoV-like viruses were isolated from two species, four out of six masked palm civets and one raccoon dog (*Nyctereutes procyonoides*). Serological data suggested that three species were positive, three out of the four masked palm civets, the raccoon dog, as well as one of the two Chinese ferret-badgers (*Melogale moschata*). Five species including three hog-badgers (*Arctonyx collaris*), three beavers (*Castor fiber*), four domestic cats (*Felis catus*), three Chinese hares (*Lepus sinensis*), and two Chinese muntjac (*Muntiacus reevesi*) were shown to be negative.

Y. Lu et al. (eds.), *Emerging Infections in Asia.*
© Springer Science+Business Media, LLC 2008

Two of the viruses from the nasal swabs of masked palm civets, SZ3 and SZ16, were completely sequenced. SZ3 and SZ16 had 18 nucleotide (nt) differences between them over the 29,709 nucleotide genome (99.94% identity), suggesting that they were closely related. The genome homology of SZ3 and SZ16 to the epidemic strain of human SARS-CoV, isolate Tor 2 (Marra et al., 2003) was 99.8%, suggesting that the animal viruses were very similar to the human epidemic strain. A 29 nt insertion was found in the ORF10 (also called open reading frame 8 or ORF8) region in these animal sequences, which was only found in some early human isolates (Guan et al., 2003; Chinese SARS Molecular Epidemiology Consortium, 2004). This 29 nt insertion was suggested as a marker for animal origin. The spike sequence of raccoon dog isolate (SZ13) was also sequenced and was found to be almost identical to the civet isolate SZ16. This led the authors to suggest that transmission or contamination from one host to the other within the market cannot be excluded (Guan et al., 2003).

The prevalence of neutralization antibody to SZ16 in humans in the same market was also evaluated. Eight out of 20 (40%) of the wild animal traders and three of 15 (20%) of those who slaughtered these animals had evidence of antibody, yet only one of 20 (5%) vegetable traders in the market was seropositive and none of the control group from individuals from outside the market (Guan et al., 2003).

Guangzhou Municipal Center for Disease Control conducted serological studies of traders from three animal markets in Guangzhou, Guangdong Province, China in May 2003 (Centers for Disease Control and Prevention (CDC), 2003). Among 508 animal traders, 66 (13%) tested positive for IgG antibody to SARS associated coronavirus by ELISA, while the control groups including hospital workers, Guangdong CDC workers, and healthy adults at clinic had an antibody prevalence of 1–3%. Among animal traders, the highest prevalence of antibody was found among those who traded primarily masked palm civets (72.7%), wild boars (57.1%), muntjac deer (56.3%), hares (46.2%), and pheasant (33.3%). Those for cat, other fowl, and snake were 18.6%, 12%, and 9.2%, respectively. None of the antibody positive traders demonstrated SARS-like disease symptoms. The prevalence of traders with IgG antibody to SARS-CoV of the three tested markets varied (6%, 11%, and 20%, respectively; $p < 0.001$). The results also provide indirect support for the hypothesis of an animal origin for SARS (Centers for Disease Control and Prevention, 2003).

A similar report investigated 635 animal traders in three animal markets (A, B, and C) in Guangzhou, Guangdong Province, China from May to June, 2003 (Xu et al., 2004a). The prevalence of IgG antibody to SARS-CoV was about 16.69% (106/635) in animal traders, significantly higher than that of the control group of vegetable traders (0.72%, 1/139). The prevalence of the traders who engaged only in masked palm civets was 58.54% (24/41), significantly higher than the 9.46% (14/148) of the traders engaged only in snakes. The prevalence of the animals traded in the three markets varied. Market A engaged mainly in the trade of wild animals, while market B engaged in domestic fowl, and market C in snakes. Market A ranked the highest prevalence of IgG positive with 25.61% (84/328), significantly higher than the 7.5% (12/160) of market B, and the 6.80% (10/147) of market C. In market A, the prevalence of IgG positive individuals occurred in traders engaged in wild animals, market managers, traders' children, traders engaged in domestic fowl, traders engaged in snakes, and traders engaged in frozen animal food was 59.34%(54/91), 20.59(7/34), 16.00% (4/25), 15.22% (7/46), 10.40% (13/125), and 9.68% (3/31), respectively. By questionnaire, it was discovered that during the SARS epidemic, the prevalence of symptoms of acute upper respiratory infection was higher in the animal markets (33.63%, 113/336) than in the vegetable markets (15.83%, 22/139). A retrospective study also indicated that in the animal markets, the prevalence of symptoms of acute upper respiratory infection was significantly higher in individuals with IgG antibody against the SARS-CoV virus 49.28% (34/69) than those who were negative (30.35%, 78/257). In the animal market, the prevalence of IgG antibody to SARS-CoV was significantly higher in those who had symptoms of acute upper respiratory infection (30.77%, 35/114) than those who were healthy (20.085, 44/218). The data indicated that infection with SARS-CoV in traders of animal markets is possibly related to their direct exposure to wild animals, particularly to masked palm civets, and during the period of the SARS epidemic, some of the traders did become infected with the SARS-CoV virus (Xu et al., 2004a).

Xu et al. (2004b) studied the early SARS epidemic in 2003 and the indexed patients in each of the seven earliest affected municipalities in Guangdong Province, China. All the indexed patients had a date of onset before 31 January 2003, with the first patient onset on 16 November 2002. In five municipalities (Foshan, Jiangmen, Zhongshan, Guangzhou, and Shenzhen), outbreaks appear to have occurred independently, but the outbreak in Heyuan may be linked to that in Shenzhen and the outbreak in Zhaoqing to that in Guangzhou. It was discovered that two of the seven indexed patients were restaurant chefs; food handlers (i.e., people who handle, kill, or butcher animals) were overrepresented among early-onset cases with no contact history; and patients with early onset were more likely than patients with late onset to live near an agricultural produce market. However, none of the early patients was a commercial farmer nor was living near a farm associated with increased risk. The authors suggest that wild animals rather than a livestock or poultry might be the original source of the SARS outbreak (Xu et al., 2004b).

Apart from the above published data, there were a couple of news reports about the investigation of animal reservoirs in China. On 24 May 2003, an animal origin investigation group from the ministry of agriculture claimed that they have collected samples from 1,700 animals including 59 species, and they had found sequences 99.9% identical to that of SARS-CoV from bats, monkeys, palm civets, and snakes. (www.chinanews.com, 24 May 2003). This research group included scientists from Harbin Veterinary Research Institute, Chinese Academy of Agriculture, Changchun University of Agriculture and Animal Sciences, South China Agriculture University, Guangdong Provincial Veterinary Station of Epidemic Prevention and Supervision, and Guangdong CDC. Another investigation result was released from Beijing Agriculture University on 19 June 2003 (The Beijing Youth Day, 19 June 2003). They claimed that 732 samples were collected from 65 animal species including 54 wild animals and 11 domestic animals. All of the samples were negative by reverse transcription–polymerase cycle reaction (RT-PCR). Among these animals there were 76 masked palm civets, including 25 from Guangdong, 10 from Yunnan, 3 from

Guangxi, 3 from Jiangxi, 20 from Shaanxi, 4 from Shanxi, and 11 from Beijing (the Beijing Youth Day, 19 June 2003). However, no detailed results of these news reports related researches have been published so far.

Investigation of the Restaurant and Market Animals and Their Relationship to the Mild SARS Cases in the Winter of 2003–2004

Between 16 December 2003 and 8 January 2004, a total of four patients were independently hospitalized in the city of Guangzhou, Guangdong Province, China, with flu-like syndromes, which were later diagnosed as SARS cases (Liang et al., 2004). All the four cases were mild and had no secondary transmission. The epidemiological information collected by the Guangdong Center for Disease Control and Prevention and the Guangzhou Center for Disease Control and Prevention indicated that although none of these patients had a contact history with previously documented SARS cases, they all had direct or indirect contact history with wild animals in geographically restricted areas. The second patient worked in a local restaurant TDLR and the fourth patient dined in the same restaurant where palm civet and other exotic dishes were served, whereas the third patient dined in a neighboring restaurant SJR. The first patient was the only patient with no contact with TDLR or SJR; however, had contact with house rats in his apartment a few days before disease onset (Song et al., 2005).

Two teams have published their results about the SARS-CoV-like viruses in civets and their links to the mild SARS cases of winter 2003–2004 (Song et al., 2005; Kan et al., 2005).

Song et al. (2005) sequenced most of the SARS-CoV viral genome from the first two of the four human patients (GZ03-01 and GZ03-02), two palm civets from the Guangzhou food market (PC4-136, PC4-227) and one sample from the palm civet cage at the restaurant TDLR (PC4-13). They were also able to sequence seven additional spike sequences (PC4-115, PC4-127, PC4-137, PC4-145, PC4-199, PC4-205, and PC4-205) from masked palm civets from the Guangzhou food market and partial spike gene from the third patient (GZ03-03).

The whole genome sequences indicated that the identities of SARS-CoV-like viruses from the civets and that of the human patients were about 99.89% homologous (Song et al., 2005). Phylogenic analysis indicated that the sequence of the masked palm civets in 2004 were closer to that of the mild human cases of winter 2003–2004 than to that of the masked palm civets found in 2003 (SZ3 and SZ16).

Kan et al. (2005) were able to get samples from Xinyuan Live Animal Market in Guangzhou, Gangdong Province, China in January 2004 just before the animals in the market were culled. They collected rectal and throat swabs from 91 civets and 15 raccoon dogs randomly selected from 18 vendors with booths located in four blocks dedicated to the sale of civets and raccoon dogs. They also collected environmental specimens from those blocks, including animal-cage swabs, cash-table swabs, and wall swabs. RT-PCR results indicated that 84 of the 91 civets were positive with both rectal and throat swabs. The other seven palm civets tested positive with throat or rectal swabs only. Of the 15 raccoon dogs, 12 tested positive with both throat and rectal swabs, while 3 tested positive with throat swabs only. Of the 24 environmental specimens, 22 tested positive.

Two whole-genome sequences (A022G and B039G) of SARS-CoV-like viruses were directly determined from palm civet samples taken from the market, and two whole-genome sequences (Civet007G and Civet020G) from the restaurant TDLR civets were obtained by Kan et al. (2005). In addition, two spike sequences from raccoon dogs (A030G and A031G) and 13 spike sequences from masked palm civets from the market were also obtained. It was found that the spike sequence of case 1 of 2003–2004 winter patients (GD03T0013) was identical to that of one of the civets in Xinyuan Live Animal Market (B012G), suggesting that this patient might have caught the virus from palm civets from Xinyuan Live Animal Market (Kan et al., 2005). The spike sequences of the two raccoon dogs (A030G and A031G) and the masked palm civet (A022G) were identical. Phylogenetic research indicated that these three sequences (A030G, A031G, and A022G) might be the original proto-type of all the sequences found in this research (Kan et al., 2005). The spike sequences of Civet007G and Civet020G from the restaurant TDLR had only five nucleotides difference from that of A030G, A031G, and A022G. In addition, the spike sequences of Civet007G and Civet020G were identical to that of other ten masked palm civets from Xinyuan Live Animal Market, including A001G, A013G, B033G, B039G, B040G, C013G, C014G, C017G, C019G, and C028G.

The 29-nt sequence that was recognized as the marker of animal origin (Guan et al., 2003; Chinese SARS Molecular Epidemiology Consortium, 2004) was detected in all of the completed sequenced viruses from masked palm civets (Guan et al., 2003; Song et al., 2005; Kan et al., 2005), with only a difference in PC4-227 that the insertion was comprised of 27 nt instead of 29 nt.

When it was found that the sequence of the first SARS case in 2004 was almost identical to that of one of the animals in the market, the local Guangdong government took aggressive action in culling all the masked palm civets in the farms and food markets (Normile, 2004; Watts, 2004). It was estimated that in January 2004, about 10,000 masked palm civets were culled in Guangdong Province, China.

If the finding in 2003 had revealed that masked palm civets are the possible origin of the SARS outbreak, the discovery of the winter 2003–2004 further confirmed that masked palm civets were the source of human infection with SARS-CoV. However, whether the masked palm civet is the primary animal reservoir or an intermediate vector of SARS-CoV remains unclear.

Investigation of Farmed Masked Palm Civets and Comparison with Market Animals

The ideal way to find out whether masked palm civets are animal reservoir of SARS-CoV is to conduct surveillance of the animals in their native habitats. However, as masked palm civets are normally solitary in nature, it is not an easy task to capture them for epidemiology study. In contrast, it was estimated that there were about 40,000 masked palm civets being raised in about 600 farms all over China in 2003 (China Daily, 6 January 2004). Also, it was reported that there were 41 civet farms in Guangdong Province at the time of the slaughter campaign in January 2004 (Tu et al., 2004). Therefore, several investigations to determine the prevalence of SARS-CoV-like virus in farmed masked palm civets were conducted.

Tu and co-workers (2004) investigated serum samples from masked palm civets in four farms and in one market in Guangdong province of China during the slaughter campaign in January 2004. Intestinal tissues and serum samples were taken from 56 animals: 38 civets from four farms in different regions of Guangdong Province (10 from Zhuhai, 10 from Shanwei, 9 from Shaoguan, and 9 from Qingyuan) and 18 civets from the Xinyuan Live Animal Market in Guangzhou. They found anti-SARS-CoV antibodies in 78% of the market animals (14 out of 18), while the overall prevalence in farm animals was ~10% (4 of 38), with the highest prevalence of 40% (4 of 10) in Farm Shanwei. SARS-CoV antibody levels in the four animals at the farm in Shanwei were lower than those from the market, and two samples found positive by a virus neutralization test failed to react on immunofluoresence antibody assay or Western blot. Intestinal tissues collected from the 56 civets including both market and farmed animals were tested by RT-PCR using nucleocapsid (N), membrane (M), or spike (S) gene specific primers, and none of the samples was positive (Tu et al., 2004).

In the same paper, Tu et al. (2004) also investigated 47 civet serum samples that had been previously collected in early June 2003 from two civet farms in Luoning City of Henan Province and Changsha City of Hunan Province. All the samples were negative by virus neutralization test and immunofluoresence antibody assay. The authors suggested that the high prevalence of SARS-CoV in market civets might be associated with trading activities, which resulted in overcrowding and the mixing of different animal species (Tu et al., 2004).

Kan et al. (2005) investigated 1,107 palm civets from 25 farms in 12 provinces in China during January and September 2004. These provinces included Anhui, Beijing, Fujian, Guangxi, Henan, Hebei, Hubei, Hunan, Jiangsu, Jiangxi, Shanxi, and Shaanxi. The criteria for the selection of farms for sampling included their sale of animals from a booth at the Xinyuan Live Animal Market and their claims to trade ~80% of their animals to Guangdong province. In contrast to the market masked palm civets and raccoon dogs, which were all positive for SARS-CoV-like viruses, all of the 1,107 civets sampled from farms tested negative for SARS-CoV-like virus by RT-PCR (Kan et al., 2005). The authors were able to trace one farmer who sold masked palm civets to Xinyuan Live Animal Market. All the seventeen masked palm civets in Xinyuan Live Animal Market from this farm tested positive for SARS-CoV like virus by RT-PCR. However, all the masked palm civets ($n = 169$) at his farm in Henan Province detected negative for SARS-CoV-like virus by the same RT-PCR method (Kan et al., 2005). The authors suggested that the palm civets were infected at the market by other palm civets or by other animals harboring the virus rather than at the farm.

If the animals were infected at the market, then new arrivals should possess a relatively low or no viral load, and the viral load should increase after arriving at

Color Plate

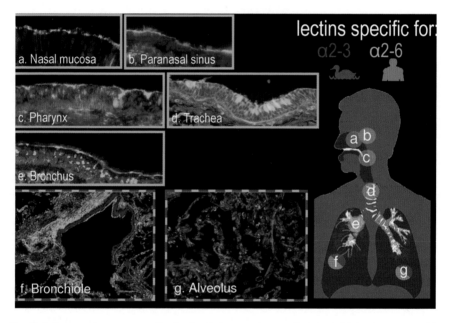

Fig. 2 Influenza virus receptor distribution in human airways. Staining with lectins that specifically recognize α2,3- or α2,6-linked sialyloligosaccharides reveals human-type receptors in the upper human airway (green), but avian-type receptors in the lower respiratory organs (red). From *Nature, 440,* 435–436. 2006

the market. Kan et al. (2005) tested viral loads in a few masked palm civets whose arrival dates were traceable. Quantitative measurement of SARS-CoV-like virus in rectal swabs taken from the masked palm civets was determined by fluorescent real-time RT-PCR based on the N gene. It was found that animals started shedding virus ($10^{3.68}$ viral copies per ml) as early as 2 days after arrival (there were no data for day 1 and that only one animal was observed at the 2-day time point). An average of $10^{4.43}$ viral copies per ml of specimen was observed for six masked palm civets which had been at the market for 4 days. The peak virus load (an average of $10^{6.91}$ viral copies per ml) was observed in animals which had been at the market for 7 days; this declined by day 15 ($10^{4.17}$ viral copies per ml). This pattern of viral load change was found similar to the results in experimentally infected masked palm civets. When palm civets were experimentally infected, the viral genome was detected by RT-PCR in throat and anal swabs from 3 to 18 days post inoculation (Wu et al., 2005). However, the viral load in rectal swabs remained relatively high in the animals that arrived at the market for 17 days ($10^{6.4}$ viral copies per ml), 52 days ($10^{6.56}$ viral copies per ml), and 180 days ($10^{5.49}$ viral copies per ml) (Kan et al., 2005), unlike the inoculated experimental masked palm civets that virus were not detectable by RT-PCR for throat or anal swabs after 18 days post inoculation (Wu et al., 2005). However, viral genomic DNA could be detected in spleen and lymph nodes up to 34 and 35 days post inoculation in experimentally infected masked palm civets (Wu et al., 2005). It is suggested that there might be a persistent viral infection or reinfection of masked palm civets in the market (Kan et al., 2005).

Hu et al. (2005) developed a multitarget real-time PCR assay for detecting SARS-CoV in clinical samples and also SARS-CoV-like viruses in masked palm civets. They used probes and primers based on sequences of the N gene, open reading frame (ORF) 3, and ORF 8. It was found that the detection of N gene was much more sensitive than that of ORF3 and ORF8. They tested seven randomly selected throat swabs of masked palm civets from a farm located in Hubei Province and found that one was positive by using three primer and probe sets, with N gene of $10^{7.99}$ copies/ml, ORF3 of $10^{2.7}$ copies/ml, and ORF8 of $10^{3.36}$ copies/ml. Two were positive by using two primer and probe sets and the other four were positive by using one primer and probe set (Hu et al., 2005).

At the moment, the data about the farmed masked palm civets are still confusing. It is quite possible that prevalence of infection in different farms varies. It could not be ruled out that in the farms, viral load is relatively lower than in the markets, and when less sensitive assays were used, the prevalence of viral infection in the farms was underestimated.

Investigation of Wild Masked Palm Civets

So far, the data of SARS-CoV prevalence in wild masked palm civets are very limited. Poon et al. (2005) trapped 21 masked palm civets from Hong Kong Special Administrative Region, China. They collected respiratory and fecal swab samples and detected the existence of coronaviruses by RT-PCR using consensus primers targeted to the conserved region of coronavirus RNA polymerase. Blood samples were taken for neutralization assay for SARS-CoV. None of the masked palm civets was positive for SARS-CoV by both serological and molecular tests (Poon et al., 2005). The authors suggested that although the result did not exclude the possibility that masked palm civet is the natural host of SARS-CoV, it at least indicated that SARS-CoV is not broadly circulating in wild masked palm civets.

Investigation of SARS-CoVs in Bats

The study of animal reservoirs of SARS-CoV was not limited on masked palm civets. As bats are an important reservoir for many zoonotic viruses including rabies virus, lyssavirus, Hendra and Nipha viruses, Menangle virus, St. Louis encephalitis virus (Halpin et al., 2000; Mackenzie et al., 2001; Mackenzie and Field, 2004), it was also one of the investigating targets for animal reservoir of SARS-CoV. An early study of bats by Poon et al. (2005) investigated 81 bats belonging to 12 different species by RT-PCR using conserved sequence of coronavirus. A novel bat coronavirus (Bat-CoV) was identified in three different species from the same genus, *Minoopterus magnater, M. pusillus, and M. schreibersii*. The Bat-CoV, from which the sequenced fragments shared 41–62% homology to that of SARS-CoV, is not a SARS-CoV-like virus and belongs to Group I coronavirus (Poon et al., 2005).

However, recently two independent research teams have published exciting results of finding SARS-CoV-like viruses in bats and suggested that the horseshoe bat is a reservoir of SARS-CoV-like viruses (Lau et al., 2005; Li et al., 2005). Lau et al. (2005) investigated bats located in Hong Kong Special Administrative Region, China. They detected 118 nasopharyngeal and anal swabs from 59 bats representing 8 species, 5 genera, and 3 families. By using RT-PCR, 23 of 59 anal swabs were found positive from Chinese horseshoe bats (*Rhinolophus sinicus*) (Lau et al., 2005) (also see Table 1).

Three genomes of bat SARS-CoV-like viruses were sequenced by Lau et al. (2005), that of B24, B43, and B41. The genomes of the bat SARS-CoV-like virus were very similar to that of SARS-CoV except for the regions of the Spike gene, ORF 3 and ORF 8. The three genomes had 88% nucleotide and 93% amino acid identity to human and civet SARS-CoVs. The 29-bp insertion was shown to exist in bat SARS-CoV like viruses, although this sequence demonstrated 12 nt substitutions. Phylogenetic analysis showed that bat SARS-CoV-like viruses formed a distinct cluster with SARS-CoVs (Lau et al., 2005) and a distantly related group 2 coronavirus (Siddell, 1995; Lai and Holmes, 2001).

Among the bats investigated, positive prevalence of the antibodies against recombinant bat-SARS-CoV N protein was 67% (12/18) by Western blot and 84% (31/37) by enzyme immunoassay, compared with only 42% (8/19) for human SARS-CoV neutralizing antibody titer ($\geq$1:20). And for those bats with neutralizing antibodies, a lower viral load was found in their anal swabs (Lau et al., 2005).

Table 1 Detection of prevalence of antibodies and RNAs of SARS-CoV like viruses in bats

Sampling location	Bat species	Antibody test against N protein: positive/total (%)	RT-PCR analysis: positive/ total (%) Fecal swabs	Respiratory swabs
Guangxi	*Rousettus leschenaulti*	1/142 (1.4%)[a]	0/165	0/55
	Rhinolophus pearsonii	13/46 (28.3%)[a]	3/30 (10%)	0/11
	Rhinolophus pussilus	2/6 (33.3%)[a]	0/6	0/2
Guangdong	*Rousettus leschenaulti*	0/42[a]	0/45	ND
	Cynopterus sphinx	0/17[a]	0/27	ND
Tianjin	*Myotis ricketti*	ND	0/21	0/21
	Rhinolophus pussilus	ND	0/15	ND
	Rhinolophus ferrumequinum	0/4[a]	1/8 (12.5%)	ND
Hubei	*Rhinolophus macrotis*	5/7 (71%)[a]	1/8 (12.5%)	0/3
	Nyctalus plancyi	0/1[a]	0/1	ND
	Miniopterus schreibersi	0/1[a]	0/1	ND
	Myotis altarium	0/1[a]	0/1	ND
Hong Kong	*Hipposideros armiger*	ND	0/12	0/12
	Miniopterus magnater	ND	0/23	0/23
	Miniopterus pusillus	ND	0/24	0/24
	Myotis chinensis	ND	0/3	0/3
	Myotis ricketti	ND	0/2	0/2
	Nyctalus noctula	ND	0/2	0/2
	Rhinolophus affinus	ND	0/2	0/2
	Rhinolophus sinicus	12/18(67%)[b]	23/59(39%)	0/59

Modified according to Lau et al., 2005 and Li et al., 2005; ND, not done
[a] Sandwich ELISA based on SARS-CoV N protein (Li et al., 2005)
[b] Western blot with recombinant N protein of bat SL-CoV (Lau et al., 2005)

Li et al. (2005) detected 402 respiratory and fecal swab samples from 408 bats representing 9 species, 6 genera, and 3 families, from four provinces in China, including Guangdong, Guangxi, Hubei and Tianjin (Table 1). Three species from the genus *Rhinolophus* (horseshoe bats) in the family *Rhinolophidae* demonstrated a high SARS-CoV antibody prevalence: 13/46 (28%) in *R. pearsonii* from Guangxi; 2/6(33%) in *R. pussilllus* from Guangxi; and 5/7 (71%) in *R. macrotis* from Hubei. A total of five positive fecal samples were detected, all of them from the genus *Rhinolophus*, three in *R. pearsonii* from Guangxi, and one each in *R. macrotis* and *R. ferrumequinum*, from Hubei (Li et al., 2005). Neutralization tests using human SARS-CoV, however, were all negative. As there is no SARS-CoV-like viral isolates from bats yet, it remains unknown whether the serum from bats can neutralize the virus from bats or not.

One virus from the fecal samples (Rp3) was completely sequenced and its genome demonstrated 92% nt identity to Tor 2 strain (Li et al., 2005). The polymerase, spike, envelope, membrane, and nucleocapsid proteins, which are present in all coronaviruses, were similarly sized in Rp3 and Tor 2, with sequence identities ranging from 96% to 100%. Partial sequences from the other four samples (Rf1, Rm1, Rp1, and Rp2) indicated that recombination occurred within the genomes of bat SARS-CoV-like viruses.

As bats are natural reservoirs of several new and reemerging viruses, it is not a surprise that it is also a reservoir of SARS-CoV-like virus. Nipah virus, for example, spread in Malaysia in 1998 and in Bangladesh in 2004, was in high-level serological prevalence in bat genus *Pteropus* and isolated from *Pteropus hypomelanus* and *P. lylei* in Malaysia, Bangladesh, and Cambodia (Chua et al., 2001; Hsu et al., 2004; Reynes et al., 2005). Nipah virus isolated in bat also showed a greater genetic diversity than that isolated in human. The discovery of bat SARS-CoV-like viruses suggests that genetic diversity exists among zoonotic viruses in bats, increasing the possibility of variants crossing the species barrier and causing outbreaks of disease in human populations. It is therefore essential to enhance our knowledge and understanding of reservoir host distribution, animal–animal and human–animal interaction. It is also interesting to find out why bats can be reservoir of so many viruses, whether there is an association with immunology or ecology of bats.

Are There Other Animal Species that Serve as Reservoirs of SARS-CoV?

So far, the sequence data showed that the average genome homology of SARS-CoV-like virus from horseshoe bat to the SARS-CoV is about 92%, while the homology of SARS-CoV-like virus of masked palm civets to the SARS-CoV is above 99.6%. This indicated that horseshoe bat is a distantly related animal reservoir of SARS-CoV-like virus, while masked palm civet can be the direct origin of SARS. Further investigations might reveal that higher homology in bats or lower homology in masked palm civets. However, it is likely that in the transmission chain between horseshoe bats and masked palm civets there are still other species(s) missing. One way is to look at the ecological circles of both bats and masked palm civets to fish out possible links and suspects. An extensive survey of wild animal species for SARS-CoV-like viruses should provide us with information about alternative animal reservoirs.

Poon et al. (2005) conducted a survey of the prevalence of coronaviruses in wild animals in Hong Kong between the summer of 2003 and the summer of 2004. They investigated small mammalian, avian, and reptile species living in natural reservoirs or city parks in Hong Kong. A total of 162 animals from 44 species were tested by RT-PCR for conserved sequences of RNA-dependent RNA polymerase, helicase-ExoN and S-encoding sequences of SARS-CoV. Apart from three species of bats, that of *Miniopterus magnater, Miniopterus pusillus, Miniopters schreibersii,* from which a new group I coronavirus was isolated, all other species were negative. However, the animal numbers for each species they investigated were limited, with only *Cynoptus sphinx* ($n = 15$), *Miniopterus magnater* ($n = 16$), *Miniopterus pusillus,* ($n = 19$), *Hystrix hodgsoni* ($n = 10$), and *Paguma larvata* ($n = 21$) over 10 animals (Poon et al., 2005). This limited sample size of animal species might not detect viruses that are circulating at a low frequency.

Rodents are another type of popular reservoir of many viral pathogens. The first patient in winter 2003–2004 had direct contact with a rat in his apartment (Liang et al., 2004). Apart from bats, Lau et al. (2005) also captured 60 rodents and 20 monkeys from summer 2004 to spring 2005 in Hong Kong Special Administrative Region, China. The 60 rodents belong to three different species, including 12 Chestnut spiny rats (*Niviventer fulvescens*), 4 Buff-bellied rats (*Rattus rattus flavipectus*), and 44 Sikkim rats (*Rattus sikkimensis*), and all samples were tested negative by RT-PCR (Lau et al., 2005).

Live-animal markets (wet markets) provide an environment for cross-species transmission of virus (Webster, 2004) and therefore it is an ideal place to look for susceptible hosts and the possible origin of SARS-CoV (Guan et al., 2003; Lau et al., 2005). Wang et al. (2005) investigated an animal market in Guangzhou, Guangdong Province, China on 5 January 2004 just before the culling of masked palm civets (Normile, 2004). Thirty one animals were sampled including 20 domestic cats (*Felis catus*), 5 red foxes (*Vulpes vulpes*), and 6 Lesser rice field rats (*Rattus losea*). Real-time PCR revealed that four cats, three red foxes, and one Lesser rice field rat were positive for SARS-CoV, indicating that the market was seriously contaminated. At the time, the environment of the market was also contaminated with SARS-CoV-like viruses (Lau et al., 2005), and it is unknown whether those positive animals were susceptible hosts rather than important reservoirs of the virus. On 20 January 2004, 2 weeks after the culling of animals and the disinfection of the market, 119 animals from the same market were tested. The animals included 6 rabbits (*Oryctolagus cuniculus*), 13 cats, 46 red jungle fowl (*Gallus gallus*), 13 spotbill duck (*Anas platyhynchos*), 10 greylag goose (*Anser anser*), and 31 Chinese francolin (*Franclnus pintadeanus*). Only a rectal swab for one greylag goose tested positive for SARS-CoV-like virus by RT-PCR, indicting the disinfection of the market was successful. Later, 102 animals including 14 greylag goose, 3 cats, 5 rabbits, 9 spotbill ducks, 2 Chinese francolins, 8 common pheasants (*Phasianus colchicus*), 6 pigeons, 9 Chinese muntjacs, 19 wild boars (*Sus scrofa*), 16 Lesser rice field rats, 5 dogs, 1 mink (*Mustela vison*), 3 goats, 2 green peafowl (*Pavo muticus*) were sampled from the market between April to November 2004. Only one rectal swab from a wild boar tested positive (Wang et al., 2005). No details were reported about the isolates from the greylag goose or the wild boar.

Experimental animal inoculation of viruses may help to identify natural viral reservoirs. Such experimental tests have indicated that SARS-CoV might be able to infect a wide-range of hosts, including masked palm civets (Wu et al., 2005), monkeys (Fouchier et al., 2003; McAuliffe et al., 2004; Rowe et al, 2004; Qin et al., 2005), cats and ferrets (Martina et al., 2003), mice (Subbarao et al., 2004; Wentworth et al, 2004; Glass et al., 2004; Roberts et al., 2005b), pigs and chickens (Weingartl et al., 2004), guinea pigs (Liang et al., 2005), and Golden Syrian Hamster (Roberts et al., 2005a). However, as most experimental tests were performed with the purpose of creating animal models for vaccine evaluation, not much is known about the transmission of the virus from the inoculated animals. Pigs and chickens, for example, may support SARS-CoV replication to a very limited degree but are not likely to play a role as an amplifying host (Weingartl et al., 2004).

Some attention was also paid to domestic animals. Chen et al. (2005) conducted a survey of SARS-CoV-like viruses in six major domestic animal species that are in close contact with humans. They surveyed 242 animals, including 108 pigs, 60 cattle, 20 dogs, 11 cats, 11 chickens, and 30 ducks in Xiqing Country of Tianjin, China, where a SARS outbreak occurred in late spring 2003. Two pigs were found antibody positive, while the other 240 animals were found antibody negative. One of the two pigs was tested positive by RT-PCR and two viral isolates were obtained from its blood and fecal samples, designed TJB and TJF, respectively. The pig was followed up for 4 weeks until its blood tested negative with RT-PCR. The genome of TJF was completely sequenced and was very close to the human epidemic strain (differing by only 18 nt from the BJ01 whole genome sequence). Because the genome of TJF does not contain the insertion marker of 29 nt, the authors suggested that TJF was transmitted from humans to the pig. As swineherds in rural areas often obtain leftovers from restaurants in the cities for use as hogwash without thoroughly fermenting, the authors suggested that the pig was most likely infected from virus-contaminated animal feed (Chen et al., 2005).

Although there are several susceptible hosts for SARS-CoV, all the above researches did not give an obvious hint to possible animal reservoirs further than horseshoe bats and masked palm civets. Also, the linkage between the horseshoe bats and masked palm civets is still missing.

Possible Factors that Contributed to the Increasing Risks of Disease Outbreaks

It remains unknown why the first SARS outbreaks appeared in the late 2002 in Guangdong, China, and whether this was the first time that SARS-CoV infected and caused disease in humans. Using immunofluorescence and neutralization assays, Zheng et al. (2004) detected antibodies to human SARS-CoV and/or an animal SARS-CoV-like virus in 17 of 938 (1.8%) healthy adults from Hong Kong in 2001, suggesting that a small proportion of healthy people in Hong Kong had been exposed to SARS-related viruses at least 2 years before the first SARS outbreak. However, Yu et al. (2005) had a different result. They used different assays to analyze 1,621 serum specimens collected from military recruits from the People's Republic of China in 2002 for SARS-CoV antibodies. Eleven samples were found positive by ELISA and six of them confirmed by IFA, but only three were confirmed by protein microarray analysis and antigen-capturing ELISA. None of the eleven samples was positive in neutralization test. The authors suggested that the people from mainland China either had only rarely been exposed to SARS-CoV before the 2003 SARS outbreak or had not been exposed to SARS-CoV at all (Yu et al., 2005).

The peak of demand of masked palm civets as a delicacy in Guangzhou, China occurred in 2000–2002; whether this provided an environment and a period for the viruses to accumulate mutations and evolve the capacity to infect humans needs further investigation.

One of the factors that might contribute to the human infection may reside in the genotypes of the virus isolated from SARS patients. Recent studies have shown that two amino acids (aa 479 and 487) might be responsible for the transmission of SARS-CoV-like virus from the masked palm civet to humans (Yang et al., 2005; Qu et al., 2005). It was demonstrated that with the mutation of either R/K479 (of masked palm civets) into N479 (of human) or S487 (of palm civets) into T487 (of human), the pseudotype viruses carrying mutated spike of civet SARS-CoV-like viruses could infect the cells expressing human receptor ACE2. On the other hand, if both N497 and T487 were mutated into R/K497 and S487, the pseudotype virus with spike of human SARS-CoV lost its infectivity to human cells (Qu et al., 2005). The mutation of N479 had been found in some of the sequenced masked palm civets from the market as well as in some of the mild human cases of winter 2003–2004 (Song et al., 2005; Kan et al., 2005). It was suggested that this mutation can cause animal to human transmission, and by further mutation such as S487T, those viruses might cause human to human transmission and a subsequent epidemic (Song et al, 2005; Qu et al., 2005). In fact, so far we have not found the original strain that caused the 2003 epidemic of SARS. The animal viruses sequenced from the Shengzhen animal market (Guan et al., 2003) had too many mutations compared to that of the human epidemic strains, suggesting that these isolates were not directly responsible for the 2003 epidemic.

The distribution of the virus in the environment and its access to humans could be another factor that contributes to the risk. Although we are not sure whether masked palm civets and raccoon dogs are natural hosts for SARS-CoV or not, their high prevalence of SARS-CoV in the wet markets certainly played an important role in the previous SARS outbreaks. Surveillance of Xinyuan Live Animal Market on 5 January 2004 revealed that 100% samples from the masked palm civets and raccoon dogs were positive for SARS-CoV by RT-PCR and 22/24 (92%) environment specimens were also positive (Kan et al., 2005). A similar surveillance indicated that 3/5 (60%) of the red foxes, 4/20 (20%) of the domestic cats, 1/6 (17%) of lesser rice-field rats were positive for SARS-CoV by RT-PCR, in the market (Wang et al., 2005). The fact that so many species and even environmental samples from animal cages, cash tables, or walls were detectable for viral RNA serves as dangerous signals for the existing of emerging SARS-CoV-like viruses in the market at that time. The coincidence of the four mild cases could be regarded as a reflection of the high risk in the winter 2003–2004. And it is believed that the culling of masked palm civets and the close of the wet markets in Guangdong in January 2004 did contribute to the absence of subsequent outbreaks.

Identification of Future Risks and Actions

After the SARS epidemic in 2003, apart from a few mild cases in the winter of 2003–2004 and laboratory contraindications, it seems that there is no evidence of the reemergence of SARS. Certain changes have been made in China.

For example, masked palm civet is hardly seen in the restaurants or markets in Guangdong China, and Xinyuan Live Animal Market has now changed into a market for frozen food. However, as we have only very limited knowledge of the ecology of the SARS-CoV virus in nature, we are unable to make accurate predictions without further scientific surveillance and research.

A wider investigation of SARS-CoV-like viruses in different animal species is still needed to fill the gaps in the transmission chain of SARS-CoVs and to understand the viral evolution. The identification of different viral genotypes in natural hosts would provide information as to the important factors in the species barrier and human infection with SARS-CoV. The culling of the masked palm civets in Guangdong in January 2004 was an urgent need at that time. However, further studies of the distribution of the SAR-CoV in the environment will provide information on its natural animal reservoirs and methods to contain its epizootic transmission.

Wet markets are an important source of emerging viruses (Webster, 2004) and therefore their surveillance can be used as an early-warning system. After the culling of masked palm civets and disinfection, only two animals were tested positive out of 221 animals from the market during the period of January to November, 2004 (Wang et al., 2005). In November and December 2004, 12 and 10 masked palm civets were sampled from Guangzhou and Shenzhen, respectively, including five of which had been at the live market for 2 days, none of them tested positive. Therefore, it was suggested that the reemergence of human infection from animal origins was low for the winter of 2004–2005 (Wang et al., 2005) and this has been proved to be the case.

For surveillance, it is important to develop a sensitive tool to detect antibody prevalence in different animals. It has been shown that the spike genes from some masked palm civets were difficult to generate neutralizing antibodies (Yang et al., 2005) and that some antibody positive sera from bats could not neutralize SARS-CoV infection (Li et al., 2005). Although recombinant N protein could be used as an antigen for detecting antibodies against SARS-CoV-like viruses in bats (Lau et al., 2005, Li et al., 2005), it may not be the case for other animals or for different viral genotypes. The relationship of different genotypes of SARS-CoV-like viruses with their serological cross-reaction needs to be further identified.

As SARS infections of humans have been controlled, much important SARS related research has been stopped due to limited resources. However, at least for the research on animal reservoir of SARS-CoV, more investigations should be made to further understand the future risks of the reemergence of SARS.

References

Center for Disease Control and Prevention (CDC). (2003). Prevalence of IgG antibody to SARS-associated coronavirus in animal traders–Guangdong Province, China, 2003. *Morbidity and Mortality Weekly Report*, 52, 986–987

Chen, W., Yan, M., Yang, L., Ding, B., He, B., Wang, Y., Liu, X., Liu, C., Zhu, H., You, B., Huang, S., Zhang, J., Mu, F., Xiang, Z., Feng, X., Wen, J., Fang, J., Yu, J., Yang, H., Wang, J. (2005).

SARS-associated coronavirus transmitted from human to pig. *Emerging Infectious Disease*, 11, 446–448

China Daily, 6 January 2004. *www.chinadaily.com.cn/en/doc/2004-01/06/content_295921.htm*

Chinese SARS Molecular Epidemiology Consortium. (2004). Molecular evolution of the SARS coronavirus during the course of the SARS epidemic in China. *Science*, 303, 1666–1669

Chua, K. B., Lam, S. K., Goh, K. J., Hooi, P. S., Ksiazek, T. G., Kamarulzaman, A., Olson, J., Tan, C. T. (2001). The presence of Nipah virus in respiratory secretions and urine of patients during an outbreak of Nipah virus encephalitis in Malaysia. *Journal of Infection*, 42, 40–43

Fouchier, R. A., Kuiken, T., Schutten, M., van Amerongen, G., van Doornum, G. J., van den Hoogen, B. G., Peiris, M., Lim, W., Stohr, K., Osterhaus, A. D. (2003). Aetiology: Koch's postulates fulfilled for SARS virus. *Nature*, 423, 240

Glass, W. G., Subbarao, K., Murphy, B., Murphy, P. M. (2004). Mechanisms of host defense following severe acute respiratory syndrome-coronavirus (SARS-CoV) pulmonary infection of mice. *Journal of Immunology*, 173, 4030–4039

Guan, Y., Zheng, B. J., He, Y. Q., Liu, X. L., Zhuang, Z. X., Cheung, C. L., Luo, S. W., Li, P. H., Zhang, L. J., Guan, Y. J., Butt, K. M., Wong, K. L., Chan, K. W., Lim, W., Shortridge, K. F., Yuen, K. Y., Peiris, J. S., Poon, L. L. (2003). Isolation and characterization of viruses related to the SARS coronavirus from animals in southern China. *Science*, 302, 276–278

Halpin, K., Young, P. L., Field, H. E., Mackenzie, J. S. (2000). Isolation of Hendra virus from pteropid bats: A natural reservoir of Hendra virus. *Journal of General Virology*, 81, 1927–1932

Hsu, V. P., Hossain, M. J., Parashar, U. D., Ali, M. M., Ksiazek, T. G., Kuzmin, I., Niezgoda, M., Rupprecht, C., Bresee, J., Breiman, R. F. (2004). Nipah virus encephalitis reemergence, Bangladesh. *Emerging Infectious Disease*, 10, 2082–2087

http://www.chinanews.com, May 24, 2003

http://www.chinanews.com/n/2003-05-24/26/306472.html

Hu, W., Bai, B., Hu, Z., Chen, Z., An, X., Tang, L., Yang, J., Wang, H., Wang, H. (2005). Development and evaluation of a multitarget real-time taqman reverse transcription PCR for detection of Severe Acute Respiratory Syndrome-associated coronavirus and surveillance for an apparently related coronavirus found in masked palm civets. *Journal of Clinical Microbiology* 43, 2040–2046

Kan, B., Wang, M., Jing, H., Xu, H., Jiang, X., Yan, M., Liang, W., Zheng, H., Wan, K., Liu, Q., Cui, B., Xu, Y., Zhang, E., Wang, H., Ye, J., Li, G., Li, M., Cui, Z., Qi, X., Chen, K., Du, L., Gao, K., Zhao, Y. T., Zou, X. Z., Feng, Y. J., Gao, Y. F., Hai, R., Yu, D., Guan, Y., Xu, J. (2005). Molecular evolution analysis and geographic investigation of severe acute respiratory syndrome coronavirus-like virus in palm civets at an animal market and on farms. *Journal of Virology*, 79, 11892–11900

Lai, M. M. C., Holmes, K. V. (2001). Coronaviruses. In Fields Virology. Knipe, D. M., Howley, P. M., eds. Lippincott, Philadelphia, PA, pp. 1163–1185

Lau, S. K., Woo, P. C., Li, K. S., Huang, Y., Tsoi, H. W., Wong, B. H., Wong, S. S., Leung, S. Y., Chan, K. H., Yuen, K. Y. (2005). Severe acute respiratory syndrome coronavirus-like virus in Chinese horseshoe bats. *Proceedings of the National Academy Sciences of the United States of America*, 102, 14040–10405

Li, W., Shi, Z., Yu, M., Ren, W., Smith, C., Epstein, J. H., Wang, H., Crameri, G., Hu, Z., Zhang, H., Zhang, J., McEachern, J., Field, H., Daszak, P., Eaton, B. T., Zhang, S., Wang, L. F. (2005). Bats are natural reservoirs of SARS-like coronaviruses. *Science*, 310, 676–679

Liang, G., Chen, Q., Xu, J., Liu, Y., Lim, W., Peiris, J. S., Anderson, L. J., Ruan, L., Li, H., Kan, B., Di, B., Cheng, P., Chan, K. H., Erdman, D. D., Gu, S., Yan, X., Liang, W., Zhou, D., Haynes, L., Duan, S., Zhang, X., Zheng, H., Gao, Y., Tong, S., Li, D., Fang, L., Qin, P., Xu, W.; SARS Diagnosis Working Group. (2004). Laboratory diagnosis of four recent sporadic cases of community-acquired SARS, Guangdong Province, China. *Emerging Infectious Disease*, 10, 1774–1781

Liang, L., He, C., Lei, M., Li, S., Hao, Y., Zhu, H., Duan, Q. (2005). Pathology of guinea pigs experimentally infected with a novel reovirus and coronavirus isolated from SARS patients. *DNA Cell Biology*, 24, 485–490

Mackenzie, J. S., Chua, K. B., Daniels, P. W., Eaton, B. T., Field, H. E., Hall, R. A., Halpin, K., Johansen, C. A., Kirkland, P. D., Lam, S. K., McMinn, P., Nisbet, D. J., Paru, R., Pyke, A. T., Ritchie, S. A., Siba, P., Smith, D. W., Smith, G. A., van den Hurk, A. F., Wang, L. F., Williams, D. T. (2001). Emerging viral diseases of Southeast Asia and the Western Pacific. *Emerging Infectious Disease*, 7, 497–504

Mackenzie, J. S., Field, H. E. (2004). Emerging encephalitogenic viruses: Lyssaviruses and henipaviruses transmitted by frugivorous bats. *Archives of Virology Supplement*, 18, 97–111

Marra, M. A., Jones, S. J., Astell, C. R., Holt, R. A., Brooks-Wilson, A., Butterfield, Y. S., Khattra, J., Asano, J. K., Barber, S. A., Chan, S. Y., Cloutier, A., Coughlin, S. M., Freeman, D., Girn, N., Griffith, O. L., Leach, S. R., Mayo, M., McDonald, H., Montgomery, S. B., Pandoh, P. K., Petrescu, A. S., Robertson, A. G., Schein, J. E., Siddiqui, A., Smailus, D. E., Stott, J. M., Yang, G. S., Plummer, F., Andonov, A., Artsob, H., Bastien, N., Bernard, K., Booth, T. F., Bowness, D., cCzub, M., Drebot, M., Fernando, L., Flick, R., Garbutt, M., Gray, M., Grolla, A., Jones, S., Feldmann, H., Meyers, A., Kabani, A., Li, Y., Normand, S., Stroher, U., Tipples, G. A., Tyler, S., Vogrig, R., Ward, D., Watson, B., Brunham, R. C., Krajden, M., Petric, M., Skowronski, D. M., Upton, C., Roper, R. L. (2003). The Genome sequence of the SARS-associated coronavirus. *Science*, 300, 1399–1404

Martina, B. E. E., Haagmans, B. L., Kuiken, T., Fouchier, R. A. M., Rimmelzwaan, G. F., Amerongen, G. V., Peiris, J. S. M., Lim, W., Osterhaus, A. D. M. E. (2003). SARS virus infection of cats and ferrets. *Nature*, 425, 915

McAuliffe, J., Vogel, L., Roberts, A., Fahle, G., Fischer, S., Shieh, W. J., Butler, E., Zaki, S., St Claire, M., Murphy, B., Subbarao, K. (2004). Replication of SARS coronavirus administered into the respiratory tract of African green rhesus and cynomolgus monkeys. *Virology*, 330, 8–15

Normile, D. (2004). Infectious diseases. Viral DNA match spurs China's civet roundup. *Science*, 303, 292

Poon, L. L., Chu, D. K., Chan, K. H., Wong, O. K., Ellis, T. M., Leung, Y. H., Lau, S. K., Woo, P. C., Suen, K.Y., Yuen, K. Y., Guan, Y., Peiris, J. S. (2005). Identification of a novel coronavirus in bats. *Journal of Virology*, 79, 2001–2009

Qin, C., Wang, J., Wei, Q., She, M., Marasco, W. A., Jiang, H., Tu, X., Zhu, H., Ren, L., Gao, H., Guo, L., Huang, L., Yang, R., Cong, Z., Guo, I., Wang, Y., Liu, Y., Sun, Y., Duan, S., Qu, J., Chen, L., Tong, W., Ruan, L., Liu, P., Zhang, H., Zhang, J., Zhang, H., Liu, D., Liu, Q., Hong, T., He, W. (2005). An animal model of SARS produced by infection of *Macaca mulatta* with SARS coronavirus. *Journal of Pathology* 206, 251–259

Qu, X. X., Hao, P., Song, X. J., Jiang, S. M., Liu, Y. X., Wang, P. G., Rao, X., Song, H. D., Wang, S.Y., Zuo, Y., Zheng, A. H., Luo, M., Wang, H. L., Deng, F., Wang, H. Z., Hu, Z. H., Ding, M. X., Zhao, G. P., Deng, H. K. (2005). Identification of two critical amino acid residues of the severe acute respiratory syndrome coronavirus spike protein for its variation in zoonotic tropism transition via a double substitution strategy. *Journal of Biological Chemistry*, 280, 29588–29595

Reynes, J. M., Counor, D., Ong, S., Faure, C., Seng, V., Molia, S., Walston, J., Georges-Courbot, M. C., Deubel, V., Sarthou, J. L. (2005). Nipah virus in Lyle's flying foxes, Cambodia. *Emerging Infectious Disease*, 11, 1042–1047

Roberts, A., Vogel, L., Guarner, J., Hayes, N., Murphy, B., Zaki, S., Subbarao, K. (2005a). Severe acute respiratory syndrome coronavirus infection of golden Syrian hamsters. *Journal of Virology*, 79, 503–511

Roberts, A., Paddock, C., Vogel, L., Butler, E., Zaki, S., Subbarao, K. (2005b). Aged BALB/c mice as a model for increased severity of severe acute respiratory syndrome in elderly humans. *Journal of Virology*, 79, 5833–5838

Rowe, T., Gao, G., Hogan, R. J., Crystal, R. G., Voss, T. G., Grant, R. L., Bell, P., Kobinger, G. P., Wivel, N. A., Wilson, J. M. (2004). Macaque model for severe acute respiratory syndrome. *Journal of Virology*, 78, 11401–11404

Siddell, S. G. (1995). The Coronaviridae. In the Viruses. Fraenkel-Conrat, H., Wagner, R. R., eds. Plenum Press, New York

Subbarao, K., McAuliffe, J., Vogel, L., Fahle, G., Fischer, S., Tatti, K., Packard, M., Shih, W.-J., Murphy, B. (2004). Prior infection and passive transfer of neutralizing antibody prevent replication of severe acute respiratory syndrome coronavirus in the respiratory tract of mice. *Journal of Virology,* 78, 3572–3577

Song, H. D., Tu, C. C., Zhang, G. W., Wang, S. Y., Zheng, K., Lei, L. C., Chen, Q. X., Gao, Y. W., Zhou, H. Q., Xiang, H., Zheng, H. J., Chern, S. W., Cheng, F., Pan, C. M., Xuan, H., Chen, S. J., Luo, H. M., Zhou, D. H., Liu, Y. F., He, J. F., Qin, P. Z., Li, L. H., Ren, Y. Q., Liang, W. J., Yu, Y. D., Anderson, L., Wang, M., Xu, R. H., Wu, X. W., Zheng, H. Y., Chen, J. D., Liang, G., Gao, Y., Liao, M., Fang, L., Jiang, L.Y., Li, H., Chen, F., Di, B., He, L. J., Lin, J. Y., Tong, S., Kong, X., Du, L., Hao, P., Tang, H., Bernini, A., Yu, X. J., Spiga, O., Guo, Z. M., Pan, H. Y., He, W. Z., Manuguerra, J. C., Fontanet, A., Danchin, A., Niccolai, N., Li, Y. X., Wu, C. I., Zhao, G. P. (2005). Cross-host evolution of severe acute respiratory syndrome coronavirus in palm civet and human. *Proceedings of the National Academy Sciences of the United States of America*, 102, 2430–2435

Tu, C. C., Crameri, G., Kong, X. G., Chen, J. D., Sun, Y. W., Yu, M., Xiang, H., Xia, X. Z., Liu, S. W., Ren, T., Y. D., Eaton, B. T., Xuan, H. & Wang, L. F. (2004). Antibodies to sars coronavirus in civets. *Emerging Infectious Diseases* 10, 2244–2248

The Biejing Youth Day, http://english.qianlong.com/7778/2003–6–26/207@912977.htm

Wang, M., Jing, H. Q., Xu, H. F., Jiang, X. G., Kan, B., Liu, Q. Y., Wan, K. L., Cui, B. Y., Zheng, H., Cui, Z. G., Yan, M. Y., Liang, W. L., Wang, H. X., Qi, X. B., Li, Z. J., Li, M. C., Chen, K., Zhang, E. M., Zhang, S. Y., Hai, R., Yu, D. Z., Xu, J. G. (2005) Surveillance on severe acute respiratory syndrome associated coronavirus in animals at a live animal market of Guangzhou in 2004. *Zhonghua Liu Xing Bing Xue Za Zhi*, 26, 84–87

Watts, J. (2004). China culls wild animals to prevent new SARS threat. *Lancet*, 363, 134

Webster, R. G. (2004). Wet markets – A continuing source of severe acute respiratory syndrome and influenza? *Lancet*, 363, 234–236

Weingartl, H. M., Copps, J., Drebot, M. A., Marszal, P., Smith, G., Gren, J., Andonova, M., Pasick, J., Kitching, P., Czub, M. (2004). Susceptibility of pigs and chickens to SARS coronavirus. *Emerging Infectious Disease* 10, 179–184

Wentworth, D. E., Gillim-Ross, L., Espina, N., Bernard, K. A. (2004). Mice susceptible to SARS coronavirus. *Emerging Infectious Disease*, 10, 1293–1296

Wu, D., Tu, C., Xin, C., Xuan, H., Meng, Q., Liu, Y., Yu, Y., Guan, Y., Jiang, Y., Yin, X., Crameri, G., Wang, M., Li, C., Liu, S., Liao, M., Feng, L., Xiang, H., Sun, J., Chen, J., Sun, Y., Gu, S., Liu, N., Fu, D., Eaton, B. T., Wang, L. F., Kong, X. (2005). Civets are equally susceptible to experimental infection by two different severe acute respiratory syndrome coronavirus isolates. *Journal of Virology*, 79, 2620–26255

Xu, H. F., Wang, M., Zhang, Z. B., Zou, X. Z., Gao, Y., Liu, X. N., Lu, E. J., Pan, B. Y., Wu, S. J., Yu, S.Y. (2004a). An epidemiologic investigation on infection with severe acute respiratory syndrome coronavirus in wild animals traders in Guangzhou. *Zhonghua Yu Fang Yi Xue Za Zhi*, 38, 81–83

Xu, R. H., He, J. F., Evans, M. R., Peng, G. W., Field, H. E., Yu, D. W., Lee, C. K., Luo, H. M., Lin, W. S., Lin, P., Li, L. H., Liang, W. J., Lin, J. Y., Schnur, A. (2004b). Epidemiologic clues to SARS origin in China. *Emerging Infectious Disease*, 10, 1030–1037

Yang, Z. Y., Werner, H. C., Kong, W. P., Leung, K., Traggiai, E., Lanzavecchia, A., Nabel, G. J. (2005). Evasion of antibody neutralization in emerging severe acute respiratory syndrome coronaviruses. *Proceedings of the National Academy Sciences of the United States of America*, 102, 797–801

Yu, S., Qiu, M., Chen, Z., Ye, X., Gao, Y., Wei, A., Wang, X., Yang, L., Wang, J., Wen, J., Song, Y., Pei, D., Dai, E., Guo, Z., Cao, C., Wang, J., Yang, R. (2005). Retrospective serological investigation of severe acute respiratory syndrome coronavirus antibodies in recruits from mainland China. *Clinical and Diagnostic Laboratory Immunology*, 12, 552–554

Zheng, B. J., Wong, K. H., Zhou, J., Wong, K. L., Young, B. W., Lu, L. W., Lee, S. S. (2004). SARS-related virus predating SARS outbreak, Hong Kong. *Emerging Infectious Disease*, 10, 176–178

SARS Epidemic: SARS Outbreaks in Inner-land of China

Li Ruan and Guang Zeng

Overview

Severe Acute Respiratory Syndrome (SARS), also known in China as Infectious Atypical Pneumonia (IAP), is the 21st century's first infectious disease to severely threaten the public health of the human population (WHO, 2003a). A respiratory transmitted disease caused by a virus, SARS is highly infectious and is rapidly transmitted, inflicting severe complications and a high case fatality rate. The first round of the SARS pandemic led to global panic and billions of dollars economic losses, for due to lack of effective SARS drugs, governments throughout the world had to take rigid steps toward prevention and treatment of the disease.

The SARS epidemic began with the first reported case in Guangzhou, China (Wang et al., 2004), on 16 November 2002. Eight months later, the disease had spread to 26 countries in Asia, America, and Europe, resulting in a reported 8,096 cases and 774 deaths (WHO, 2004). In this global epidemic, China, with 7,429 cases and 685 deaths, accounted for 91.8% of the world's reported cases and 88.5% of the deaths (5,327 SARS cases and 349 deaths were reported in 24 provinces in the inner-land of China – mostly in Beijing and Guangzhou, which, with a combined 4,033 cases, accounted for 75.7% of the total number in the inner-land of China; Hong Kong had 1,755 cases, 299 deaths; Taiwan: 346 cases, 37 deaths; Macao: 1 case, 0 deaths) (He et al., 2003; Peng et al., 2003; Yang et al., 2003; Leadership Group of SARS Prevention and Control in Beijing, 2003; Chinese Center for Disease Control and Prevention, 2003).

The second round of the SARS epidemic broke out locally in various areas of Guangdong province where, from December 2003 until February 2004, four laboratory-confirmed cases were reported but did not result in death (Liang et al., 2004). Singapore (WHO, 2003c), Taiwan (WHO, 2003d), and inner-land of China (Ministry of Health, People's Republic of China, 2004) each had one laboratory infection (total three lab infection events). The laboratory infections from inner-land of China resulted in the third round of the SARS outbreak, infecting nine patients and resulting in one death. These outbreaks, having forced the realization that the prevention of laboratory infections is an important component to avoid a SARS

Y. Lu et al. (eds.), *Emerging Infections in Asia*.
© Springer Science+Business Media, LLC 2008

outbreak, soon came under effective control after firm measures of prevention and treatment were taken.

During the first round of the SARS pandemic, Chinese scientists excluded many common causes of the disease and focused on the exploration of a "new pathogen." The WHO established a global laboratory network on 17 March 2003, and scientists from China and other nations began to work together on finding the causative pathogen of SARS. They conducted research through approaches of viral morphology, molecular biology, serology, and animal studies in 13 network laboratories throughout nine countries (five were in China). On April 16th, the WHO declared that a new coronavirus, dubbed "SARS-CoV," was the pathogen causing SARS (WHO, 2003b). Although epidemiology and experimental results have shown that SARS-CoV comes from animals, further research is necessary to determine the major animal reservoir from which the pathogen derives.

Research has made it clear that SARS is an acute infectious pneumonia caused by SARS-CoV (Drosten et al., 2003; Hong et al., 2003; Zhu et al., 2003; Rota et al., 2003). SARS cases have tended to cluster by family and hospital, mainly transmitted by close contact via droplet transmission. Clinically manifested as fever, pulmonary progressive inflammation, and dyspnea, SARS is characterized by symptomatic infection and there is no transmissibility within the incubation period of 1–12 days (Ministry of Health, People's Republic of China, 2005). Studies show that bodily fluids, such as blood, saliva, and feces, as well as patho-anatomical tissues of patients, contain SARS viruses (Lau et al., 2005).

There are currently no effective therapeutic drugs for SARS. Epidemiological data showing that reinfections have not occurred in recovered patients reveal that SARS patients can have strong immunity after recovery, thus suggesting that an effective vaccine, which is still in clinical study, would be able to prevent SARS infection (Weidong et al., 2006). There has also been significant progress in developing SARS diagnostic reagents. Combining the application of approved reagents, including the detection of viral nucleic acid, protein antigen, and serum viral antibody, the SARS infection could be detected in its early stages (i.e., within approximately 1 week of infection) (Ministry of Health, People's Republic of China, 2005; Che et al., 2004). Until effective vaccine and therapeutic drug research have reached fruition, the comprehensive prevention and treatment remain the basic principle to control the SARS infection.

Epidemiological Features

Current Status of Epidemic

Since 2002, SARS has broken out three times: the first epidemic spread worldwide from November 2002 to July 2003 (WHO, 2004); the second spread locally in Guangdong province between December 2003 and February 2004 (Liang et al.,

2004); and the third developed on a small scale from laboratory infection in the inner-land of China from March to April 2004 (Ministry of Health, People's Republic of China, 2004). Furthermore, two other laboratory infections occurred in Singapore (WHO, 2003c) and Taiwan (WHO, 2003d), although they did not result in an epidemic.

Features of the First Epidemic

Geographic Distribution

The first case of SARS was discovered in Fushan city, Guangdong province, with onset date of 16 November 2002 (Wang et al., 2004). The last case occurred in Taiwan on 15 June 2003 (WHO, 2004). After starting in Guangdong, the epidemic in China then spread to Shanxi, Xichuan, and Beijing, followed by further expansion to other regions of China. Altogether, in accordance with the outbreak and transmission, China can be divided into the following four regional categories (He et al., 2003; Peng et al., 2003; Yang et al., 2003; Leadership Group of SARS Prevention and Control in Beijing 2003; Chinese Center for Disease Control and Prevention, 2003):

• Regions with a localized epidemic (Guangdong)
• Regions where an introduced case induced a localized epidemic (Beijing, Inner Mongolia, Shanxi, Hebei, Tianjin, et al.)
• Regions where a case was introduced but did not lead to a localized epidemic (Shanghai, Shandong, Hunan, Liaoning, Ningxia, et al.)
• Regions without reported cases (Hainan, Yunnan, Guizhou, Qinghai, Tibet, Xinjiang, Hei Longjiang et al.)

Time Distribution

SARS had caused worldwide epidemic as SARS cases were reported in China (including Hong Kong), Vietnam, Singapore, and Canada from November 2002 to February 2003. The disease was effectively under control by June 2003. During these 7 months, the period from mid-March to mid-May of 2003 witnessed the highest number of reported cases.

The localized outbreak in China's Guangdong province lasted from January to February of 2003, and then rapidly expanded to other regions in China until the last case of disease was reported on June 11. The incidence of SARS in Guangdong province peaked in February, while in other regions it peaked between early April and mid-May, reflecting the earlier appearance of cases in Guangdong. Although primary cases appeared in the cities of Fushan and Heyuan in Guangdong province and in Hechi city in Guangxi province, there is no evidence of intertransmission of these primary cases among the different cities (He et al.,

2003; Peng et al., 2003; Yang et al., 2003; Leadership Group of SARS Prevention and Control in Beijing, 2003; Chinese Center for Disease Control and Prevention, 2003).

Population Distribution

Youths and those in the prime age group make up the majority of SARS patients. According to data collected from 5,327 SARS cases in China, the main age group for onset infection ranges from 20 to 60 years old, accounting for 85% of the total cases. While those aged 20–29 years account for 30% of the total number of cases, those under the age of 15 show a low incidence of SARS; children under the age of 9 show an even lower incidence (He et al., 2003; Peng et al., 2003; Yang et al., 2003; Leadership Group of SARS Prevention and Control in Beijing. Epidemiological features of severe acute respiratory syndrome in Beijing, 2003; Chinese Center for Disease Control and Prevention, 2003; Liang et al., 2004).

No significant differences have been found between men and women with regards to SARS infection. A comparison of incidence rates in different professions shows that, as one might assume, medical personnel have a higher incidence of SARS. Up to 20% of SARS cases were in medical staff (in some provinces, up to 50%); the number of cases in medical staff declined in the later stages of the epidemic, largely due to effective preventive measures of medical staffs. Students made up 8.6% of the total number of cases; however, the cases were sporadic, with no cases occurring as school clusters. A study in Guangdong found SARS cases among people, such as restaurant cooks and meat animal's vendors or purchasers, who had no history of contact with SARS patients but had been in contact with wild animals (He et al., 2003; Peng et al., 2003; Yang et al., 2003; Leadership Group of SARS Prevention and Control in Beijing, Epidemiological features of severe acute respiratory syndrome in Beijing, 2003; Chinese Center for Disease Control and Prevention, 2003).

Distribution Features of Death Cases

The WHO reported that in the epidemic of 2002–2003, the case-fatality rate of SARS ranged from 0%–50%, with different age groups with different fatality rates. The case-fatality rate of those under the age of 24 is lower than 1%; that of those between 24 and 44 years-old is 6%; 45–66 years-old is 15%; 65 years and older is over 50% (WHO, 2004). In China, the case-fatality rate of SARS is 6.6% (He et al., 2003; Peng et al., 2003; Yang et al., 2003; Leadership Group of SARS Prevention and Control in Beijing, 2003; Chinese Center for Disease Control and Prevention, 2003) and the death rate of SARS in whole population is 0.024/100,000; elderly patients account for a higher proportion of SARS fatalities (approximately 44% of all SARS deaths), with the fatality rate of patients who are above 60 years of age being 11%–14%. Generally, the fatality rate increases with age. SARS patients who also have other diseases such as high blood pressure, diabetes, heart disease, emphysema, or tumors have a high fatality rate.

Features of the Second Outbreak

From 5 January to 2 February of 2004, Guangzhou city in Guangdong province reported four mild SARS cases with confirmed laboratory tests (Liang et al., 2004). The four patients did not experience severe clinical conditions and no clear sources of infection were found. They did not infect others and had no history of travel or activities in the wild, although two of them may have had contact history with wild animals.

Features of the Third Outbreak

From 25 March to 17 April of 2004, Anhui and Beijing reported a total of nine cases, which were later confirmed to have derived from research laboratories conducting SARS research (Ministry of Health, People's Republic of China, 2004). Anhui reported two cases and one death; Beijing reported seven cases, none of which resulted in death. Two of the nine cases resulted from direct contact with the infectious virus in the research laboratory, while the remaining seven were secondary infections of one laboratory infection.

Other Infections

Since the WHO declared on 5 July 2003 that the first global SARS epidemic had ended, two other research laboratory-related infections later occurred in addition to the aforementioned outbreaks. Both of these later infections (one in Singapore (WHO, 2003c) on 8 September 2003; the other in Taiwan (WHO, 2003d) on 17 December 2003) were confirmed to have resulted from laboratory accidents; neither of these infections brought about a SARS epidemic.

Source of Infection, Routes of Transmission, Population Susceptibility

Sources of Infection

SARS patients are the main source of infection, because the disease is communicable as soon as patients exhibit symptoms of the disease, growing more infectious as the disease manifests itself through apparent symptoms such as fever and coughing, and even more so when patients develop acute respiratory distress syndrome (ARDS). The disease likewise becomes less infectious as fever declines (Ministry of Health, People's Republic of China, 2005).

Although SARS patients compose the main source of infection, patients in the incubation period (1–12 days after the time of infection) and patients released from hospitals have not been found to be infectious to others (Ministry of Health, People's Republic of China, 2005).

SARS-CoV infection is characterized by symptomatic infection; however, mild cases, such as the cases in the second outbreak, and nonsymptomatic infection may exist. For instance, people who breed or sell wild animals in Guangdong province show a significant number of SARS-CoV infection with no apparent clinical symptoms. These subclinical cases have not been found to be infectious (Ministry of Health, People's Republic of China, 2005).

Polymerase chain reactions (PCR) or serological tests of various animal species, such as the civet cat, wild pig, rabbit, snake, badger, bat, and jungle fowl, have shown positive results, which suggest that the SARS virus may come from animals (Chinese SARS Molecular Epidemyology Consortium, 2004; Song et al., 2005; Kan et al., 2005; Li et al., 2005); however, further evidence is needed to confirm this hypothesis.

In addition to SARS patients and various animal species, research institutes that conduct SARS research, testing, and production of diagnostic reagents and vaccines may become sources of SARS infection under certain circumstances, depending on these institutes' safety regulations, management, staff quality, health monitoring, and whether they have designated health care centers (WHO, 2003c,d; Ministry of Health, People's Republic of China, 2004).

Routes of Transmission

The major and most important route of SARS transmission is respiratory droplet transmission through close contact (short distance transmission) with a patient (Yang et al., 2003; Ministry of Health, People's Republic of China, 2005). The recipient then inhales droplets containing viral particles coughed out by the patient. However, transmission via aerosol without close contact is also reported as the route of SARS transmission, which led to the outbreaks in hospitals in severely-infected areas and in certain communities. Direct contact such as hand-to-hand contact is another important route of SARS transmission. There have also been reports of the viral isolation from bodily fluid – like teardrops. There is no epidemiological proof for blood, sex, and vertical transmissions, but the possibility of intestinal transmission can not be excluded.

Population Susceptibility

Although the general population is susceptible to SARS infection, infection rates differ among population subgroups. For reasons yet unknown, children have a lower infection rate than the rest of the population. Those in close contact with SARS symptomatic patients and those without effective protection in a SARS treatment environment (i.e., medical staff, patients' relatives and friends) form a high-risk population, as do SARS laboratory researchers and those who work with wild animals such as civet cats.

It has been proven that the human body can generate a protective antibody after SARS infection, and maintain the antibody at a high level for 2 years after the onset of the disease (Li et al., 2006). Consequently, no SARS patients have been reported to become reinfected after recovery. These data indicate the possibility of generating an effective immunity after infection with SARS; however, since SARS is chiefly a symptomatic infection, those who have not yet been infected are still susceptible after a SARS epidemic.

Clinical Manifestations, Diagnostic Criteria, and Treatment Principles of SARS

Major Clinical Manifestations of SARS (Ministry of Health, People's Republic of China, 2005)

Major clinical manifestations of SARS include fever, progressive pulmonary inflammation, and dyspnea. The disease may be classified as occurring in five successive periods.

1. Incubation period: The first 1–12 days (usually 1–7 days) after infection; not infectious to others in this period.
2. Initial period: The first 1–3 days of the onset of the disease. Most patients show clinical manifestations such as fever, a nonreceding body temperature, and increased pulse rate. The disease progresses very quickly in some patients, manifesting itself in dry coughing, short breaths or obstruction of breathing, and abnormal chest X-rays.

Fever is the first symptom, with body temperature reaching over 38°C. More than half of the patient population exhibit other symptoms such as headache, joint and muscular soreness and debilitation, dry coughing, chest pain, and diarrhea. Few cases have symptoms of upper respiratory catarrh with unclear pulmonary signs, and moist rale can be heard in some of them.

3. Progression period: The period usually occurring between the 4th and 7th days of the course of disease, during which the disease further progresses in most patients. Fever and toxic symptoms of infection continue; pulmonary affliction, usually manifested as a progressive development of chest distress, tachypnea, and dyspnea, worsens – particularly after physical movement; saturation of blood oxygen declines; and chest X-rays show more abnormalities.
4. Acme period: The period between the 8th and 14th days after the onset of disease. Patients continue showing the aforementioned symptoms, although body temperatures further reach unusual levels. Most patients keep this high temperature if they are not hospitalized; however, even with hospitalization,

some severe patients are unable to return to a normal body temperature. Patients show acute lung injury and even ARDS, with chest X-rays demonstrating leafy pulmonary infiltration or severe hypoxemia. Some show impairment of multi-organs, with severe cases showing multi-organ functional defects.

5. Convalescence period: The period between the 15th and 28th days after the onset of disease. Body temperature gradually declines, clinical manifestations lessen, pulmonary pathological damages begin to be absorbed, fever and toxic symptoms disappear prior to other symptoms, followed by a gradual decline and ultimate disappearance of such anoxia symptoms as chest distress, shortness of breath, and breath obstruction; saturation of blood oxygen of lymphocytes, and X-rays of the chest return to normal. Most patients can meet the standards of hospital release after 2 weeks of recovery; however, absorption of lung shadow (lung damage shown in X-ray) requires further recovery time. A few severe cases may retain restrictive ventilatory disorder and declining pulmonary diffusion for a short period, but most usually convalesce within 2–3 months after leaving the hospital.

Diagnostic Criteria of SARS (Ministry of Health, People's Republic of China, 2005)

Diagnosis of SARS

Suspected Cases

Those who have clinical manifestation of the disease and pathological changes in their pulmonary X-rays but show no history of being in close contact with SARS patients or other epidemiological evidence can be regarded as suspected cases. For them, further epidemiological investigation and etiological and serological tests are needed. Those who are suspected of being infected based on epidemiological evidence and certain clinical manifestations, but without pathological changes in their pulmonary X-rays, are also considered suspected cases.

Clinically Diagnosed Cases

If the possible diagnoses of other diseases have been excluded, clinical diagnoses of SARS may be given to those with SARS epidemiological connection, related clinical manifestations, and pathological changes in pulmonary X-rays.

Confirmed Diagnosis

On the basis of suspected and clinical diagnosis, confirmed SARS diagnosis may be given if any of the following conditions is met:

- SARS-CoV RNA testing of secretion or serum is positive
- SARS-CoV-specific nucleocapsid antigen testing of serum (or blood plasma) is positive
- Anti-SARS-CoV antibody conversion test is positive
- Antibody titer in recovery period is four times higher than that in early period.

Laboratory Diagnosis

The available laboratory detection techniques and studies of the etiological and serological features of SARS patients now make it possible to conduct tests at different periods in the course of the SARS disease. When supplemented with clinical manifestations, these tests can positively diagnose SARS.

Early Diagnosis

Within 5 days of the onset of disease, serum and a nasopharynx swab of a patient need to be collected to test the nucleocapsid protein (protein N) and nucleate of SARS virus in serum, and then the viral nucleates in patients' nasopharynx to assist the serum test. If the serum protein N and nucleates in the serum or nasopharynx are positive, the patient may be diagnosed with SARS.

Routinely taking SARS-CoV protein N testing with serum sample of causative-agent uncleared pneumonia patients in early period may enable early detection of SARS in this particular group.

Metaphase Diagnosis

Conducted 6–10 days after the onset of disease. Patients' nasopharynx swab, feces, anal swab, blood, and urine are collected and tested first for SARS viral nucleates. Meanwhile, a patient's serum is tested for viral nucleocapsid protein, nucleic acid, and antibodies of IgG and IgM as supporting proof. Positive test results or antibody conversion warrant the diagnosis of SARS.

Late Stage Diagnosis

Conducted anytime after the tenth day since the onset of disease. Patients' serum, nasopharynx swab, anal swab, feces, and urine are collected and SARS IgG and IgM are tested with serum samples first and then viral nucleocapsid protein in serum and viral nucleates in the other samples as supporting proofs. If antibodies become positive or increase fourfold, or if viral nucleates and nucleocapsid protein tests are positive, then the patient can be diagnosed with SARS.

Thus far, China has had ELISA testing reagents for serum nucleocapsid protein of the SARS virus, IgM and IgG antibody testing reagents (ELISA and fluorescence) on the serum of SARS patients, and real-time PCR reagents to SARS viral nucleic acid in various samples. All of these reagents have obtained approval from the government. Isolation of viral samples which are etiologically positive (nucleocapsid protein and nucleates) and SARS viral neutralization experiments on samples which are antibody positive are useful for further clarified diagnosis. Regarding the use and interpretation of other testing methods for blood-lymphocytes and X-rays, "Consensus of the management of Severe Acute Respiratory Syndrome" published by MOH of China can be referenced (Ministry of Health, People's Republic of China, 2005).

Differential Diagnosis

Early SARS diagnosis, to a certain extent, is an exclusive diagnosis. Prior to SARS diagnosis, other diseases that cause similar clinical manifestations must be excluded. Especially, some manifestations being negative in SARS can help differentiate the diseases. For instance, SARS does not cause lung necrosis; therefore, emphysema of the chest or cavity will not occur if the disease is, indeed, SARS. Moreover, although SARS is a viral infection, it rarely leads to rash (excluding drug rash) or lymphadenectasis. Symptoms of upper respiratory catarrh are scarcely seen in SARS. All that has mentioned can be considered as criteria to rule out other diseases. The many other pneumonias with fever, low WBC, and pulmonary infiltration, which are caused by non-SARS pathogens such as atypical pathogen, virus, fungus, and common bacteria, and so on, need to be carefully differentiated. However, in addition, some other diseases, such as TB, tumor, pulmonary vasculitis, allergic pneumonia, and acute interstitial pneumonia, also need to be considered in an exclusive diagnosis.

Treatment Principles of SARS

Although the pathogen of SARS has been identified, the mechanism by which the virus causes disease is not clear. Thus far, no effective anti-viral treatment has been scientifically and clinically approved. Consequently, symptomatic supportive treatment and treatment targeting various disease complications remain the main treatment of the disease, including the use of glucocorticoids. It is necessary to correctly implement mechanical ventilation, treat complications positively, and actively develop a combination therapy of Western and traditional Chinese medicine. Large doses of long-term blind drug therapy – especially the combination of multiple drugs such as antibiotics, antiviral drugs, immunomodulators, and glucocorticoids – must be rejected as a form of treatment. Detailed treatment regimens may be consulted in "Consensus of the management of Severe Acute Respiratory Syndrome" published by MOH of China (Ministry of Health, People's Republic of China, 2005).

Lessons Learned from SARS Epidemic and Experiences Based on Successful Control of SARS in Inner-Land of China

Lessons Learned from SARS Epidemic

Characteristics of the Spread of SARS (Chinese Center for Disease Control, 2003)

During the SARS epidemic in the inner-land of China, 24 provinces, autonomous regions, and municipalities submitted SARS case reports, while seven provinces and autonomous regions (Hainan, Guizhou, Yunnan, Hei Longjiang, Tibet, Qinghai, and Xinjiang) did not. The epidemic was concentrated in six areas, including Beijing (2,521 cases), Guangdong (1,512 cases), Shanxi (448 cases), Inner Mongolia (282 cases), Hebei (215 cases), and Tianjin (175 cases), making up 96.7% (5,153 cases) of the nation's cases and 94.3% (329 deaths) of the nation's deaths from SARS. Of the other regions of China, six provinces had between 10 and 35 cases and 12 provinces had less than 10 cases.

The epidemiological investigation showed that SARS outbreaks in 24 provinces of inner-land of China have apparent applications. The survey study indicated that Guangdong and Beijing were the most important sources of transmission for China's SARS epidemic. From Guangdong, the disease spread to Xichuan, Hunan, Inner Mongolia, Shanxi, Beijing, Anhui, Shanghai, and Fujian; then from Beijing, it spread to Gansu, Jilin, Liaoning, Shanxi, Chongqing, Hubei, Zhejiang, Tianjin, and Hebei.

Lessons Drawn from the SARS Spread

Two months after the first case was reported on 16 November 2002, Guangdong had a SARS outbreak. During the 2-month period of the outbreak, medical staffs and local government officials in Guangdong had learned of the severity of the disease and had acquired a basic knowledge of the clinical manifestations, major routes of transmission, and response measures to the disease.

By early February 2003, Guangdong province had managed to contain the outbreak by formulating and implementing a series of effective public health measures. Unfortunately, Guangdong's experience did not help the rest of China to control the further spread of SARS. What happened in Guangdong between December 2002 and January 2003 recurred many times in a worse manner in many other provinces. There are disputes about whether Guangdong's efforts to contain the SARS epidemic in February were strong enough. Objectively, one can offer the explanation that a new infectious disease necessitates a learning process such as Guangdong's; however, this explanation fails with regard to Beijing's repetition of Guangdong's process, which resulted in a high number of infections among medical staffs in March 2003 – 2 months after the outbreak in Guangdong. The consequences of this mistake have resulted in an important lesson worthy of reflection.

1. The consideration that should accord severe infectious diseases the top priority in emergency public health events was inadequate. Nowadays, infectious diseases – especially acute and severe ones transmitted via respiratory and intestinal tracts – may appear as either newly emerged infectious diseases or weapons in biological terrorism. Since such diseases usually emerge in an explosive and indiscriminate manner and have wide spread impact, they often lead to panic, social disorder, and economic trauma. Historically, severe epidemics had sometime changed war outcomes, wreaked social disorder, and altered political regimes. Considering these grave potential impacts, the establishment of a response system to severe infectious diseases should be given significant priority in the response system of sudden public health incidents. Acute and severe viral infectious diseases generally do not have specific and effective prevention and treatment measures; therefore, emergency response, prevention, and control need to be given the top priority.

2. The most significant revelation from the SARS outbreaks is that the response system to emergency public health events is inadequate. In the epidemics, weaknesses in China's command system, information system, prevention and treatment teams, and corresponding material storages were completely exposed. For the past two decades, the public health service in China has lagged behind, primarily due to inadequate funding. To solve these problems is an essential step for China to build a harmonious modern society with long-term lasting and equilibrating economic development. The establishment of China's CDC-centered nationwide laboratory monitor network, epidemic information network, emergency teams, and material storage is an essential component in building up the national response to public health emergencies.

3. No consummate public reporting institution of epidemic is observed. In the beginning of the epidemic, the policy of "strict inward while loose outward" concerning SARS blocked the epidemic information. The mystery of epidemic disease hovered among the public. Information was not transparent and blocked between related CDCs and researchers, even among departments of government including China and international organizations. This delayed the timely control of the epidemic and even initiated a confidence crisis among the public. It is essential to develop a complete system to announce and report epidemics – a scientific system to analyze and explain epidemics so that various departments can coordinate control of the epidemic and so that the public can correctly understand the epidemic and positively support the measures that the government takes to contain the epidemic.

4. The cognition needed to promptly tackle key problems in science and technology when a new infectious disease occurs is deficient. In early February 2003, common belief held that SARS was caused by a "new etiological agent." So as to "keep the outbreak confidential," only a few research institutions independently began to organize teams to try to identify the new etiological agent. (National Institute for Viral Disease Control and Prevention, 2003a) Unclear about the details of the outbreak and the lack of a mechanism of collaborative research, each research institute worked independently, making the much-needed national cooperation impossible. At the end of February and beginning of March, a national program proposal requesting collaboration in etiology, epidemiology, and clinical remedy finally reached the related departments of government (National Institute for Viral Disease Control and Prevention, 2003). However, collaborative research, organized by the government, did not start until mid-April of 2003. In this regard, it is understandable that, although scientists in inner-land of China had observed "coronavirus" in autopsies of SARS patients by the end of February, which was one month earlier than the discovery made by a group of Hong Kong scientists, their work was never publicly released. Scientific and technological sectors in China learn from this lesson the importance of establishing a systematic scientific and research response to emergencies when threatened by a new disease.

Experiences Based on Successful Control of SARS

China has a responsible government, which took timely and effectively measures nationwide in the face of severe SARS outbreaks. Without reliable diagnostic reagents, effective drugs, or vaccines, "four early" steps stressing "early detection, early report, early quarantine, early treatment" were adopted in early-April of 2003 according to basic principles of containing infectious diseases and targeting major clinical manifestations and transmission features of SARS. Within the 2 months following "four early" steps, SARS transmission was controlled and blocked nationwide. To offer scientific support for the implementation of the "Four Early Steps," the experiences could be summarized as follows:

- Publicize the epidemic to get understanding, support, and cooperation from the public to facilitate government efforts to contain the epidemic
- Disseminate knowledge of SARS to promote the public's ability of self-protection
- Establish a network system of reporting the epidemic to actively monitor the epidemic so that prevention and control measures can be most effectively focused
- Develop designated hospitals with strict quarantines of patients and medical monitors on those in close Contact with patients and improve the preventive and protective condition and ability of doctors and nurses
- Strengthen aid and treatment to patients to minimize the number of deaths

- Promptly launch scientific and technological research and intensify studies on etiology, epidemiology, and medical treatment

Drawing lessons and experiences from the SARS outbreaks, the Chinese government, and its health workers have further acknowledged the important position of prevention and control infectious diseases in the public health cause. In May of 2003, the Chinese government formulated the "Regulations on Preparedness for and Response to Emergent Public Health Hazards" (People's Republic of China, 2003) and revised the "Law of the People's Republic of China on the Prevention and Treatment of Infectious Diseases" (People's Republic of China, 2004). All provincial governments activated components of the "Emergency Preparedness Plan for Emergent Public Health Hazards" and prepared the needed personnel, materials, technology, and grounds. China's capacity to respond to emergency public health events has improved significantly with a broad variety of improvements for such keynote infectious diseases as SARS during the past few years, including the following:

- Establishment of a nationwide direct report network of epidemic diseases,
- An epidemic-publicizing institution
- Identification of fever clinics in designated infectious disease hospitals
- Operation of monitor networks on severe infectious diseases
- Cooperative efforts in handling problems of diagnostic techniques, prevention and control measures.

The experiences in controlling the first SARS outbreak played a crucial role in the response to four mild SARS cases that appeared in Guangdong in early 2004. The diagnoses of these four cases were fast and accurate, conforming to check result from WHO network laboratories (Liang et al., 2004). No epidemic formed, largely due to the developed firm means of preventing the outbreak. The same prevention and control measures were applied in nine laboratory SARS infections in Beijing. Upon learning that two suspected SARS cases in Anhui came from a certain research institute in Beijing, related experts were quickly sent to Anhui on 21st April. Beijing also found SARS suspected cases at the same day. That afternoon, Beijing SARS network laboratory test results confirmed the clinical diagnosis of SARS. Meanwhile, epidemiological analyses suggested connections between Anhui and Beijing cases, and additionally circled the potential range of those who had come into close contact with the infected patients. The Beijing government publicized the outbreak according to emergency preparedness planning on 23rd April and followed up with decisive measures to close up the epidemic sites, quarantine close contact persons with patients, and give quick treatments to patients (Government of Xuan Wu Qu, Beijing, 2004). The firm reactions blocked successfully the transmission of SARS. The experience showed that China had remarkably improved its response to acute and severe infectious diseases after its previous "SARS accident," and its response measures to the emergency proved efficient. The same improvement was later evident in the prevention and control of avian flu and pig streptococcal infection in China (Yu et al., 2006).

Why, then, did a SARS laboratory infection transmit to the public in April of 2004? If the world's largest epidemic of streptococcal infection in pigs (Yu et al., 2006) could be spread among the public, what would the result be? Evidently, there is still much to be done to develop prevention and control response systems to outbreak emergencies.

Main Factors Contributing to SARS Epidemic in China and China's Prevention and Control Strategies

It may not be an accident that SARS first broke out in China. Hong Kong (China) reported in 1997 for the first time that humans could be infected by avian flu (H5N1). Of flu viruses that caused worldwide pandemic four times, two originated in China – H2N2 in Guizhou in 1957 and H3N2 in Hong Kong in1968. In recent years, avian flu has broken out in Asia (including China) and spread. Not long ago, the world's largest epidemic of streptococcal infection in pigs was seen in Sichuan, China (Yu et al., 2006). Furthermore, in the past two decades, new diseases have emerged in other countries of Asia. It seems that Asia has become a significant origin for new infectious diseases – but why? Perhaps this issue must be placed in the context of China – even, to a larger extent, of Asia – for a solution.

Main Factors Contributing to SARS Epidemic in China

1. For the past 30 years, Asia, particularly China, has experienced rapid social and economic development. A large population on weak foundations, in combination with rapid progress, has severely polluted the environment and damaged ecological balance. This has enhanced the opportunities for pathogenic microorganisms that had been previously blocked and limited to hit larger populations, and also augmented the risk of a trans-genus spread of microorganisms, thereby presenting social and economic surroundings advantageous for new diseases.

Studies illustrate that SARS-CoV derives from animals, showing that during long periods of frequent contact with people, the virus evolves from nonpathogenic to pathogenic. An unregulated breeding industry of wild animals in Guangdong provided the womb to the evolution of this microorganism.

2. Rapid economic development has caused significant changes in human communication and lifestyles, which have consequently accelerated the rapid transmission of infectious diseases via respiratory and intestinal tracts. This accelerated transmission was witnessed in the rapid spread of the SARS epidemic from the original outbreak in Guangdong (in China) to cases in 26 countries in Asia, North America, and Europe within the course of 2 months. Although, from this

data, it may seem that the infectivity of SARS is very high, it is still far weaker than that of influenza. At present, if no effective measures are taken with the emergence of an influenza pandemic, its coverage might greatly surpass that of the devastating flu pandemic of 1918.

Moreover, the cognition of the negative impacts of infectious diseases on social development is far from enough. The initial position of infectious diseases, especially highly pathogenic ones, in emergency public health hazards has been neglected. The funds invested in laboratory test networks and networks monitoring infectious diseases are ultimately inadequate. Confronted with the epidemic, its related information is unclear and responses are not powerful. These factors facilitate chaos and loss of control in epidemic situations.

China's Prevention and Control Strategies

1. To practice the "concept of scientific development" in all around and prioritize the public health within social and economic development. The development of public health services is a critical standard by which to measure social and economic progress. In China, while the national economy had doubled in the two decades before 2002, the investments in public health services had conversely dropped by approximately 45% compared with that in 1980s, nearly destroying the already weak disease prevention and control network. Therefore, it is no wonder that SARS could so easily penetrate the hospital defense lines and rapidly spread throughout the nation. The lessons learned from the SARS outbreaks are not exclusively related to SARS, but are rather far-reaching and applicable to future scientific endeavors.

   To strategically practice the "concept of scientific development," one must make the development of public health services, which is directly related to public life and health, a significant standard by which to measure social and economic progress. To effectively and tactfully respond to new infectious diseases such as SARS, the prevention and control of infectious diseases need to be accorded top priority in the development of a response system to public health emergencies. Therefore, one must build and improve upon a response commanding system, a monitoring network, an information-reporting network, a technical platform, prevention and treatment teams, and a storage system of materials for infectious disease emergencies.

2. To keep ecological balance and protect the environment are important measures to reduce the emergence of new diseases and prevent their further expansion. In analyzing human social development, it is apparent that the occurrence of new diseases is always accompanied by ecological imbalance and environmental damages caused by social and economic development. For example, the infamous infectious disease smallpox appeared after humans shifted from a nomadic lifestyle to live in agricultural settlements that made the original ecology and

environment obvious change. In monitoring ecological balance, a society must practice strict regulations in handling wild animals, for many diseases may be transmitted from animals to humans. Livestock and poultry, for instance, live in close contact with human beings and thereby create multiple areas for the transmission of common diseases such as the flu and Japanese B encephalitis. The casual capture and breeding of wild animals also offer grounds for the occurrence of the SARS virus. To ensure sustainable stability and development in a society in which the economy progresses at a high rate, it is critical to establish a harmony between humans and nature so as to protect the environment, maintain an ecological balance, decrease the occurrence of new diseases, and create enjoyable surroundings for human life and health.

Strategies and Measures of SARS Prevention and Treatment (Wang et al., 2003)

General Principles of Prevention and Treatment

SARS has been included in the "Law of the PRC on the Prevention and Treatment of Infectious Diseases" (People's Republic of China, 2004) as one of the severe infectious diseases that require key prevention and treatment for management. Although there have been no effective therapeutic and preventative drugs for SARS thus far, there are satisfactory diagnostic reagents. Thus, the general principle of SARS prevention and treatment may be defined as a system of comprehensive prevention and treatment measures aimed at three key points of infectious sources, transmission routes, and susceptible populations, which focus mainly on managing and containing infectious sources, and preventing and controlling transmissions within hospitals. Efforts must be made to implement the "Four Early" policy that calls for "early detection, early report, early quarantine, early treatment," especially during the period of SARS epidemic, and to emphasize local quarantine and local treatment to avoid a long-distance transmission.

Measures of Prevention and Treatment

Avoid or Reduce Viral Infections of Humans from the External Environment

Prevent and Control Animals from Contracting the SARS Viral Infection

We are still unclear about animals' infection of SARS-CoV, infection components, and the impacts. Monitoring studies need to be strengthened on animal hosts in high risk areas such as Guangdong province, followed by steps to reduce or avoid animal infections or spread SARS virus.

Prevent SARS-CoV Infections Transmitted from Animals to Humans

According to a study on the economic values of infected animals, the procedures requiring the management of infectious animal sources to kill or quarantine wild animal species should be adapted to dwindle their chances of contact with humans instead of terminating the infection among the animals. Thus, when the management should have eliminated the sources of infection and consequently eliminate the possibility of transmission to humans, it instead only reduced the chances of animal-to-human transmission.

Strengthen the Safety of Laboratories

Strengthen the biological safety management of all institutions concerning SARS research, testing, and reagent and vaccine manufacturing. In the condition that possible profits and risks were fully demonstrated, the topics and contents of SARS-related pathogenic studies were carefully selected and only the qualified laboratories and researchers could be authorized to launch studies. To prevent the spread of laboratory infection to the public, it was needed to improve the management organization for severe infectious diseases, formulate and improve technique operation standards of biological safety in severe infectious disease labs, strengthen the biological safety training of related professionals who may be exposed to the SARS virus or potential infectious materials, and establish a system to report suspect symptoms, such as fever, among laboratory staff to ensure they can get treatment in designated hospitals in time.

Prevent and Control Human-to-Human Transmission

Management of Infectious Sources

- Management of patients: Try to detect early, report early, quarantine early, and treat early. It is extremely important to establish precautionary measures and a SARS protective and clinical treatment system.
- Management of those in close contact with patients: Establish systems of medical monitoring and follow-up investigation for people in close contact with SARS patients.

Cut-Off Routes of Transmission

- Strengthen the control of in-hospital infections: A prerequisite of avoiding in-hospital infections is choosing hospitals and wards that meet standards to receive SARS patients. During an outbreak, designated hospitals and fever clinics must be set up in accordance with standardized requirements – equipped with essential preventative and disinfection facilities, and with utilities bearing obvious, eye-catching labels. Specialized patient areas, wards, elevators, and passages must be established specifically to receive SARS patients.

- Practice good self-protection: Individual precautionary equipment includes a shielding face mask, gloves, protective clothing, eyewear or veil, and shoe covers. Of these precautions, the shielding face mask and gloves are the most important.

Protection of Susceptible Population

Research for a SARS vaccine is now underway. China started the first trial of a SARS inactivated vaccine on humans in May of 2004 (Jiang-Tao Lin et al., 2007). Although global research on a SARS vaccine has seen great progress, it still has a long way to go before it can produce a vaccine for real practice on humans. Studies show that the correct use of interferon has certain preventive effects for SARS infection; however, there have been no effective vaccines or drugs for prevention, leaving the strengthening of self-protection as the main measure to protect susceptible populations.

Other Prevention and Treatment Measures

1. Collaborate multi-departmentally for good prevention and treatment of SARS in joint efforts; it is vital for the control of a SARS outbreak to establish a powerful organizing and commanding system supported by the coordination and collaboration of multiple departments.
2. Disinfection and management of infectious sources: Abide by the principle of "early, exact, strict, and real" in the management of epidemic foci or epidemic areas, i.e., take early steps with exact targets, execute measures strictly and put them into real practice, and disinfect epidemic foci seriously. In most cases, it is not necessary to disinfect the extended surrounding areas of the foci of an epidemic.
3. Quarantine and manage public places: If SARS breaks out or spreads with a trend of further expansion, emergency steps should be taken according to either "Frontier Health and Quarantine Law of People's Republic of China" and "Regulations on Domestic Communications Health Quarantine" or the 25th and 26th rules in "Law of the PRC on the Prevention and Treatment of Infectious Diseases."
4. Intensify health education, social care, and psychological intervention: Publicize knowledge of SARS prevention and treatment in a wide range and through various media. Educate the public so as to raise awareness of self-protection and support the current prevention and treatment work; adjust the education focus to cater to the changes of the epidemic; take full advantage of the role and function of the media and direct public opinion by utilizing the media to focus on

disseminating knowledge of prevention and treatment; make the public understand the measures of mass prevention and mass treatment; and clarify the public's
responsibilities and obligations. The reports must adhere to the truth, and try to
reduce any reports that may lead to a sense of panic among the public.

Priority on SARS Prevention and Treatment in China

1. Intensify the development of SARS testing laboratories: To provide reliable and
   powerful technique back-ups to the "Four Early" policy, we need to put into
   serious practice the hardware construction and management of laboratories,
   testing plans, storage of reagents, and working staff. As well, we have to ensure
   biological safety and reliable test result.
2. Intensify the management of key susceptible animals: Set up monitoring and
   testing systems of the SARS virus in susceptible animals in high risk regions to
   allow the issuance of a prompt precaution warning of the possibility of a SARS
   outbreak.
3. Intensify the management of SARS laboratories to ensure that laboratories are
   not sources of SARS infections.
4. Upgrade early precautionary systems that report SARS cases so as to detect
   SARS patients as soon as possible and take immediate actions of prevention and
   control in cases of detected infections.
5. Improve the clinical treatment and prevention system so as to raise the recovery
   rate, reduce the fatality rate, and block inter-hospital infections and transmission
   to the public.
6. Update medical quarantine and observation systems so that a SARS outbreak
   can be blocked and controlled on a smallest scale in the shortest time.

This article was finished in 2005. During the 3 years from 2004, no SARS cases have
been reported. Since SARS is featured by symptomatic infection (Ministry of Health,
People's Republic of China, 2005), it is impossible that SARS-CoV could be hidden
in population without disease. The results from monitoring of SARS-CoV of animals
in recent 2 years in different provinces, especially in Guangdong province, did not
show that SARS-CoV existed. These results indicated the SARS-CoV causing the
epidemic in 2003 might disappear in nature and reemergence of SARS seems to be
depended on a new SARS virus derived from mutation. However, the four confirmed
SARS cases with mild manifestations and caused by a SARS-CoV differentiated
from the SARS-CoV in 2003 (Liang et al., 2004) told us the "mild" SARS-CoV may
be still hidden in animal hosts. Since the mild SARS case is difficult to be differentiated from other atypical pneumonia, it gives the mild SARS-CoV a chance to become
an epidemic strain through further trans-genus mutation. Thus, the possibility of
SARS outbreak is still there. Although this article was finished 2 years ago, we
believe the main points and contents in this article will be still valuable for prevention
and control of reemerging of SARS.

References

Che XY, Qiu LW, Pan YX, Wen K, Hao W, Zhang LY, Wang YD, Liao ZY, Hua X, Cheng VC, Yuen KY. Sensitive and specific monoclonal antibody-based capture enzyme immunoassay for detection of nucleocapsid antigen in sera from patients with severe acute respiratory syndrome. J Clin Microbiol, 42:2629–2635, 2004

Chinese Center for Disease Control and Prevention. Document: Primary analysis of severe acute respiratory syndrome epidemic in China, 2003

Chinese SARS Molecular Epidemiology Consortium. Molecular evolution of SARS coronavirus during the course of the SARS epidemic in China. Science, 303:1666–1669, 2004

Drosten C, Günther S, Preiser W, van der Werf S, Brodt HR, Becker S, Rabenau H, Panning M, Kolesnikova L, Fouchier RA, Berger A, Burguière AM, Cinatl J, Eickmann M, Escriou N, Grywna K, Kramme S, Manuguerra JC, Müller S, Rickerts V, Stürmer M, Vieth S, Klenk HD, Osterhaus AD, Schmitz H, Doerr HW. Identification of a novel coronavirus in patients with severe acute respiratory syndrome. N Engl J Med, 348:1967–1976, 2003

Government of Xuan Wu Qu, Beijing. Affiche: Isolation and Control of Institute for Viral Disease Control and Prevention, China CDC, April 23, 2004

He JF, Pen GW, Zheng HZ, Luo HM, Liang WJ, Li LH, Guo RN, Deng ZH. An epidemiological study on the index cases of severe acute respiratory syndrome occurred in different cities among Guangdong province. Chin J Epidemiol, 24(5):347–349, 2003

Hong T, Wang JW, Sun YL, Duan SM, Chen LB, Qu JG, Ni AP, Liang GD, Ren LL, Yang RQ, Guo L, Zhou WM, Chen J, Li DX, Xu WB, Xu H, Guo YJ, Dai SL, Bi SL, Dong XP, Ruan L. Chlamydia-like and coronavirus-like agents found in dead cases of atypical pneumonia by electron microscopy. Natl Med J China, 83(8):632–636, 2003

Kan B, Wang M, Jing H, Xu H, Jiang X, Yan M, Liang W, Zheng H, Wan K, Liu Q, Cui B, Xu Y, Zhang E, Wang H, Ye J, Li G, Li M, Cui Z, Qi X, Chen K, Du L, Gao K, Zhao YT, Zou XZ, Feng YJ, Gao YF, Hai R, Yu D, Guan Y, Xu J. Molecular evolution analysis and geographic investigation of severe acute respiratory syndrome coronavirus-like virus in palm civets at an animal market and on farms. J Virol, 79(18):11892–11900, 2005

Lau SK, Che XY, Woo PC, Wong BH, Cheng VC, Woo GK, Hung IF, Poon RW, Chan KH, Peiris JS, Yuen KY. SARS coronavirus detection methods. Emerg Infect Dis, 11(7):1108–1111, 2005

Leadership Group of SARS Prevention and Control in Beijing. Epidemiological features of severe acute respiratory syndrome in Beijing. Chin J Epidemiol, 24(12):1096–1099, 2003

Li W, Shi Z, Yu M, Ren W, Smith C, Epstein JH, Wang H, Crameri G, Hu Z, Zhang H, Zhang J, McEachern J, Field H, Daszak P, Eaton BT, Zhang S, Wang LF. Bats Are Natural Reservoirs of SARS-Like Coronaviruses, Sciencexpress (www.sciencexpress.org), Page1–8/10.1126/ science. 1118391, 29 September, 2005

Li T, Xie J, He Y, Fan H, Baril L, Qiu Z, Han Y, Xu W, Zhang W, You H, Zuo Y, Fang Q, Yu J, Chen Z, Zhang L. Long-term persistence of robust antibody and cytotoxic T cell responses in recovered patients infected with SARS coronavirus. PLoS ONE (www.plosone.org), 1:e24, 2006

Liang G, Chen Q, Xu J, Liu Y, Lim W, Peiris JS, Anderson LJ, Ruan L, Li H, Kan B, Di B, Cheng P, Chan KH, Erdman DD, Gu S, Yan X, Liang W, Zhou D, Haynes L, Duan S, Zhang X, Zheng H, Gao Y, Tong S, Li D, Fang L, Qin P, Xu W; SARS Diagnosis Working Group. Laboratory diagnosis of four recent sporadic cases of community acquired SARS-CoV infection in Guangdong Province, China. Emerg Infect Dis, 10:1774–1781, 2004

Ministry of Health, People's Republic of China. News release: Breaking off of no SARS case report by Ministry of Health, People's Republic of China. 1 June 2004

Ministry of Health, People's Republic of China. Consensus of the management of Severe Acute Respiratory Syndrome (version 2004), 2005

National Institute for Viral Disease Control and Prevention, China CDC. Document: Decision for establishing the joined scientists group for tackling key problem of etiology of causative-unclear pneumonia recently occurring in Gongdong Province. 12 February 2003a

National Institute for Viral Disease Control and Prevention, China CDC. Document: National program proposal for tackling key problem of causative-unclear pneumonia recently occurring in Gongdong Province. 25 February 2003b

Peng GW, He JF, Lin JY, Zhou DH, Yu DW, Liang WJ, Li LH, Guo RN, Luo HM, Xu RH. Epidemiological study on severe acute respiratory syndrome in Guangdong province. Chin J Epidemiol, 24(5):350–352, 2003

People's Republic of China. State Department Order No. 376: Regulations on Preparedness for and Response to Emergent Public Health Hazards, http://www.gov.cn/zwg/2005-05/content_145.htm, May 5, 2003

People's Republic of China. Chairman Order No. 17: Law of the People's Republic of China on the Prevention and Treatment of Infectious Diseases, http://www.gov.cn/ziliao/flfg/2005-08/05/conter_20946.htm, Aug 28, 2004

Rota PA, Oberste MS, Monroe SS, Nix WA, Campagnoli R, Icenogle JP, Peñaranda S, Bankamp B, Maher K, Chen M-H, Tong S, Tamin A, Lowe L, Frace M, DeRisi JL, Chen Q, Wang D, Erdman DD, Peret TC, Burns C, Ksiazek TG, Rollin PE, Sanchez A, Liffick S, Holloway B, Limor J, McCaustland K, Olsen-Rassmussen M, Fouchier R, Günther S, Osterhaus AD, Drosten C, Pallansch MA, Anderson LJ, Bellini WJ. Characterization of a novel coronavirus associated with severe acute respiratory syndrome. Science, 300:1394–1399, 2003

Song HD, Tu CC, Zhang GW, Wang SY, Zheng K, Lei LC, Chen QX, Gao YW, Zhou HQ, Xiang H, Zheng HJ, Chern SW, Cheng F, Pan CM, Xuan H, Chen SJ, Luo HM, Zhou DH, Liu YF, He JF, Qin PZ, Li LH, Ren YQ, Liang WJ, Yu YD, Anderson L,Wang M, Xu RH, Wu XW, Zheng HY, Chen JD, Liang G, Gao Y, Liao M, Fang L, Jiang LY, Li H, Chen F, Di B, He LJ, Lin JY, Tong S, Kong X, Du L, Hao P, Tang H, Bernini A, Yu XJ, Spiga O, Guo ZM, Pan HY, He WZ, Manuguerra JC, Fontanet A, Danchin A, Niccolai N, Li YX, Wu CI, Zhao GP. Cross-host evolution of severe acute respiratory syndrome coronavirus in palm civet and human. Proc Natl Acad Sci USA, 102(7):2430–2435, 2005

Wang L. Reflections on SARS outbreak and recent works on prevention and treatment of SARS. Natl Med J China, 83(20): 1753–1756, 2003

Wang DM, Feng ZJ, Yang WZ, Zhang YM, Luo HM, Yu HJ. Analysis of the first clinical-diagnosed SARS cases in 24 provinces, municipalities and autonomous regions in China. Chin J Epidemiol, 25(1):29–30, 2004

Jiang-Tao Lin, Jian-San Zhang, Nan Su, Jian-Guo Xu, Nan Wang, Jiang-Ting Chen, Xin Chen, Yu-Xuan Liu, Hong Gao, Yu-Ping Jia, Yan Liu, Rui-Hua Sun, Xu Wang, Dong-Zheng Yu, Rong Hai, Qiang Gao, Ye Ning, Hong-Xia Wang, Ma-Chao Li, Biao Kan, Guan-Mu Dong, Qi An, Ying-Qun Wang, Jun Han, Chuan Qin, Wei-Dong Yin and Xiao-Ping Dong. Safety and immunogenicity from a Phase I trial of inactivated severe acute respiratory syndrome corona-virus vaccine. Antiviral Therapy 12:1107–1113, 2007

WHO. Update 1 – Severe Acute Respiratory Syndrome (SARS). 16 March, 2003a

WHO. Update 31 – Coronavirus Never Before Seen in Humans is the Cause of SARS, Unprecedented Collaboration Identifies New Pathogen in Record Time. 16 April, 2003b

WHO. Severe Acute Respiratory Syndrome (SARS) in Singapore. 10 September, 2003c

WHO. Severe Acute Respiratory Syndrome (SARS) in Taiwan, China. 17 December, 2003d

WHO. Summary of Probable SARS Cases with Onset of Illness from 1 November 2002 to 31 July 2003., 21 April, 2004

Yang W, Wang HZ, Zhang J, Yu HJ, Luo HM, Ni DX, Huang YY, Wang MW, Yan JY, Li LM. Primary analysis of infectivity of severe acute respiratory syndrome and its control measures. Chin J Epidemiol, 24(6):432–433, 2003

Yu H, Jing H, Chen Z, Zheng H, Zhu X, Wang H, Wang S, Liu L, Zu R, Luo L, Xiang N, Liu H, Liu X, Shu Y, Lee SS, Chuang SK, Wang Y, Xu J, Yang W; Streptococcus Suis Study Groups. Human Streptococcus suis outbreak, Sichuan, China. Emerg Infect Dis, 12(6):914–920, 2006

Zhu QY, Qin ED, Wang CE, Yu M, Si BY, Fan BC, Chang GH, Peng WM, Yang BA, Jiang T, Li YC, Deng YQ, Liu H, Gan YH. Isolation and identification of a novel coronavirus from patients with SARS. China Biotechnol, 23(4):106–112, 2003

The 2003 SARS Outbreak In Singapore: Epidemiological and Clinical Features, Containment Measures, and Lessons Learned

Annelies Wilder-Smith and Kee Tai Goh

The Evolution of the SARS Outbreak in Singapore

The Beginning of the Outbreak at Tan Tock Seng Hospital

On 6 March 2003, the Singapore Ministry of Health was notified of a cluster of atypical pneumonia in three patients with a history of travel to Hong Kong (Hsu et al., 2003). These three female travelers had stayed at the Metropole Hotel on the same floor as a Chinese physician later diagnosed with severe acute respiratory syndrome (SARS) (Hsu et al., 2003; Peiris et al., 2003). After returning to Singapore, one of the travelers (index A) who developed fever on February 25 was hospitalized at Tan Tock Seng Hospital on March 1, and was managed initially for straightforward community-acquired pneumonia. The other two travelers were also admitted with similar symptoms. Shortly thereafter, clusters of cases emerged in three separate wards, all traceable to the first imported case. By the time index A was isolated on March 6, she had already infected 22 persons, comprising ten health care workers, two inpatients, seven visitors, and three family members. One of the infected health care workers (index case B), with onset of symptoms on March 7 and a provisional diagnosis of dengue fever, was later admitted on March 10 to Ward 8A. At the ward she in turn infected 21 persons, including an inpatient with ischemic heart disease and diabetes mellitus, before she was isolated on March 13 (Wilder-Smith et al., 2004b). The inpatient (index case C) had been admitted on March 10 with fever, community-acquired pneumonia, and gram-negative bacteremia. When she developed heart failure on March 12, she was transferred to Ward 6A (the coronary care unit) and mechanically ventilated. However, she was isolated only on March 20 when SARS was suspected. By that time, 21 health care workers and 5 family members had become infected (Wilder-Smith et al., 2004b). A total of 109 cases were epidemiologically linked to index A. Intra-hospital transmission at Tan Tock Seng Hospital was interrupted by April 12, the date of onset of the hospital's last case. Despite the institution of very rigorous infection control measures at Tan Tock Seng Hospital, SARS spread to four other health care institutions (Singapore General Hospital, National University Hospital, Changi General Hospital, and Orange Nursing Home – the last two are

Y. Lu et al. (eds.), *Emerging Infections in Asia.*
© Springer Science+Business Media, LLC 2008

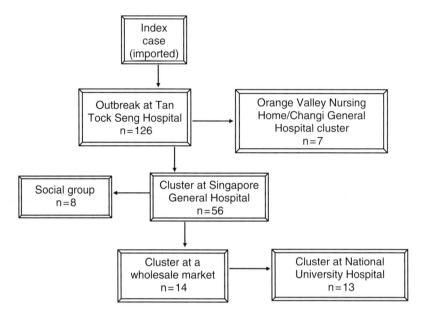

Fig. 1 Inter-hospital and community spread of the SARS outbreak in Singapore in 2003

grouped together in Fig. 1 and a vegetable wholesale market (Gopalakrishna et al., 2004) (Fig. 1).

Spread to Singapore General Hospital

Index case D was a 60-year-old ex-patient of Tan Tock Seng Hospital with multiple medical problems, including ischemic heart disease and diabetes mellitus with kidney damage. He was admitted on March 5 to Tan Tock Seng Ward 5A (the same ward as index case A) and discharged on March 20 with no clinical manifestations of SARS. He was later admitted to an open ward (Ward 57) at Singapore General Hospital on March 24 for steroid-induced gastrointestinal bleeding and a diabetic foot ulcer (Chow et al., 2004). Although he had a low-grade fever on March 26, four consecutive chest X-rays were normal. His blood culture grew *E. coli* (Tan et al., 2004). He was transferred to another open ward (Ward 58) where he stayed from March 29 to April 2. On April 4, a cluster of 13 febrile health care workers from the two wards he had occupied was identified. It was only on April 5 when chest X-ray showed evidence of pneumonia that he was clinically diagnosed as a probable SARS case. A total 40 cases were directly linked to him, with the date of onset of the last probable case on April 17. All the exposed health care workers and inpatients were transferred to Tan Tock Seng Hospital, where eight subsequently developed probable SARS.

Outbreak at National University Hospital

Index case E at National University Hospital was a 63-year-old man with a history of hypertension, ischemic heart disease, and chronic atrial fibrillation. He was infected with SARS when he visited his brother, index case D, at Singapore General Hospital on March 31. He developed a fever on April 5, was seen at the National University Hospital Accident and Emergency Department on April 8, and was admitted 4 h later to an open ward for cardiac failure (Fisher et al., 2003b; Ooi and Tambyah, 2004). When his condition deteriorated rapidly over the next 8 h, he was isolated in the intensive care unit (ICU). As soon as SARS was suspected, the patient was immediately transferred to Tan Tock Seng Hospital where he died on April 12. A total of 13 SARS cases at National University Hospital were epidemiologically linked to him, with the date of onset of the last case on April 25.

Outbreak at Orange Valley Nursing Home/Changi General Hospital

A 90-year-old woman (index case F) with pneumonia and a urinary tract infection who had been warded next to a SARS patient in Ward 7D at Tan Tock Seng Hospital from March 16–17 was discharged to a private nursing home (Orange Valley Nursing Home) and then admitted to Changi General Hospital on March 25 when she fell ill again with breathing difficulty (Tee et al., 2004). This led to a small cluster of seven cases linked to the nursing home and Changi General Hospital. The dates of onset of the last cases at the nursing home and Changi General Hospital were April 2 and April 4, respectively.

Community Outbreaks

Index case E at National University Hospital worked as a vegetable seller at the Pasir Panjang wholesale market. He worked there for a few hours each day on April 5, 7, and 8. It was only on April 19 that two additional SARS cases (a taxi driver who transported index E to work and another worker at the market) were epidemiologically linked to the market. Index E started a cluster of 14 cases, including eight in a family linked to the market. Another cluster of eight cases in the community was started by a febrile health care worker (index case G) at Singapore General Hospital who was given medical leave to stay at home. Transmission occurred through social contact in a Chinese card game.

There were two local cases whose sources of infection could not be determined despite intensive epidemiological investigations. Three of 32 probable cases retrospectively diagnosed to have SARS could not be linked to any of the clusters.

Summary of Epidemiological Features

The SARS outbreak in Singapore was mainly perpetuated in seven clusters related to five index cases, with a fireworks-like pattern of spread (Fig. 2). A total of 206 probable SARS cases, including eight imported cases, with illness onset dates between 25 February and 11 May 2003 were reported. Of these, 58 cases were detected among 12,194 persons that had previously been on home quarantine (7,863) or telephone surveillance (4,331). Of 600 clinically suspected cases who were admitted to Tan Tock Seng Hospital and had laboratory tests conducted during the post-outbreak period, an additional 32 probable cases were picked up, for a final figure of 238 probable cases, including 33 deaths. None of the 700 patients admitted for observation tested positive.

The demographic characteristics of the reported cases and deaths are shown in Table 1. The majority (79.4%) were Singaporeans, and 67.6% were females. About half (46.6%) of the cases were in the 25–44-year-old age group. The ethnic distribution among the Singaporean cases was proportionate to that of the population of Singapore. Health care workers constituted 40.8%; family members, friends, social contacts, and visitors, 37.4%; and inpatients, 13%. Transmission within health care and household settings accounted for over 90% of the cases.

The epidemic curve of the SARS outbreak is shown in Fig. 3.

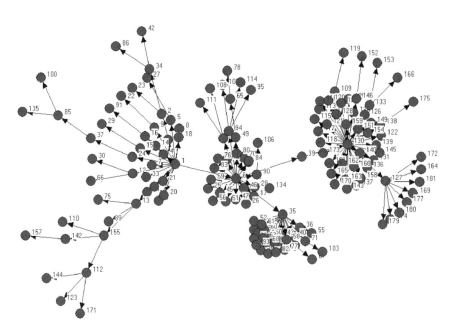

Fig. 2 The "fireworks effect" of several clusters related to five index cases in Singapore (Centers for Disease Control and Prevention, 2003)

Table 1 Demographic characteristics of the 238 SARS cases in Singapore, March–May 2003

Characteristics	Number of Cases (Deaths)			
	Male	Female	Total	%
Age group (yrs)				
0–4	2 (0)	3 (0)	5 (0)	2.1
5–14	0 (0)	5 (0)	5 (0)	2.1
15–24	8 (1)	29 (0)	37 (1)	15.5
25–34	13 (2)	53 (2)	66 (4)	27.7
35–44	21 (4)	24 (1)	45 (5)	18.9
45–54	11 (2)	22 (5)	33 (7)	13.9
55–64	11 (4)	14 (2)	25 (6)	10.5
65+	11 (6)	11 (4)	22 (10)	9.2
Nationality				
Singaporean	66 (14)	123 (17)	189 (31)	79.4
Filipino	5 (0)	17 (1)	22 (1)	9.2
Chinese	3 (0)	7 (0)	10 (0)	4.2
Indonesian	1 (0)	6 (0)	7 (0)	2.9
Malaysian	1 (0)	4 (0)	5 (0)	2.1
Indian	1 (0)	3 (0)	4 (0)	1.7
Sri Lankan	0 (0)	1 (0)	1 (0)	0.4
Ethnic group (among 189 Singaporeans)				
Chinese	53 (9)	85 (15)	138 (24)	73.0
Malay	21 (0)	4 (3)	25 (3)	13.2
Indian	14 (2)	8 (2)	22 (4)	11.6
Other	3 (0)	1 (0)	4 (0)	2.1
Occupational group				
Health care workers	13 (3)	84 (2)	97 (5)	40.8
Nonhealth care workers[a]	64 (16)	77 (12)	141 (28)	59.2
Source of infection				
Imported	1 (0)	7 (1)	8 (1)	3.4
Healthcare institution	50 (16)	125 (8)	175 (24)	73.5
Household	17 (1)	24 (5)	41 (6)	17.2
Community/Workplace[b]	6 (2)	2 (0)	8 (2)	3.4
Undefined	3 (0)	3 (0)	6 (0)	2.5
Total	77 (14)	161 (19)	238 (33)	238 (33)

[a] Family members, friends or visitors (37.4%), inpatients (13%), others (8.8%)
[b] wholesale market (3), taxi (3), and airplane (1)

The last probable SARS patient, whose illness began on May 5, was isolated at Tan Tock Seng Hospital on May 11. The World Health Organization (WHO) removed Singapore from its list of areas with local SARS transmission on May 31. However, intensive case-finding efforts continued, particularly among patients with chronic medical conditions and with atypical clinical presentation. They were repeatedly tested for SARS-associated coronavirus (SARS-CoV) prior to discharge from the hospital. In view of the improved situation globally and locally, SARS prevention and control measures were progressively stepped down beginning in mid-July 2003. Unfortunately, a laboratory-acquired case of SARS was diagnosed at Singapore General Hospital on 8 September 2003 (Lim et al., 2004).

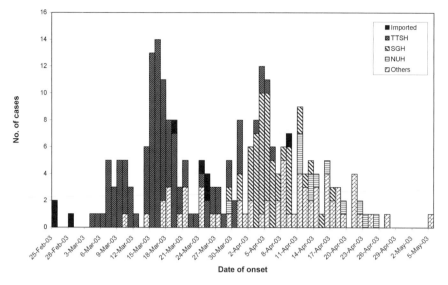

Fig. 3 Epidemic Curve of the SARS outbreak in Singapore in 2003

Laboratory-Acquired SARS Case

The patient with laboratory-acquired SARS was a 27-year-old Chinese Singaporean in his third year of a doctoral program in microbiology at the National University of Singapore. He was working on the West Nile virus at a University microbiology laboratory. He also did some work at the Environmental Health Institute (EHI) laboratory of the National Environment Agency; he last visited this laboratory on August 23. He had no history of travel to SARS-affected areas and no known contact with SARS patients. The date of onset of his illness was August 26. When he was admitted to Singapore General Hospital on September 3, he complained of fever, muscle aches, and joint pains, but he did not have any significant respiratory symptoms. He developed a dry cough after admission, but his fever resolved 2 days later. Three serial chest X-rays done at Singapore General Hospital were all normal. On September 8, his stool and sputum specimens tested positive for SARS-CoV by reverse-transcriptase polymerase chain reaction (RT-PCR). Three serial serological tests done on September 3, 4, and 8 showed a rising titer of SARS-CoV antibodies. He was immediately transferred to the Communicable Disease Centre at Tan Tock Seng Hospital for further management.

A repeat of his PCR tests in two other laboratories in Singapore on September 9 confirmed positive results. Blood samples also tested positive for antibodies to SARS-CoV in another laboratory in Singapore. Results from the Centers for Disease Control, Atlanta, corroborated Singapore's PCR and serological results.

Subsequent investigations of the chest on September 13 showed that he had radiological evidence of pneumonic changes in his left lung. Tests for a whole range of other pathogens, including two human coronaviruses (OC 43 and 229 E), were negative. The patient was discharged on September 16 and placed on a 14-day home quarantine.

Investigations by an 11-member review panel, comprising local and international experts, revealed that the patient worked in the EHI laboratory 3.5 days prior to the onset of his illness. Although the patient reported only working with West Nile virus, the laboratory was doing live SARS-CoV work around that time. Poor record keeping made it difficult to ascertain whether there was live SARS-CoV in the laboratory on the day of his visit, but it was there 2 days before. The frozen specimen that the patient worked with on August 23 was positive by RT-PCR for the SARS-CoV and West Nile virus, suggesting contamination. As the laboratory had only worked on one strain of the SARS-CoV, the laboratory strain and the patient strain were sequenced for comparison. Approximately 91% of the genome was sequenced from the patient's strain and found to be most closely related to the sequence of the laboratory strain. Minor differences were likely the result of natural mutations of the virus (Lim et al., 2004).

Clinical Features of SARS

The clinical and radiological manifestations of SARS in Singapore were consistent with those reported elsewhere (Hsu et al., 2003; Lee et al., 2003; Poutanen et al., 2003). The median incubation period was determined based on the records of 50 SARS cases who, prior to onset of illness, had a single and specific close contact history with another person who had been diagnosed with probable SARS. Of the 50 cases reviewed, 15 were hospital visitors, 20 were health care workers, and 15 were family and social contacts. The median age of the cases was 42 years (range 22–84 years) and 56% were females. The mean (standard deviation) and median incubation periods were estimated to be 5.1 (2.2) and 5 days, respectively. The 95th percentile for the incubation period was 9 days. None of the 50 cases studied had an incubation period longer than 10 days. (Kuk and Ma, 2005).

In the Singapore cohort, the case-fatality rate increased with age from 2.7% in the 15–24-year age group to 45.5% in those 65 years and older. The overall case-fatality rate was 13.9% (33/238). The median days from symptom onset to ICU admission was 8 days (range 6–10); the median length of hospital stay was 23.5 days (range 15–36); and the median length of stay in the ICU was 14.5 days (range 7–22) (Tai et al., 2003). Among SARS patients, 20.2% required ICU care. Predictors for ICU admission were comorbidities (especially diabetes mellitus and heart disease), advanced age, peaked lactate dehydrogenase, and high absolute neutrophil counts (Tai et al., 2003).

The WHO case definition for SARS was revised on 1 May 2003 after laboratory tests for SARS-CoV became available. Locally validated assays for SARS-CoV by

RT-PCR (available as of the first week of April) and serology (available as of the first week of May) were used for all suspected and probable cases as well as for cases under observation in whom SARS could not be excluded.

We conducted a seroepidemiological cohort study amongst 80 health care workers exposed to SARS patients prior to the implementation of infection control measures (Wilder-Smith et al., 2005). Of these, 45 (56%) were SARS-positive by serology. Of these 45, 37 (82%) were classified as having pneumonic SARS, 2 (4%) as subclinical SARS, and 6 (13%) as having asymptomatic SARS-CoV infection. The overall incidence of asymptomatic SARS-CoV infection was 7.5% (6 out of 80), and was higher than that reported elsewhere. This was most likely due to the fact that this cohort had unprotected exposure. The median titer of SARS antibodies was 1:6,400 (range 1:1,600–1:6,400) for pneumonic SARS, 1:4,000 (range 1:1,600–1:6,400) for subclinical SARS cases, and 1:4,000 (range 1:400–1:6,400) for asymptomatic cases. In univariate analysis, none of the variables for gender, age, use of gloves, hand-washing, index case, distance to index case, or contact time were associated with asymptomatic SARS. However, a higher proportion of those who had asymptomatic SARS (50%) had used masks compared to those who developed pneumonic SARS (8%) ($p = 0.025$). Although the extent to which cases with asymptomatic SARS-CoV infection contributed to the ongoing transmission during the outbreak is unknown, our data from Singapore suggest that they did not constitute a major source of transmission.

The diagnosis of SARS is difficult early in the illness as presentation and laboratory features resemble other nonspecific viral fevers, such as dengue. Dengue fever is endemic in Singapore. One of the index cases was misdiagnosed as having dengue and therefore not isolated, which led to subsequent SARS transmissions. We did a study to identify simple laboratory features to differentiate SARS from dengue (Wilder-Smith et al., 2004a). Multivariate analysis identified three laboratory features that together are highly predictive of a diagnosis of dengue and able to rule out the possibility of SARS: platelet count $<140 \times 10^9$ L^{-1}, white-blood-cell count $<5 \times 10^9$ L^{-1}, and aspartate aminotransferase >34 IU L^{-1} (Wilder-Smith et al., 2004a). The application of the combination of these parameters can identify dengue 75% of the time and rule out SARS 100% of the time. This approach can help to rationalize the use of isolation rooms for patients presenting with nonspecific fever. Dengue PCR is helpful in the early diagnosis of dengue and was used during the SARS outbreak in Singapore.

Containment Measures

Following the WHO's global alert on 12 March 2003, all health care institutions were advised to notify their Health Ministries of every patient who met the WHO's case definition of a suspected or probable case of SARS. Health care institutions were also directed to notify contacts of suspected and probable cases. Prevention and control measures were initiated by the Singapore Ministry of Health (MOH)

SARS Task Force, which was formed on 15 March 2003 and chaired by the Director of Medical Services. Its members included the chief executive officers of all hospitals, chairmen of medical boards, infectious disease physicians, epidemiologists, and virologists. Strategies to contain the rapid nosocomial transmission were discussed, formulated, and effectively implemented across all health care institutions through the Infectious Diseases Act and Private Hospitals and Medical Clinics Act. The Ministerial Committee on SARS (chaired by the Minister for Home Affairs) was established on April 7 to provide political guidance and quickly make strategic decisions to minimize the socioeconomic impacts of SARS. The Executive Group, comprising permanent secretaries of the relevant ministries, was responsible for the overall coordination and implementation of strategies to address multi-agency issues outside the health care setting, while an Inter-Ministry SARS Operations Committee ensured that cross-ministry operational issues on SARS were well coordinated. A Ministerial SARS Combat Unit was also appointed on April 20. This Unit worked closely with public and private hospitals and other health care institutions to prevent and control SARS transmission in these facilities. Key measures implemented in Singapore were directed at the prevention and control of SARS in health care institutions, in the community, and at borders.

Containment of SARS in Health Care Institutions

SARS transmission was quickly established to occur mainly via droplets and contact (Seto et al., 2003). A case–control study done early in the outbreak found that N95 masks and hand washing after each patient contact were independently associated with a significantly decreased risk of infection, with adjusted odds ratios of 0.1 and 0.07, respectively (Teleman et al., 2004). Contact with a patient's nasal secretions before infection control measures were implemented was independently associated with a 22-fold increased risk of infection. Enhanced personal protective measures were progressively instituted in tandem with growing understanding of this novel disease. From March 6, health care workers were employing N95 masks for personal protection when nursing the first index case and her contacts. By the end of week 2, personal protective equipment (PPE) against contact, droplet, and respiratory transmissions had been adopted by health care workers attending to patients in areas involved in SARS screening or treatment (ICU, emergency department, and communicable disease wards). On March 22, Singapore's second largest general hospital, Tan Tock Seng, was designated as the central referral, screening, and treatment center for SARS. The Communicable Disease Centre (which is part of Tan Tock Seng Hospital) is a specialist facility with a national role, staffed by experts in clinical infectious diseases, hospital infection control, and public health. By March 22, N95 masks were required when treating any patient in the hospital. On April 6, the wearing of gloves, gowns, and N95 masks was enforced during contact with all patients in the hospital, with visitors additionally advised for procedures with a risk of splashing. On April 25, goggles were made mandatory for all patient contact. Later, powered air purifying respirators for high-risk or aerosol-generating procedures were also required. With all of these measures in place, no further intra-hospital transmission to health care workers at Tan Tock Seng occurred after March 22. However, with the new outbreak at Singapore General Hospital, health care workers were affected again. Prompt institution of strict measures in all hospitals nationwide curbed in-hospital transmissions, and the last such case occurred on April 13.

Triage and Surveillance

At the first point of contact with health care facilities (accident and emergency departments and specialist outpatient clinics), triage was carried out to separate febrile patients. To widen the surveillance net, the WHO's definition for suspected and probable SARS was expanded to include any health care worker with fever and/or respiratory symptoms (particularly in a cluster of three or more febrile cases), inpatients (>16 years old) with atypical pneumonia under investigation, sudden unexplained deaths with respiratory symptoms, and inpatients with unexplained fever (>38°C) of more than 72 h who also had relevant travel history. Case-finding was further intensified with the introduction of thrice daily temperature surveillance of all health care workers in every institution and active surveillance for clusters of febrile patients and for staff working in the areas occupied by these patients. Special attention was paid to immunocompromised patients who tended to have atypical clinical presentations. Health care workers' sick leave was centrally monitored. Audits were periodically conducted to ensure that the directives and guidelines issued by MOH were strictly enforced.

Three separate hospital containment strategies were implemented. Tan Tock Seng Hospital was designated as a SARS hospital and non-SARS patients were diverted to other hospitals (Gopalakrishna et al., 2004). The strategy at Singapore General Hospital was ring fencing and transfer of the exposed group (patients and health care workers) to Tan Tock Seng Hospital. At National University Hospital, the strategy was management of the exposed cohort in situ. These containment strategies were supported by strict enforcement of the proper use of PPE (test-fitted N95 masks, gowns, gloves, and goggles/protective eye gear if managing suspicious cases, and powered air purifying respirator for high-risk procedures such as intubation), control of visitors, restriction of movements of health care workers (including being confined to practice at one institution) and patients (readmission to the same hospital if within 21 days after discharge), and close monitoring of discharged patients from SARS-affected wards. In view of the risk posed by atypical SARS cases, all inpatients at Tan Tock Seng and Singapore General Hospitals with chronic medical conditions were placed on home quarantine for 10 days upon discharge.

The Infectious Diseases Act was amended to ensure that all necessary measures were taken to control the outbreak, e.g., handling and disposing of bodies within 24 h after SARS-related death.

Containment of SARS in the Community

Isolation, Contact Tracing, and Quarantine

There was a significant correlation between the length of time taken to isolate a case and the number of secondary cases that arose. A total of 159 cases who did not transmit had a mean time to isolation of 3 days, compared with those with who were isolated after 4–10 days and infected 15–40 secondary cases each. For the prevention and control of SARS within the community in Singapore, the key strategy was to detect persons with suspected or probable SARS as early as possible and isolate them at Tan Tock Seng Hospital. Early identification of SARS cases was achieved in several ways, including active tracing of all contacts within 24 h of notification of a case, mandatory home quarantine enforced through the use of electronic cameras, and intensive education of health care professionals and the public. The effectiveness of these strategies was reflected in the progressive reduction in the time to isolation of cases over the course of the outbreak. During the week of March 3, the average interval between the onset of symptoms and isolation in the hospital was 6.8 days. This interval was reduced to 2.9 days by the week of March 31 and 1.3 days by the week of April 21. Reducing the time to isolation of cases was one of the main contributing factors for interrupting transmission and curbing the outbreak in Singapore.

Contact tracing, initiated within 24 h of notification of a case, was carried out by trained medical and health officers in hospitals, nursing homes and other health care institutions, and the community, including residential homes, places of work or school, hostels, food centers, markets, places of worship, and factories. Following the spread of infection to a wholesale market in April, 200 staff members from the Peoples' Association were mobilized and trained on the spot to trace the large number of contacts. On April 23, 250 army personnel were deployed to the MOH for 2 months to strengthen its operational capability, especially the development of the IT system to support epidemiological investigations, contact tracing, and quarantine operations. Contacts included health care workers who did not wear personal protective gear while attending to a case of SARS, family members, visitors to health care institutions, school teachers, classmates, workplace colleagues, and commuters in close proximity to a SARS case in the public transport system (taxi, bus, train, ship, aeroplane). These contacts were assessed for the likelihood of exposure to SARS. Those who were febrile were immediately transported by a delegated ambulance service to Tan Tock Seng Hospital. Contacts who were apparently well were quarantined for 10 days either at home or at a specific quarantine center where their temperatures were monitored twice daily for early signs of SARS. Any person who developed a fever (>38°C) during the quarantine period was isolated at Tan Tock Seng Hospital for further investigations. As a precautionary measure, contacts assessed to have a low risk of developing SARS (e.g., inpatients with no chronic comorbid conditions discharged from Tan Tock Seng Hospital) were not quarantined but put on daily telephone surveillance for SARS symptoms for 21 days by a team of 100 health staff.

Secondary household transmission of SARS was studied in 114 households involving 417 contacts. The attack rate was low (6.2%) (Goh et al., 2004).

The Pasir Panjang wholesale market was closed for 15 days from April 19, and a total of 2,007 workers and regular visitors to the market from April 5–19 were put on mandatory home quarantine. Teams of nurses visited all those under quarantine to check their temperatures and to ensure that they were well. The infection did not spread to other wet markets.

To allay the concerns of parents, all preschools, primary, and secondary schools were closed for 2–3 weeks from the end of March to early-mid-April 2003.

Containment of SARS at Border Checkpoints

International travel was responsible for the rapid intercontinental spread of SARS. The outbreak in Singapore can be traced to the first imported case. To prevent further importation of SARS, a number of measures were taken at the air- and sea-ports and road entry points into Singapore. As of 30 March 2003, Health Alert Notices were issued to air passengers arriving from affected areas. On March 31 visual screening was instituted for all passengers arriving from SARS affected areas; this measure was replaced by temperature screening a few days later. Passengers who appeared to be unwell or had a temperature of >37.5°C were sent by a special ambulance to Tan Tock Seng Hospital, which had been singly designated to perform SARS screening. From April 7 onward, passengers arriving from SARS-affected countries were asked to complete health declaration cards. The information collected on these cards included recent travel, contact history, and symptoms suggestive of SARS, as well as address in Singapore and flight seat numbers to facilitate contact tracing. On April 23, thermal scanners were installed at Changi Airport and at the road entry points to check temperatures for all departing and arriving passengers. Temperature checks were introduced to all of the Singapore's ferry terminals on April 28. SARS screening was progressively extended to all arriving flights from April 29 onwards.

Of the seven imported cases, which all occurred before screening measures were implemented at the airport, only the first resulted in extensive secondary transmission (Wilder-Smith and Paton, 2003). None of the imported cases resulted in in-flight transmission. Of 442,973 air passengers screened after measures were implemented, 136 were sent to Tan Tock Seng Hospital for further SARS screening; none were diagnosed with SARS (Wilder-Smith and Paton, 2003). After implementation of screening methods, no further importation of patients with SARS occurred (March 31–May 31). The absence of transmission from the other six imported cases was likely a result of their relatively prompt identification and isolation together with a low potential for transmission. New imported SARS cases therefore need not lead to major outbreaks if systems are in place to identify and isolate them early. Screening at entry points is costly, has a low yield, and is not sufficient as a single containment strategy, but may be justified in light of the major economic, social, and international impact that even a single imported SARS case may have (Wilder-Smith and Paton, 2003).

Between 25 February and 31 May 2003, nine passengers who were later diagnosed as suffering from probable SARS (based on the WHO criteria) arrived in Singapore on seven flights: three were from Hong Kong (with five cases of SARS), one from Beijing, one from New York, one from East Malaysia, and one from Indonesia. Six of the nine travelers imported SARS to Singapore (from Hong Kong and Beijing) and three had acquired SARS in Singapore and were returning to Singapore (from New York, East Malaysia, and Indonesia) (Wilder-Smith et al., 2003b). However, only three of the airplanes (carrying four of the passengers with probable SARS) had symptomatic cases of SARS on board; the passengers of the other flights developed symptoms within the first 2 days after arrival in Singapore (Wilder-Smith et al., 2003b). In-flight transmission occurred in only one of the three airplanes with symptomatic SARS patients on board. This transmission was to only one person, a stewardess who had served and cleaned the tray of the passenger with SARS on the flight from New York to Singapore via Frankfurt (March 14) (Wilder-Smith et al., 2003a). The passenger was a doctor who had treated the first admitted case of SARS in Singapore at a time when the new disease had not yet been identified and no infection control measures were in place. At disembarkation, the passengers were briefed on the symptoms of SARS and advised to seek prompt health care should they develop symptoms. None of the 82 passengers who disembarked in Frankfurt, or the 28 who disembarked in Singapore developed SARS. Very stringent steps were taken to minimize the possibility of exporting cases to other countries. These measures included rapid containment of outbreaks in Singapore, and mandatory temperature screening of all outgoing travelers from Singapore. In addition, special bilateral arrangements on the exchange of information necessary to conduct contact tracing and quarantine was set up with both Malaysia and Indonesia. Singapore also initiated a similar multilateral agreement among the ten member countries of the Association of Southeast Asian Nations plus China, Japan, and the Republic of Korea (ASEAN + 3) in view of the possible spread of infection by travelers.

SARS and the Public

During the outbreak of SARS in Singapore from 1 March to 11 May 2003, various measures were undertaken at the national level to control and eliminate the transmission of the infection. During the initial period of the epidemic, communication with the public was achieved through press releases and media coverage of the epidemic. About a month into the epidemic, a public education campaign was mounted to educate Singaporeans on SARS and the adoption of appropriate social behavior to prevent the spread of the disease. Rigorous preventive measures were implemented by various ministries. For example, the Ministry of Education issued a personal thermometer to every student, taught students about SARS and how to check their temperatures, and required students and staff to declare their travel history. Standard operating procedures for screening children at child-care centers and kindergartens were implemented. The Ministry of Defense conducted daily screening of all recruits and national servicemen who were undergoing in-camp training, and issued personal thermometers to all personnel, including the Singapore Armed Forces. The Ministry of Environment checked sewerage systems and required environmental workers and market stallholders to take their temperatures twice a day. The government of Singapore disseminated information on SARS and encouraged the general public to adopt good health practices, such as measuring body temperature and restraining "socially irresponsible habits," such as spitting in public. During the SARS outbreak in Singapore, "fighting SARS" as a "shared responsibility" was a central message. Prime Minister Goh's open letter in the front page of the Singapore main newspaper (Straits Times) urged all Singaporeans to practice social responsibility and civic consciousness in order to be "good citizens." Singaporeans were also urged to give health care workers on the front line battling SARS their utmost support and not ostracize them. Contributions to the SARS Courage Fund, in aid of health care workers and victims of SARS exceeded US$10 million by the end of May 2003. A survey was conducted in late April 2003 to assess Singaporeans' knowledge of SARS and infection control measures, and their concerns and anxiety in relation to the outbreak (Deurenberg-Yap et al., 2005). The survey also sought to assess their confidence in the ability of various institutions to deal with SARS and their opinion on the seemingly tough measures enforced. The study involved 853 adults selected from a telephone-sampling frame. Stratified sampling was used to ensure adequate representation from major ethnic groups and age groups. The study showed that the overall knowledge of SARS and control measures undertaken was low (mean score of 24.5% ± 8.9%). While 82% of respondents expressed confidence in measures undertaken by Tan Tock Seng Hospital (the hospital designated to manage SARS), only 36% had confidence in nursing homes. However, >80% of the public agreed that the preventive and control measures instituted were appropriate. Despite the low knowledge score, the score for overall mean satisfaction with the government's response to SARS was 4.47 (out of a possible highest score of 5.00), with >93% of adult Singaporeans indicating that they were satisfied or very satisfied with the government's response to SARS. Generally, Singaporeans had a high level of public trust (satisfaction with the government, confidence in institutions, and agreement that government measures were appropriate), scoring 11.4 out of a possible maximum of 14. The disparity between low scores for knowledge and high scores for confidence and trust in the government's actions suggests that Singaporeans do not require high levels of knowledge to be confident in measures undertaken by the government to control the SARS crisis (Deurenberg-Yap et al., 2005).

A cross-sectional telephone survey of 1,201 Singaporean adults and 705 adults from Hong Kong compared the public's knowledge and perception of SARS and the extent to which various precautionary measures were adopted (Leung et al., 2004). The results showed that respondents from Hong Kong had significantly more anxiety about SARS than Singaporean respondents [State Trait Anxiety

Inventory (STAI) score, 2.06 vs. 1.77; $p < 0.001$]. The former group also reported more frequent headaches, difficulty in breathing, dizziness, rhinorrhea, and sore throat. More than 90% of respondents in both places were willing to be quarantined if they had close contact with a SARS case, and 70% or more would comply with quarantine following a social contact. Most respondents (86.7% in Hong Kong vs. 71.4% in Singapore; $p < 0.001$) knew that SARS could be transmitted via respiratory droplets, although fewer (75.8% in Hong Kong vs. 62.1% in Singapore; $p < 0.001$) knew that fomites were also a possible transmission source. Twenty-three percent of respondents in Hong Kong and 11.9% of those in Singapore believed that they were "very likely" or "somewhat likely" to contract SARS during the outbreak ($p < 0.001$). There were large differences between respondents in Hong Kong and Singapore in the adoption of personal precautionary measures. Respondents with higher levels of anxiety, better knowledge of SARS, and greater risk perceptions were more likely to take comprehensive precautionary measures against the infection, as were older, female, and more educated individuals (Leung et al., 2004).

Lessons Learned from the SARS Outbreak in Singapore

The SARS outbreak in Singapore can be traced to the first imported index case that was imported from Hong Kong before this new disease had been identified and before appropriate measures had been put in place to prevent transmission. Progressive understanding of the clinical manifestations and modes of transmission led to the progressive implementation of infection control and public health measures and the successful containment of the outbreak, even without an early diagnostic test for this novel viral agent. Because of the rapid institution of measures to quickly identify and isolate SARS cases, more than 80% of the cases did not transmit the infection to their contacts. Unrecognized cases of SARS in Singapore were rare, but were the main cause of perpetuation of the national outbreak because they were not isolated early enough. Unrecognized cases were either due to atypical presentations in patients with comorbidities (Fisher et al., 2003b) or to concomitant infection (Wilder-Smith et al., 2004b). The WHO definition for probable SARS states: "A case should be excluded if an alternative diagnosis can fully explain their illness" (definition from 2003 before sensitive and specific diagnostic tests were available). Whilst this definition is reasonable for epidemiological surveillance purposes, our cases show that it should not be the basis on which infection control measures are implemented during an outbreak (Wilder-Smith et al., 2004b). Discharged patients from a hospital with known SARS cases should be kept under surveillance for at least 14 days after discharge, and readmitted to the original hospital should medical problems arise within this time-frame. All patients with fever, even when there is another known etiology, should be isolated in times of a hospital-related SARS outbreak. In response to the experience of the index cases in Singapore, these policies were implemented and contributed to the successful containment of the outbreak. Nationwide enforcement of infection control measures for the care of any patients (SARS or non-SARS) combined with temperature surveillance of all health care workers are thought to be the other major factors that interrupted the chain of transmission in Singapore. Although there were further imported cases of SARS to Singapore, none of them led to secondary transmission due to early identification and isolation. New imported cases need not lead to major outbreaks if systems are in place to identify and isolate them efficiently (Wilder-Smith and Paton, 2003). Although screening at entry points may be justified in the light of the severe socioeconomic and public health consequences of a single imported case, strengthening screening and infection control capacities at points of entry into the health care system should be prioritized over investing in airport screening measures to detect a rare infectious disease (St. John et al. 2005).

The rapid containment of the outbreak in Singapore was due to a combination of strong political leadership, effective control and coordination at all levels, prompt and coordinated inter-agency responses, good communication with the public (Menon and Goh, 2005), and collaboration with international agencies such as the WHO and US Centers for Disease Control.

Post SARS Surveillance and Preparedness

Based on the lessons learned, Singapore has further strengthened its operational readiness and laboratory safety measures to respond to SARS. A center has been established to undertake community contact tracing as well as coordinate and assist with contact tracing efforts undertaken by hospitals and government agencies. All matters related to quarantine operations, e.g., the issue and enforcement of home quarantine orders (HQOs), phone surveillance, ambulance services, allowances, and alternate housing facilities for those on HQOs, will be centrally managed. New SARS Information Technology infrastructure has been developed and consolidated to support the surveillance and management of SARS. It provides MOH and other agencies with the ability to access integrated information about all SARS cases in Singapore in a timely fashion. For medical surveillance, there is the Infectious Disease Alert and Clinical Database System, which integrates critical clinical, laboratory, and contact tracing information on SARS. In addition, the Health Check System enables health care professionals in hospitals and clinics to identify patients who may have been exposed to SARS. For contact tracing and quarantine operations, the Contact Tracing System is in place to capture SARS cases, contact history, and HQO status. This will facilitate speedier generation of HQO reports, contact listings, and listings for external agencies automatically. An e-Quarantine Management System has also been developed for better management in the processing and enforcement of HQOs by a Singapore security agency.

The MOH was reorganized with the incorporation of an Operations Group, which serves as the main operational linkage between the MOH and all health care providers. This group is responsible for the prevention and control of outbreaks of major infectious diseases, including bioterrorism events, planning for crisis management and coordination of health services and operations during peacetime, and command and control of all medical resources during a crisis. A three-pronged strategy comprising the establishment of a disease outbreak and response system, the strengthening of the public health system, and the development of national biosafety standards was formulated. As a result, Singapore's surveillance and analysis capacity has been enhanced, a command and communication network has been put in place, contingency plans for all health care institutions and agencies have been developed and coordinated, preparedness exercises and audits are periodically conducted, and emergency procurement and stockpiling of critical medical supplies such as PPE for up to 6 months has been undertaken. Professional manpower has been reviewed and additional isolation facilities in all hospitals, including Tan Tock Seng Hospital's Communicable Disease Centre 2 with 39 isolation and 18 intensive care beds, have been built. A national center for infectious diseases and emergency preparedness is being reviewed. Legislative framework for biosafety, including licensing for Biosafety Level 3 laboratories, has been finalized.

A SARS response framework with three levels corresponding to local SARS transmission levels and the severity of threat to the public's health has been formalized. This framework serves as a platform for coordinating the responses of various agencies. There are three color-coded alert levels, which are also adopted by the hospitals: yellow (no cases or sporadic imported cases with no local transmission); orange (local transmission confined to close contacts in health care settings or households); and red (outbreak in the community where local transmission is no longer confined to close contacts in health care settings or households).

At the yellow SARS alert level, the main focus is to prevent imported cases and detect any SARS cases that do occur early. Active surveillance and enhanced protection at high-risk areas in health care settings underpin the prevention strategy. Temperature screening of inbound visitors will be instituted at all border entry points. Within the health care setting, active surveillance for atypical pneumonia as well as fever clusters will be carried out. For prevention, health care workers in high-risk areas such as accident and emergency departments, isolation facilities, ICUs, and triaging areas will be required to don full PPE. Workflow changes to separate febrile and non-febrile patients at hospitals and health care institutions will be enforced. To reduce the prevalence of acute respiratory viral infections due to influenza, health care workers and those traveling to temperate countries are encouraged to receive influenza vaccination. Influenza vaccination is mandatory for long-term patients in nursing homes.

At the orange alert level, the focus is on containment. Additional measures will be introduced to contain the spread of SARS in Singapore as well as to prevent the export of cases. Infection control measures in health care institutions will be enhanced to break the chain of transmission. This will include the restriction of hospital visitation and the movement of health care workers and patients between health care institutions. Contact tracing and quarantine efforts will be stepped up. Community surveillance through daily temperature-taking at workplaces and schools will also be instituted. Outbound screening and "not-to-depart" restrictions will be implemented at the border checkpoints to prevent the export of cases. Health declaration cards will also be required for inbound travelers.

At the red alert level, the strategy is to suppress the outbreak. More stringent measures will be added to gain control of community spread in Singapore and prevent the export of cases. Such measures could include the selective closure of schools, foreign workers' dormitories, factories, and places of mass gatherings, and the suspension of selected public events. Contact tracing and quarantine measures will be strictly enforced.

The robustness of the response system was demonstrated in the early detection, isolation, and contact tracing of all contacts in the workplace, health care setting, and the community when the laboratory-acquired SARS case was diagnosed in September 2003.

Singapore is now better prepared to respond to the reemergence of SARS and other emerging infectious diseases spread by the respiratory route. An avian influenza/influenza pandemic preparedness plan was developed based on the SARS response framework to prevent and control an impending health emergency.

References

Centers for Disease Control and Prevention. (2003). Severe acute respiratory syndrome-Singapore, 2003. *Morbidity and Mortality Weekly Report*, 52, 405–411

Chow, K. Y., Lee, C. E., Ling, M. L., Heng, D. M., Yap, S. G. (2004). Outbreak of severe acute respiratory syndrome in a tertiary hospital in Singapore linked to an index patient with atypical presentation: Epidemiological study. *BMJ*, 328, 195

Deurenberg-Yap, M., Foo, L. L., Low, Y. Y., Chan, S. P., Vijaya, K., Lee, M. (2005). The Singaporean response to the SARS outbreak: Knowledge sufficiency versus public trust. *Health Promot Int*, 20, 320–326

Fisher, D. A., Lim, T. K., Lim, Y. T., Singh, K. S., Tambyah, P. A. (2003b). Atypical presentations of SARS. *Lancet*, 361, 1740

Goh, D. L., Lee, B. W., Chia, K. S., Heng, B. H., Chen, M., Ma, S., Tan, C. C. (2004). Secondary household transmission of SARS, Singapore. *Emerg Infect Dis*, 10, 232–234

Gopalakrishna, G., Choo, P., Leo, Y. S., Tay, B. K., Lim, Y. T., Khan, A. S., Tan, C. C. (2004). SARS transmission and hospital containment. *Emerg Infect Dis*, 10, 395–400

Hsu, L. Y., Lee, C. C., Green, J. A., Ang, B., Paton, N. I., Lee, L., Villacian, J. S., Lim, P. L., Earnest, A., Leo, Y. S. (2003). Severe acute respiratory syndrome (SARS) in Singapore: Clinical features of index patient and initial contacts. *Emerg Infect Dis*, 9, 713–717

Kuk, A. Y., Ma, S. (2005). The estimation of SARS incubation distribution from serial interval data using a convolution likelihood. *Stat Med*, 24, 2525–2537.

Lee, N., Hui, D., Wu, A., Chan, P., Cameron, P., Joynt, G. M., Ahuja, A., Yung, M. Y., Leung, C. B., To, K. F., Lui, S. F., Szeto, C. C., Chung, S., Sung, J. J. (2003). A major outbreak of severe acute respiratory syndrome in Hong Kong. *N Engl J Med*, 348, 1986–1994

Leung, G. M., Quah, S., Ho, L. M., Ho, S. Y., Hedley, A. J., Lee, H. P., Lam, T. H. (2004). A tale of two cities: Community psychobehavioral surveillance and related impact on outbreak control in Hong Kong and Singapore during the severe acute respiratory syndrome epidemic. *Infect Control Hosp Epidemiol*, 25, 1033–1041

Lim, P. L., Kurup, A., Gopalakrishna, G., Chan, K. P., Wong, C. W., Ng, L. C., Se-Thoe, S. Y., Oon, L., Bai, X., Stanton, L. W., Ruan, Y., Miller, L. D., Vega, V. B., James, L., Ooi, P. L., Kai,

C. S., Olsen, S. J., Ang, B., Leo, Y. S. (2004). Laboratory-acquired severe acute respiratory syndrome. *N Engl J Med*, 350, 1740–1745

Menon, K.U., Goh, K.T. (2005). Transparency and trust: Risk communications and the Singapore experience in managing SARS. *J Commun Manage*, 9, 375–383

Ooi, S. B., Tambyah, P. A. (2004). Transmission of severe acute respiratory syndrome in an emergency department. *Am J Med*, 116, 486–489

Peiris, J. S., Yuen, K. Y., Osterhaus, A. D., Stohr, K. (2003). The severe acute respiratory syndrome. *N Engl J Med*, 349, 2431–2441

Poutanen, S. M., Low, D. E., Henry, B., Finkelstein, S., Rose, D., Green, K., Tellier, R., Draker, R., Adachi, D., Ayers, M., Chan, A. K., Skowronski, D. M., Salit, I., Simor, A. E., Slutsky, A. S., Doyle, P. W., Krajden, M., Petric, M., Brunham, R. C., McGeer, A. J.; National Microbiology Laboratory, Canada; and Canadian Severe Acute Respiratory Syndrome Study Team (2003). Identification of Severe Acute Respiratory Syndrome in Canada. *N Engl J Med*, 348, 1995–2005

Seto, W. H., Tsang, D., Yung, R. W., Ching, T. Y., Ng, T. K., Ho, M., Ho, L. M., Peiris, J. S.; Advisors of Expert SARS group of Hospital Authority (2003). Effectiveness of precautions against droplets and contact in prevention of nosocomial transmission of severe acute respiratory syndrome (SARS). *Lancet*, 361, 1519–1520

St. John R. K., King, A., de Jong, D., Bodie-Collins, M., Squires, S., Tam, T. (2005). Border screening for SARS. *Emerg Infect Dis*, 11, 6–10

Tai, D. Y., Lew, T. W., Loo, S., Earnest, A., Chen, M. I. (2003). Clinical features and predictors for mortality in a designated national SARS ICU in Singapore. *Ann Acad Med Singapore*, 32, S34–S36

Tan, T. T., Tan, B. H., Kurup, A., Oon, L. L., Heng, D., Thoe, S. Y., Bai, X. L. Chan, K. P., Ling, A. E. et al. (2004). Atypical SARS and *Escherichia coli* bacteremia. *Emerg Infect Dis*, 10, 349–352

Tee, A. K., Oh, H. M., Lien, C. T., Narendran, K., Heng, B. H., Ling, A. E. (2004). Atypical SARS in geriatric patient. *Emerg Infect Dis*, 10, 261–264

Teleman, M. D., Boudville, I. C., Heng, B. H., Zhu, D., Leo, Y. S. (2004). Factors associated with transmission of severe acute respiratory syndrome among health-care workers in Singapore. *Epidemiol Infect*, 132, 797–803

Wilder-Smith, A., Paton, N. I. (2003). Severe acute respiratory syndrome: Imported cases of severe acute respiratory syndrome to Singapore had impact on national epidemic. *BMJ*, 326, 1393–1394

Wilder-Smith, A., Leong, H. N., Villacian, J. S. (2003a). In-flight transmission of severe acute respiratory syndrome (SARS): A case report. *J Travel Med*, 10, 299–300

Wilder-Smith, A., Paton, N. I., Goh, K. T. (2003b). Low risk of transmission of severe acute respiratory syndrome on airplanes: The Singapore experience. *Trop Med Int Health*, 8, 1035–1037

Wilder-Smith, A., Earnest, A., Paton, N. I. (2004a). Use of simple laboratory features to distinguish the early stage of severe acute respiratory syndrome from dengue fever. *Clin Infect Dis*, 39, 1818–1823

Wilder-Smith, A., Green, J. A., Paton, N. I. (2004b). Hospitalized patients with bacterial infections: A potential focus of SARS transmission during an outbreak. *Epidemiol Infect*, 132, 407–408

Wilder-Smith, A., Teleman, M. D., Heng, B. H., Earnest, A., Ling, A. E., Leo, Y. S. (2005). Asymptomatic SARS coronavirus infection among healthcare workers, Singapore. *Emerg Infect Dis*, 11, 1142–1145

The 2003 SARS Outbreaks in Taiwan

Yi-Ming Arthur Chen

Introduction

Severe acute respiratory syndrome (SARS) is caused by SARS-associated coronaviruses (SARS-CoVs) (Drosten et al., 2003; Fouchier et al., 2003; Peiris et al., 2003b; Ksiazek et al., 2003). The first known outbreak of SARS occurred in China's Guangdong province in November, 2002 (Chinese SARS Molecular Epidemiology Consortium, 2004). By August 7 of the following year, SARS had spread to more than 30 countries, affecting 8,096 people and resulting in 774 deaths worldwide (World Health Organization, 2004). In 2003, Taiwan experienced a series of SARS outbreaks and the Municipal Hoping Hospital (referred to hereafter as HP) in Taipei City suffered the first and the most serious outbreak of SARS-CoV nosocomial infections: 137 probable cases and 26 deaths (Division of Surveillance and Investigation, Center for Disease Control, Taiwan, 2003; Lan et al., 2005b). According to the Center for Disease Control (CDC) in Taiwan, 364 of the 664 probable Taiwanese SARS cases reported to the World Health Organization were confirmed by reverse transcriptase-polymerase chain reaction (RT-PCR) and/or neutralizing antibody tests (Center for Disease Control, 2003a). In this chapter, we will discuss the molecular and clinical epidemiology of SARS infection in Taiwan during 2003.

The First and Second Waves of SARS Infections

In Taiwan, the first SARS case was diagnosed on 14 March 2003 (Center for Disease Control and Prevention, 2003b). This index case involved a Taiwanese businessman who had visited Guangdong province from February 5–21. After he came back to Taiwan, he transmitted the disease to his wife, his son (SARS-CoV-TW1), and the doctor who treated his son (SARS-CoV-TW3). On 15 March 2003, seven employees from a Taiwanese construction company flew from Hong Kong to Beijing. Four of them developed SARS symptoms on March 26, several days after returning to Taiwan (Olsen et al., 2003).

Y. Lu et al. (eds.), *Emerging Infections in Asia.*
© Springer Science+Business Media, LLC 2008

The Third Wave of SARS Infection: A Series of Nosocomial Infections

On 26 March 2003, a male resident of the Amoy Gardens housing complex in Hong Kong flew to Taiwan; he stayed overnight in a small hotel in Taipei and took a train from Taipei to Taichung City to visit his younger brother the following day. The visitor returned to his Hong Kong home on March 28 after experiencing fever the preceding evening. His younger brother, who developed symptoms on March 31, became Taiwan's first SARS-related fatality (TC1).

On April 6, a 47-year-old Taiwanese female (TW-HP1) suffering from fever and coughing for several days visited the emergency room at the municipal Hoping hospital. On April 9, this patient was transferred to another private hospital where she was diagnosed to have SARS. Although patient TW-HP1 stayed only in the emergency room of Hoping hospital for 3 days, seven employees including a laundry worker (the index case) developed SARS after she left. In all, 137 probable SARS cases and 26 mortalities resulted from this nosocomial infection.

On April 24, for the reason of quarantine, the Taipei City government shut down Hoping hospital without warning. All the employees of the hospital were asked to return to the hospital and stay with the patients and their visitors during the quarantine. On April 28, the Taiwan government imposed mandatory quarantines on all air travelers from China, Hong Kong, Singapore, Macau, and Toronto, but nosocomial SARS infections continued to be reported in many hospitals island-wide. More than ten hospitals experienced outbreaks of nosocomial SARS-CoV infec-

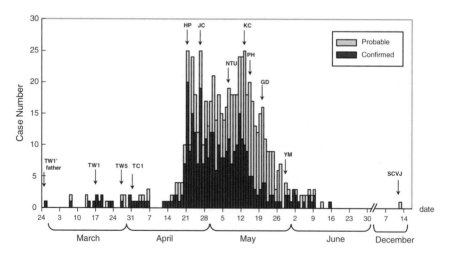

Fig. 1 Epidemiological curves of probable (*gray color*) and confirmed (*darker color*) SARS cases in Taiwan. Confirmed cases were validated by the Taiwan's Center for Disease Control using RT-PCR and serological tests. Arrows mark dates of outbreaks of nosocomial infections in HP, JC, NYU, KC, PH, GD, and YM hospitals and of diagnoses of SARS in several key patients

tions in Taiwan. The following hospitals were marked on the epidemiological curve chronologically (Fig. 1): Taipei Municipal Hoping Hospital (HP), Jenchi Hospital (JC), National Taiwan University Hospital (NTU), Kaohsiung Chang-Gung Hospital (KC), Taipei Municipal Guando Hospital (GD), and Taipei Municipal Yangming Hospital (YM) which had the most severe outbreaks of nosocomial SARS infections.

Development of a New Tool for the Phylogenetic Analysis of SARS-CoV Infections

The SARS-CoV genome size has been measured as 29.7 kb (Marra et al., 2003; Rota et al., 2003). A comparative analysis of SARS-CoV isolates has identified two distinct clades belonging to the early and late epidemics, respectively (Lan et al., 2005a). Conventionally, phylogenetic SARS-CoV analyses require full genome sequences (Lan et al., 2005a). Because of the limited amount of specimens for full-length sequencing, some researchers have used the SARS-CoV spike gene for this purpose, but most results have been less than satisfactory (Guan et al., 2003; Guan et al., 2004). Therefore, we developed a new phylogenetic analytical tool by combining nucleotide sequences from six variable regions, 5.6-kb in total, of a SARS-CoV genome and validated the robustness of the method (Lan et al., 2005b). Since this new method requires only seven RT-PCR reactions to obtain the nucleotide sequences for phylogenetic tree analysis, it is less time-consuming and more efficient than conventional methods. To facilitate future molecular epidemiological studies of SARS outbreaks in other laboratories, we have made the nucleotide sequences alignment file of 80 SARS-CoV reference strains available on our center's website: http://www.ym.edu.tw/aids/Molepi/.

Molecular Epidemiology of SARS-CoV Infections in Taiwan

We applied the new method mentioned above to elucidate the origin and dissemination pathways of SARS CoV infections collected from different hospitals in Taiwan. Phylogenetic analyses demonstrated that the Taiwanese SARS-CoVs were distributed in three clusters: B1, B2, and B3 (Fig. 2). After considering the epidemiological data of the SARS patients, it is clear that Taiwan experienced five infection waves in 2003. The first wave, in early March 2003, was composed of one imported case, two intra-familiar transmission cases (TW1), and one nosocomial infection (TW3). In cluster B1, both TW1 and TW3 SARS-CoVs were clustered with other SARS-CoVs linked to Hotel M in Hong Kong (Center for Disease Control and Prevention, 2003b). The second wave consisted of four Taiwanese (TW5) who contracted the disease as they flew from Hong Kong to Beijing, and then carried it back to Taiwan in mid-March 2003 (Olsen et al., 2003). The third wave, which

Phylogenetic Clusters   Epidemic Waves

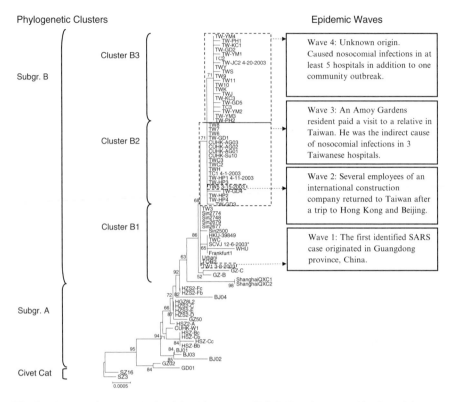

Fig. 2 Phylogenetic tree analysis of 39 Taiwanese SARS-CoVs using a combination of the proposed strategy and neighbor-joining method. A summary of the five infectious waves of SARS infection, corresponding to each phylogenetic cluster, was demonstrated on the right side of the figure. Node numbers indicate bootstrap value (%). Scale bar shows estimated genetic distance using Kimura's two-parameter substitution model. (Adapted from Lan et al., 2005b)

began in late March, consisted of an infection that occurred on a train (TW-HP1), an intra-familiar transmission (TC1), as well as multiple nosocomial infections (all TW-HPs and TW-GD1, TW-GD-3, and TW-GD4). In cluster B2, all the SARS-CoVs mentioned above clustered with the SARS-CoVs from the Amoy Gardens housing complex in Hong Kong (CUHK-AG01, CUHK-AG02, and CUHK-AG03) (Chim et al., 2003). Additionally, we identified a fourth wave of SARS infection (cluster B3), which started in late April and ended in mid-June, that contained SARS-CoVs not only from hospitals JC, KC, PH, GD [TW-GD2 and TW-GD5], and YM, but also from sporadic community outbreaks (TW10 and TW11).

The fifth wave happened in early December 2003 with a laboratory contamination case-SCVJ. It clustered with a SARS-CoV isolate used in the laboratory HKU-39849 and another isolate from Taiwan CDC-TWC (Lan et al., 2005b).

The first and second waves were in different phylogenetic clusters, suggesting they had different origins. Neither the first, nor the second wave led to serious outbreaks, but the third wave – originating with a visitor to Taiwan from the Amoy Gardens housing complex – led to one transmission on a train (TWC3), one intra-familiar transmission (TC1), and nosocomial infections in at least two hospitals (HP and GD) in the northern region of Taiwan. It is worthy to note that there is only one nucleotide difference between SARS-CoV strains TC1 and TWC3. In addition, TWC3 shared an identical sequence with CUHK-AG01 (Chim et al., 2003), an Amoy Gardens isolate, even though patient TW-HP1 (SARS-CoV strain TC1) never left Taiwan at any time during the epidemic. An epidemiological investigation showed that the Hong Kong visitor and this female patient sat in different cars during their train ride. This is the first documented case with molecular proof of transmission of SARS-CoV infection on a train (Lan et al., 2005b).

If we assume that the CUHK-AG01 represents the first generation virus in the transmission link, then both TC1 and TWC3 were the second generation viruses and TWH was the third generation virus. According to the nucleotide variation analysis, the number of nucleotide change in the SARS-CoV genome per number of intermediate hosts was extremely low (less than 1 nucleotide change per host).

Community-Based Epidemiological Study of SARS in the Wan-Hwa District of Taipei City

In 9 May 2003, one month after the outbreak of a nosocomial infection in the Hoping hospital, there was an outbreak of SARS infection in the Hwa-Chung Residential Complex located in the same district as the Hoping hospital (Fig. 3). Four residents living in the complex had SARS and one of them died. In July, we conducted a sero-epidemiological study to understand the extent and risk factors associated with the infection. The results showed that 2 of 103 (1.9%) residents from Hwa-Chung Residential Complex and none of 76 people who lived in the same neighborhood were seropositive for SARS infection (Fig. 3). In terms of risk factors, one male had contact history (his wife died of SARS), while another female who lived in a different building from that of other cases did not have any contact history.

Clinical Epidemiology of SARS in Taiwan

The transmission of SARS is thought to occur primarily via respiratory droplets or direct contact. Contaminated sewage is believed to be responsible for the first major SARS outbreak in Hong Kong's Amoy Garden housing complex, with over 300 residents affected (Peiris et al., 2003a). Two months after the final outbreak of the SARS nosocomial infection, we recruited 658 employees from Hoping hospital that suffered the first and most severe SARS infections to help us investigate the epidemiological and genetic factors associated with SARS-CoV. SARS-CoV infections were detected using enzyme immunoassays and confirmed by a combination

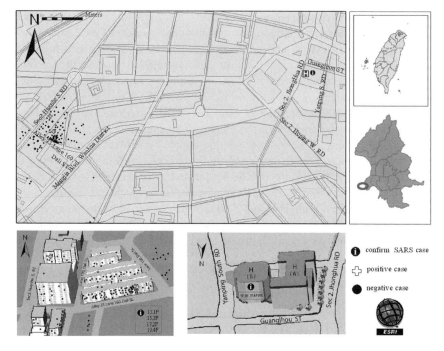

Fig. 3 Geographic locations of Hoping hospital and the Hwa-Chung housing complex in the Wah-Hwa District of Taipei City. Individuals participated in the sero-epidemiological study in the Hwa-Chung housing complex were marked on the map 2006. (Chen YM, unpublished data)

of Western blot assays, neutralizing antibody tests, and commercial SARS tests. Risk factors were analyzed via questionnaire responses and sequence-specific oligo-nucleotide probes of human leukocyte antigen (HLA) alleles. Our results indicate that 3% (20/658) of the study participants were seropositive, with one female nurse identified as a subclinical case. Identified SARS-CoV infection risk factors include working in the same building as the hospital's emergency room and infection ward, providing direct care to SARS patients, and carrying a Cw*0801 HLA allele (Fig. 3). Three SARS-CoV-infected nursing aides and one infected occupational therapist claimed that they had no direct contact with SARS patients; they may have come into contact with patient specimens or contact with infected bedclothes.

HLA Alleles Associated with SARS-CoV Infection

We found evidence of a link between HLA-Cw*0801 and SARS-CoV infection susceptibility. One of the cases was HLA-Cw*0801-homozygous; we observed that relative risk of infection increased from 3.3 for heterozygous individuals to 6 for homozygous individuals (95% confidence intervals of 0.9–11.6 and 0.2–188.7, respectively). The odds ratio for contracting a SARS-CoV infection among persons with either a homozygous or heterozygous Cw*0801 genotype was 4.4 (95% confidence interval, 1.5–12.9; $p = 0.007$) (Chen et al., 2006). We also compared our data with data from a normal group provided by a separate Taiwanese research team (Chung et al., 2004) and obtained similar results (OR = 4.1, 95% CI = 1.4–12.0, $p = 0.01$).

The human leukocyte antigen (HLA) complex plays an important role in determining susceptibility to infectious diseases. HLA class I gene products present antigenic peptides to T cells, initiating an immune response and the removal of foreign material (Segal and Hill, 2003). Researchers have demonstrated that specific HLA alleles are associated with susceptibility to and outcomes from such viral infections as HIV-1, HTLV-1, and HCV (Jeffery et al., 2000; Carrington and O'Brien, 2003; Khakoo et al., 2004). During their study of potential SARS patients and high-risk health care workers (HCWs), Lin et al. (2003) observed an association between HLA-B*4601 and SARS-CoV infections. However, their definition of a SARS patient was based on clinical diagnosis rather than serological evidence, and HCWs may not have been a suitable control group. In contrast, 14.6% of our 80-member control group and 5% of the 20 seropositive participants carried the HLA-B*4601 allele (no statistical significance) (Chen et al., 2006). In a Hong Kong study that used bone marrow donors as a control, Ng et al. described HLA-B*0703 and HLA-DRB1*0301 as susceptible and resistant alleles for SARS-CoV infection, respectively. However, they did not collect or analyze HLA-Cw allelic frequencies among their participants (Ng et al., 2004). In our study, the seropositive group had a lower HLA-DRB1*0301 frequency than the seronegative group, but not at a statistically significant level ($p = 0.22$) (Chen et al., 2006).

Previous reports have stated that individuals carrying HLA-Cw*0801 are at significantly higher risk of contracting adult periodontitis (OR = 6.2) (Machulla et al., 2002) and that a link exists between HLA-Cw*04 and persistent hepatitis C viral infection (Thio et al., 2002). A research team in Beijing found that the total numbers of natural killer (NK) and CD158b + NK cells were significantly lower in SARS patients compared to healthy patients (National Research Project for SARS, Beijing Group, 2004). NK cells play a central role in innate antiviral immune response. In vivo, their activity is controlled via inhibitory and activation receptors for major histocompatibility complex class I molecules (Bauer et al., 1999; Ahmad et al., 2001). Therefore, we postulated that HLA-Cw*0801 may affect SARS-CoV susceptibility via its interaction with the killer-cell immunoglobulin-like receptors (KIR) of NK cells.

Subclinical Cases

Very few subclinical cases of SARS-CoV infection have been identified to date (Leung et al., 2004; Woo, et al., 2004; Chen et al., 2006). Of the 242 asymptomatic participants in our study who had close contact with SARS patients, only 1 (0.41%) had a subclinical infection. The anti-SARS-CoV antibody reactivity of the asymptomatic nurse (case no. HP613) was verified by all available serological assays. Her neutralizing antibody (NA) titer was measured at 32 in June of 2003 and it dropped to 2 in December 2003. As an internal medicine ward employee, she had frequent contact with SARS patients. She claimed that she took her own body temperature twice a day for more than 1 month during the nosocomial infection outbreak and that it was slightly above normal (37.4°C) only once. We tried to isolate the SARS-CoV from a nasopharyngeal swab in order to refute the possibility that she was an asymptomatic SARS-CoV carrier, but the results were negative.

The single asymptomatic case was unusual in several respects. In addition to carrying the heterozygous HLA-Cw*0801, she also carried a HLA haplotype (HLA-A*0101/2402, -B*4006/5701, -Cw*0801/0602, -DRB1*0701/0803, and -DQB1*0303/0601) considered rare among the Chinese (Fig. 4). Her HLA allelic frequencies were relatively low compared to the majority of Taiwanese: 1%, 2%, and 2.9% for HLA-A*0101, -B*4006, and -Cw*0602, respectively (http://www.allelefrequencies.net/). On the other hand, all of her HLA class I alleles were heterozygous, which is consistent with the hypothesis of a heterozygote advantage against infectious disease (Carrington and O'Brien, 2003; Doherty and Zinkernagel, 1975).

Public Health Control Measures

In Taiwan, during the SARS epidemic in 2003, different control measures including wearing masks (first only among medical personnel then among all citizens), inclusion of SARS in the infectious disease control law, home quarantine, and taking body temperature (first only among travelers, then among all the citizens) were implemented (Twu et al., 2003; Huang et al., 2005). Some measures were quite innovative, e.g., providing funding for hospitals to build a screening station outside the main building for patients with fever. Some may not have been so effective and needed to be modified, e.g., home quarantine. During the period, more than 150,000 persons were quarantined and 24 of whom were found later to have SARS (Hsieh et al., 2005). Furthermore, instead of using "home quarantine," the Taiwan CDC made a mistake and used "home isolation" in the mass media communication. Fear, stigma, and discrimination were generated among the general public towards SARS patients as well as persons under home quarantine. A mental health coalition composed of different nongovernmental organizations was formed, and they provided counseling through hot lines and radio programs.

Lesson Learned and Future Perspectives

Currently, highly pathogenic avian influenza viruses of the H5N1 subtype are circulating in eastern Asia with unprecedented epizootic and epidemic effects (Li et al., 2004). In 2004, the Council of Agriculture of Taiwan conducted a survey

HLA								
	Cw			A	B	Cw	DRB1	DQB1
0801	0801	0303	0102	0101	4006	0801	0701	0303
&	&	&	&	&	&	&	&	&
0801	1402	1203	0304	2402	5701	0602	0803	0601

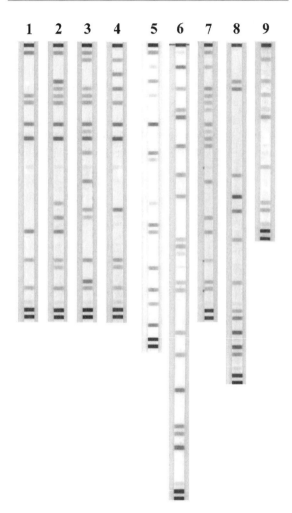

Fig. 4 HLA typing of several anti-SARS-CoV antibody-positive cases. *Lane 1*, case with homozygous HLA-Cw*0801; *lane 2*, case with heterozygous HLA-Cw*0801; *lanes 3 and 4*, two cases with HLA-Cw*0801 null genotype; *lanes 5–9*, the HLA-A, HLA-B, HLA-Cw, HLA-DRB1, and HLA-DQB1 genotypes of the lone asymptomatic case (HP613). Allele typing was performed via polymerase chain oligonucleotide probing (Dynal Biotech Ltd., Wirral, UK, 2006)

on migratory binds, chickens, ducks, geese, and pigs and found a H5N2 strain in poultry (Bureau of Animal and Plant Health Inspection and Quarantine, 2007). Facing the threats of the pandemic bird flu, Taiwan CDC has built multiple surveillance systems to detect patients infected with avian flu. Twelve virology laboratories belonging to medical centers in different regions have joined the laboratory surveillance system.

The SARS pandemic in 2003 is a metaphor for global public health interconnectivity. It is difficult to draw a conclusion regarding whether better outbreak control would be achieved by placing fewer persons in quarantine or by concentrating on improving the efficiency of detection and isolation procedures. In fact, each area may become more efficient without jeopardizing the other's improvement. It also showed us that international cooperation especially among regional cities is vital to the control of communicable diseases. Balanced aggressive public health measures should be combined with stringent hospital infection control practices. Although the governments should inform the public as soon and as thoroughly as they can, they must take caution in raising awareness without stigmatizing those infected.

Acknowledgment I thank Dr. Yu-Ching Lan and Mr. Yuan-Ming Lee for their help in preparing the figures of this chapter. This study is partially supported by the following two grants: No. 93004-62-007 from the Department of Health, Taipei City Government and NSC 92-2751-B-010-001-Y from the Taiwan's National Science Council.

References

Ahmad, R., Sindhu, S. T., Tran, P., Toma, E., Morisset, R., Menezes, J., Ahmad A. (2001). Modulation of expression of the MHC class I-binding natural killer cell receptors, and NK activity in relation to viral load in HIV-infected/AIDS patients. *Journal of Medical Virology*, 65, 431–440

Bauer, S., Groh, V., Wu, J., Steinle, A., Phillips, J. H., Lanier, L. L., Spies, T. (1999). Activation of NK cells and T cells by NKG2D, a receptor for stress-inducible MICA. *Science*, 285, 727–729

Bureau of Animal and Plant Health Inspection an Quarantine. (2007). Council of Agriculture, Executive Yuan, Republic of China. Animal health inspection: Accomplishment. http://www.baphiq.gov.tw/ct.asp?xItem = 296&CtNode = 1701&mp = 2 (accessed January 29, 2007)

Carrington, M., O'Brien, S. J. (2003). The influence of HLA genotype on AIDS. *Annual Review of Medicine*, 54, 535–551

Center for Disease Control and Prevention (CDC). (2003a). Severe acute respiratory syndrome-Taiwan, 2003. *Morbidity and Mortality Weekly Report*, 52, 461–466

Center for Disease Control and Prevention. (2003b). Update: Outbreak of severe acute respiratory syndrome-Worldwide, 2003. *Morbidity and Mortality Weekly Report*, 52, 241–248

Chen, Y. M., Liang, S. Y., Chu, D. C., Lee, Y. M., Chang, L., Jung, S. Y., Chen, H. Y., Chjan, Y. J., Ho, M. S., Liang, K. Y., Jang, Y. J., Chu, T. C. (2006). Epidemiological and genetic correlates of SARS coronavirus infection in a hospital with the highest nosocomial infection rate in Taiwan in 2003. *Journal of Clinical Microbiology*, 44, 359–362

Chim, S. S., Tsui, S. K., Chan, K. C., Au, T. C., Hung, E. C., Tong, Y. K., Chiu, R. W., Ng, E. K., Chan, P. K., Chu. C.M., Sung, J. J, Tam, J. S., Fung, K. P., Waye, M. M., Lee, C. Y., Yuen, K. Y., Lo, Y. M., CUHK Molecular SARS Research Group. (2003). Genomic characterization of the severe acute respiratory syndrome coronavirus of Amoy Gardens outbreak in Hong Kong. *Lancet*, 362, 1807–1808

Chinese SARS Molecular Epidemiology Consortium. (2004). Molecular evolution of the SARS coronavirus during the course of the SARS epidemic in China. *Science*, 303, 1666–1669

Chung, W. H., Hung, S. I., Hong, H. S., Hsih, M. S., Yang, L. C., Ho, H. C., Wu, J. Y., Chen, Y. T. (2004). Medical genetics: A marker for Stevens-Johnson syndrome. *Nature*, 428, 486

Doherty, P. C., Zinkernagel, R. M. (1975). Enhanced immunological surveillance in mice hetero-zygous at the H-2 gene complex. *Nature*, 256, 50–52

Division of Surveillance and Investigation, Center for Disease Control, Taiwan. (2003) SARS probable cases in Taiwan-reclassified on 15 September 2003. In: Su IJ, editor. Memoir of severe acute respiratory syndrome control in Taiwan. Republic of China Center for Disease Control, Taipei

Drosten, C., Gunther, S., Preiser, W., van der Werf, S., Brodt, H. R., Becker, S., Rabenau, H., Panning, M., Kolesnikova, L., Fouchier, R. A., Berger, A., Burguiere, A. M., Cinatl, J., Eickmann, M., Escriou, N., Grywna, K., Kramme, S., Manuguerra, J. C., Muller, S., Rickerts, V., Sturmer, M., Vieth, S., Klenk, H. D., Osterhaus, A. D., Schmitz, H., Doerr, H. W. (2003) Identification of a novel coronavirus in patients with severe acute respiratory syndrome. *The New England Journal of Medicine*, 348, 1967–1976

Fouchier, R. A., Kuiken T., Schutten, M., van Amerongen, G., van Doornum, G. J., van den Hoogen, B. G., Peiris, M., Lim, W., Stohr, K., Osterhaus, A. D. (2003). Aetiology: Koch's postulates fulfilled for SARS virus. *Nature*, 423, 240

Guan, Y., Peiris, J. S., Zheng, B., Poon, L. L., Chan, K. H., Zeng, F. Y., Chan, C. W., Chan, M. N., Chen, J. D., Chow, K. Y., Hon, C. C., Hui, K. H., Li, J., Li, V. Y., Wang, Y., Leung, S. W., Yuen, K. Y., Leung, F. C. (2004). Molecular epidemiology of the novel coronavirus that causes severe acute respiratory syndrome. *Lancet*, 363, 99–104

Guan, Y., Zheng, B. J., He, Y. Q., Liu, X. L., Zhuang, Z. X, Cheung, C. L., Luo, S. W., Li, P. H., Zhang, L. J., Guan, Y. J., Butt, K. M., Wong, K. L., Chan, K. W., Lim, W., Shortridge, K. F., Yuen, K. Y., Peiris, J. S., Poon, L. L. (2003). Isolation and characterization of viruses related to the SARS coronavirus from animals in southern China. *Science*, 302, 276–278

Hsieh, Y. H., King, C. C., Chen, C. W. S., Ho, M. S., Lee, J. Y., Liu, F. C., Wu, Y. C., Wu, J. S. (2005). Quarantine for SARS, Taiwan. *Emerging Infectious Diseases*, 11, 278–282

Huang, C. Y., Sun, C. T., Hsieh, J. L., Chen, Y. M., Lin, H. (2005). A novel small-world model: Using social mirror identities for epidemic simulations. *Simulation*, 81, 671–699

Jeffery, K. J., Siddiqui A. A., Bunce, M., Lloyd, A. L., Vine, A. M., Witkover, A. Izumo, D. S., Usuku, K., Welsh, K. I., Osame, M., Bangham, C. R. (2000). The influence of HLA class I alleles and heterozygosity on the outcome of human T cell lymphotropic virus type I infection. *Journal of Immunology*, 165, 7278–7284

Khakoo, S. I., Thio, C. L., Martin, M. P., Brooks, C. R., Gao, X., Astemborski, J., Cheng, J., Goedert, J. J., Vlahov, D., Hilgartner, M., Cox, S., Little, A. M., Alexander, G. J., Cramp, M. E., O'Brien, S. J., Rosenberg, W. M., Thomas, D. L., Carrington, M. (2004). HLA and NK cell inhibitory receptor genes in resolving hepatitis C virus infection. *Science*, 305, 872–874

Ksiazek, T. G., Erdman, D., Goldsmith, C. S., Zaki, S. R., Peret, T., Emery, S., Tong, S., Urbani, C., Comer, J. A., Lim, W., Rollin, P. E., Dowell, S. F., Ling, A. E., Humphrey, C. D., Shieh, W. J., Guarner, J., Paddock, C. D., Rota, P., Fields, B., DeRisi, J., Yang, J. Y., Cox, N., Hughes, J. M., LeDuc, J. W., Bellini, W.J., Anderson, L. J., SARS Working Group. (2003). A novel coronavirus associated with severe acute respiratory syndrome. *New England Journal of Medicine*, 348, 1953–1966

Lan, Y. C., Liu, H. F., Shih, Y. P., Yang, J. Y., Chen, H. Y., Chen, Y. M. (2005a). Phylogenetic analysis and sequence comparison of structural and non-structural SARS coronavirus protein in Taiwan. *Infection, Genetics, and Evolution*, 5, 261–269

Lan, Y. C., Liu, T. T., Yang, J. Y., Lee, C. M., Chen, Y. J., Chan, Y. J., Lu, J. J., Liu, H. F., Hsuing, C. A., Ho, M. S., Hsiao, K. J., Chen, H. Y., Chen, Y. M. (2005b). Molecular epidemiology of severe acute respiratory syndrome-associated coronavirus infections in Taiwan. *Journal of Infectious Diseases*, 191, 1478–1489

Leung, G. M., Chung, P. H., Tsang, T., Lim, W., Chan, S. K., Chau, P., Donnelly, C. A., Ghani, A. C., Fraser, C., Riley, S., Ferguson, N. M., Anderson, R. M., Law, Y. L., Mok, T., Ng, T., Fu, A., Leung, P. Y., Peiris, J. S., Lam, T. H., Hedley, A. J. (2004). SARS-CoV antibody prevalence in all Hong Kong patient contacts. *Emerging Infectious Diseases*, 10, 1653–1656

Li, K. S., Guan, Y., Wang, J., Smith, G. J., Xu, K. M., Duan, L., Rahardjo, A. P., Puthavathana, P., Buranathai, C., Nguyen, T. D., Estoepangestie, A. T., Chaisingh, A., Auewarakul, P., Long, H. T., Hanh, N. T., Webby, R. J., Poon, L. L., Chen, H., Shortridge, K. F., Yuen, K. Y., Webster, R. G., Peiris, J. S. (2004). Genesis of a highly pathogenic and potentially pandemic H5N1 influenza virus in eastern Asia. *Nature*, 430, 209–213

Lin, M., Tseng, H. K., Trejaut, J. A., Lee, H. L., Loo, J. H., Chu, C. C., Chen, P. J., Su, Y. W., Lim, K. H., Tsai, Z. U., Lin, R. Y., Lin, R. S., Huang, C. H. (2003). Association of HLA class I with severe acute respiratory syndrome coronavirus infection. *BMC Medical Genetics*, 4, 9

Machulla, H. K., Stein, J., Gautsch, A., Langner, J., Schaller, H. G., Reichert, S. (2002). HLA-A, B, Cw, DRB1, DRB3/4/5, DQB1 in German patients suffering from rapidly progressive periodontitis (RPP) and adult periodontitis (AP). *Journal of Clinical Periodontology*, 29, 573–579

Marra, M. A., Jones, S. J., Astell, C. R., Holt, R. A., Brooks-Wilson, A., Butterfield, Y. S., Khattra, J., Asano, J. K., Barber, S. A., Chan, S. Y., Cloutier, A., Coughlin, S. M., Freeman, D., Girn, N., Griffith, O. L., Leach, S. R., Mayo, M., McDonald, H., Montgomery, S. B., Pandoh, P. K., Petrescu, A. S., Robertson, A. G., Schein, J. E., Siddiqui, A., Smailus, D. E., Stott, J. M., Yang, G. S., Plummer, F., Andonov, A., Artsob, H., Bastien, N., Bernard, K., Booth, T. F., Bowness, D., Czub, M., Drebot, M., Fernando, L., Flick, R., Garbutt, M., Gray, M., Grolla, A., Jones, S., Feldmann, H., Meyers, A., Kabani, A., Li, Y., Normand, S., Stroher, U., Tipples, G. A., Tyler, S., Vogrig, R., Ward, D., Watson, B., Brunham, R. C., Krajden, M., Petric, M., Skowronski, D. M., Upton, C., Roper, R. L. (2003). The genome sequence of the SARS-associated coronavirus. *Science*, 300, 1399–1404

National Research Project for SARS, Beijing Group. (2004). The involvement of natural killer cells in the pathogenesis of severe acute respiratory syndrome. *American Journal of Clinical Pathology*, 121, 507–511

Ng, M. H., Lau, K. M., Li, L., Cheng, S. H., Chan, W. Y., Hui, P. K., Zee, B., Leung, C. B., Sung, J. J. (2004). Association of human-leukocyte-antigen class I (B*0703) and class II (DRB1*0301) genotypes with susceptibility and resistance to the development of severe acute respiratory syndrome. *Journal of Infectious Diseases*, 190, 515–518

Olsen, S. J., Chang, H. L., Cheung, T. Y., Tang, A. F., Fisk, T. L., Ooi, S. P., Kuo, H. W., Jiang, D. D., Chen, K. T., Lando, J., Hsu, K. H., Chen, T. J., Dowell, S. F. (2003). Transmission of the severe acute respiratory syndrome on aircraft. *New England Journal of Medicine*, 349, 2416–2422

Peiris, J. S., Chu, C. M., Cheng, V. C., Chan, K. S., Hung, I. F., Poon, L. L., Law, K. I., Tang, B. S., Hon, T. Y., Chan, C. S., Chan, K. H., Ng, J. S., Zheng, B. J., Ng, W. L., Lai, R. W., Guan, Y., Yuen, K. Y. (2003a). Clinical progression and viral load in a community outbreak of coronavirus-associated SARS pneumonia: a prospective study. *Lancet*, 361, 1767–1772

Peiris, J. S., Lai, S. T., Poon, L. L., Guan, Y., Yam, L. Y., Lim, W., Nicholls, J., Yee, W. K., Yan, W. W., Cheung, M. T., Cheng, V. C., Chan, K. H., Tsang, D. N., Yung, R. W., Ng, T. K., Yuen, K. Y., SARS Study Group. (2003b). Coronavirus as a possible cause of severe cause of severe acute respiratory syndrome. *Lancet*, 361, 1319–1325

Rota, P. A., Oberste, M. S., Monroe, S. S., Nix, W. A., Campagnoli, R., Icenogle, J. P., Penaranda, S., Bankamp, B., Maher, K., Chen, M. H., Tong, S., Tamin, A., Lowe, L., Frace, M., DeRisi, J. L., Chen, Q., Wang, D., Erdman, D. D., Peret T. C., Burns, C., Ksiazek, T. G., Rollin, P. E., Sanchez A., Liffick, S., Holloway, B., Limor, J., McCaustland, K., Olsen-Rasmussen, M., Fouchier, R., Gunther, S., Osterhaus, A. D., Drosten, C., Pallansch, M. A., Anderson, L. J., Bellini, W. J. (2003). Characterization of a novel coronavirus associated with severe acute respiratory syndrome. *Science*, 300, 1394–1399

Segal, S., Hill, A. V. (2003). Genetic susceptibility to infectious disease. *Trends in Microbiology*, 11, 445–448

Thio, C. L., Gao, X., Goedert, J. J., Vlahov, D., Nelson, K. E., Hilgartner, M. W., O'Brien, S. Karacki, J. P., Astemborski, J., Carrington, M., Thomas, D. L. (2002). HLA-Cw*04 and hepatitis C virus persistence. *Journal of Virology*, 76, 4792–4797

Twu, S. J., Chen, T. J., Chen, C. J., Olsen, S. J., Lee, L. T., Fisk, T., Hsu, K. H., Chang, S. C., Chen, K. T., Chiang, I. H., Wu, Y. C., Wu, J. S., Dowell, S. F. (2003). Control measures for severe acute respiratory syndrome (SARS) in Taiwan. *Emerging Infectious Diseases*, 9, 718–720

Woo, P. C., Lau, S. K., Tsoi, H. W., Chan, K. H., Wong, B. H., Che, X. Y., Tam, V. K., Tam, S. C., Cheng, V. C., Hung, I. F., Wong, S. S., Zheng, B. J., Guan, Y., Yuen. K. Y. (2004). Relative rates of non-pneumonic SARS coronavirus infection and SARS coronavirus pneumonia. *Lancet*, 363, 841–845

World Health Organization, Geneva. (2004). Summary of probable SARS cases with onset of illness 2002 to 31 July 2003. (Accessed April 21, 2004) http://www.who.int/csr/sars/country/table2004_04_21/en/)

Part 3
HIV/AIDS

HIV/AIDS: Lessons from a New Disease Pandemic

M. Essex and Yichen Lu

Introduction

The acquired immunodeficiency syndrome (AIDS) was first recognized about 25 years ago (Gottlieb et al., 1981; Masur et al., 1981; Siegal et al., 1981). The best available evidence suggests that HIV newly infected the human species about 50–100 years ago (Korber et al., 2000). It did not originate in Asia. It apparently moved to people from sub-human primates in Africa (Keele et al., 2006; Kanki, 1997). Because of different clinical presentations in different populations of people, and a long incubation period, it was more difficult to diagnose than SARS or avian influenza.

As a new epidemic that originated in the era of modern medicine, it taught us many lessons about the difficulties that a new infectious disease can present. Already claiming at least 60–80 million victims, AIDS seems destined to continue as a pandemic for the foreseeable future. Drugs that control HIV replication and reverse disease progression have been developed, but none eliminate the virus from the body. Sexual transmission can be prevented by abstinence or condoms, but such measures, which prevent procreation, provide only limited value.

Approaches for making a vaccine using conventional techniques have failed. Most experts believe that an effective vaccine will be made eventually, but not for at least 10–20 years. We need to learn more about the immunobiology of acute HIV infection, and about potentially protective immunoepitopes, such as conformational intermediates of the virus envelope. Until a vaccine is available, there is little or no chance that HIV can be eliminated, or even drastically reduced in prevalence. AIDS has presented scientists, political leaders, and health policy experts with unprecedented challenges.

History

The first diagnosis of AIDS occurred when small groups of homosexual men in a few US cities presented with unusual diseases. The diseases observed, particularly Kaposi's sarcoma, pneumocystis pneumonia, and *Mycobacterium avium* tuberculosis,

Y. Lu et al. (eds.), *Emerging Infections in Asia.*
© Springer Science+Business Media, LLC 2008

had not been seen previously in young men, except perhaps in very rare and sporadic cases associated with other problems such as terminal cancer or immuno-suppression associated with organ transplants. Of great importance for the initial identification of the AIDS epidemic, these outcomes occurred in unrelated young men who knew each other. Such a clustering in time and space is often the key clue to the etiology of a new infectious disease.

In the case of AIDS, however, infectious agents were not initially pursued as the most likely cause of the new disease. The first clusters of AIDS were among homo-sexual men who indulged in promiscuous recreational sex, a lifestyle associated with performance-enhancing drugs such as amyl and butyl nitrates. Early hypotheses to explain the disease often favored the use of such drugs, or autoimmune responses to antigens presented by rectal sex (Francis et al., 1983).

For most infectious disease experts who favored a microbial etiology, retrovi-ruses were not high on the list of candidates (Rogers et al., 1983). Although retroviruses were well known as a cause of leukemia, lymphoma, and even immu-nosuppression in chickens, laboratory mice, and cats, the first human retroviruses had just been described in 1980 (Poiesz et al., 1980).

The clinical characterization of the AIDS complex soon revealed that it was a disease of the immune system, particularly one where CD4 T helper responses became depleted. Ultimately, the loss of CD4 cells would be one of the most reliable ways to diagnose AIDS, along with detection of HIV.

As various investigators searched for the cause of AIDS, both the Gallo group and our own hypothesized that a human retrovirus might be involved (Essex et al., 1983a; Gallo et al., 1983; Gelmann et al., 1983). The rationale for this hypothesis was based in part on the recognition that lymphotropic feline retroviruses caused immunosuppression in cats (Essex et al., 1975), and that the recently discovered human leukemia retroviruses infected the same CD4 lymphocyte population that became depleted when people developed AIDS. Additionally, patients who devel-oped leukemia following infection with the first human lymphotropic retrovirus (HTLV-1) also experienced immunosuppression (Essex et al., 1984).

Pursuit of a Retroviral Etiology

The first attempts to link a human retrovirus to AIDS included various approaches. One approach involved the use of HTLV-1 as an antigen to search for cross-reacting antibodies in the serum of AIDS patients and people who were involved in the same epidemiological circles. Such individuals included, for example, donors who provided blood used for transfusions associated with AIDS development or blood product preparations given to hemophiliacs (Curran et al., 1984; Essex et al., 1983b). Patients from high risk categories, such as homosexual men and injection drug users, were also similarly screened when they experienced symptoms such as lymphadenopathy or oral candidiasis. A second approach to screen AIDS patients involved assays for reverse transcriptase activity using enzyme conditions that had been developed for HTLV-1 (Barre-Sinoussi et al., 1983; Gelmann et al., 1983). A third major approach was the use of electron microscopy, to determine if particles similar to retroviruses could be found in tissues from AIDS patients (Barre-Sinoussi et al., 1983). All of these approaches yielded some degree of success, but none gave consistent positivity as an indication of complete success.

Incubation Period

In retrospect, it seems clear that two aspects of HIV/AIDS made the etiology more difficult to solve. First was the long incubation period, which ordinarily lasts 5–10 years before disease develops. This obviously made the tracking and linking of clinical AIDS cases unusually difficult and disease detectives much less likely to suspect an infectious cause. The second was the wide range of lethal clinical outcomes. While it was clear that patients died from such conditions as pneumocystis pneumonia or tuberculosis, many were reluctant to accept destruction of the immune system as a common denominator.

With most cases occurring in groups that were often marginalized by discrimination, such as homosexuals and infectious drug-users, some denied the very existence of AIDS as a new disease (Duesberg, 1988). This in turn led to a substantial delay before resources were allocated in developed countries to identify the cause and attempt measures of control. Political leaders in some developing countries also pursued a course of denialism under the mistaken impression that this would conserve financial support for health care and avoid reductions in tourism.

AIDS in Africa

The first cases of what was thought to be AIDS in Africa were reported a few years after the American cases (Clumeck et al., 1983). This happened when a few Africans sought medical treatment in Europe. The earliest epidemics within Africa were from the central and eastern regions. The most severe epidemic, which is in southern Africa, came considerably later (Essex & Mboup, 2002).

In West Africa, a modest epidemic of HIV-2 preceded the invasion of HIV-1 (Kanki, 1997). HIV-2 is less virulent than HIV-1, by both the criteria of transmission and of disease development (Kanki et al., 1994; Marlink et al., 1994). Perhaps a million people became infected with HIV-2, with the highest prevalence in Guinea-Bissau and southern Senegal. Infections were also observed in other countries in West Africa, and in sites such as Mozambique, Angola, Goa, and Cape Verde, which were apparently connected by colonial trade routes. Aside from a few diagnoses in travelers or immigrants from these regions, HIV-2 never appeared to expand elsewhere in Africa, in Europe, or in the U.S.

As of 2006, almost two-thirds of the world's infections with HIV are in Africa (UNAIDS, 2006). An even higher proportion of the deaths from AIDS are in sub-Saharan Africa, in part because treatment is less likely to be available there as compared to other regions of the world. As opposed to most other regions of the world, the vast majority of infections in Africa are due to either heterosexual transmission or transmission from infected mothers to their infants. In Asia, injection drug-users represent the most important population for transmission, at least in the early stages of the epidemic.

Viral Variation

Soon after the recognition of major differences between HIV-2 and HIV-1, it became apparent that these viruses evolved more rapidly than other viruses known to cause human diseases. Some, such as the HIV-2s of West Africa, have probably had multiple entries to people from mangabey monkeys. Some HIV-1s are very closely related to viruses of chimpanzees (Keele et al., 2006) (See Fig. 1).

HIV-related viruses in subhuman primates, designated simian immunodeficiency viruses (SIVs), were actually identified in Asian monkeys before they were identified in African monkeys or apes (Daniel et al., 1985; Kanki et al., 1985). However, in retrospect it seems clear that the viruses originated in Africa, not Asia. Many species of African monkeys have evidence of infection with SIVs, whereas wild Asian monkeys do not. It appears that captive Asian monkeys in research colonies initially became infected when injected with experimental materials. Furthermore, Asian monkeys become sick with an AIDS-like illness when injected with SIVs, whereas African monkeys or apes do not become ill when injected with SIVs and/or HIVs.

HIVs have been categorized into groups and subtypes, which differ from each other by 15–30% in nucleotide and amino acid sequences. Subtypes HIV-1A, B, C,

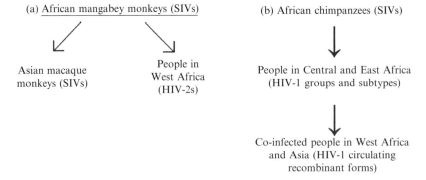

Fig. 1 Evolutionary origin of human immunodeficiency viruses

and D are particularly important because they have infected at least a million people. In the case of HIV-1C, perhaps 25 million people have become infected with the virus.

It is still not clear whether certain subtypes of HIV-1 entered people independently from subhuman primates, or diverged to form distinct subtypes after they already existed in people. In the case of HIV-1B and HIV-1D, it is most likely that they diverged in people, as these viruses are more similar than either is to other subtypes. In the case of HIV-1C and HIV-1A, it seems possible that they entered separately into the human population.

The HIV retroviruses also replicate through the use of a diploid genome that contains two complete copies of all viral genes. As a result, when a single human cell happens to get infected with two different HIVs, recombinants are created. These recombinants retain block segments from each parental virus. When the two parental viruses represent different clades or subtypes, intersubtype recombinants develop. Some of the new recombinants, or chimeras, represent circulating recombinant forms (CRFs) that themselves infect large populations of people.

In places such as Tanzania, where high rates of multiple subtypes such as A, C, and D are already present, up to one-third of the infectious viruses found in infants infected from their mothers were new intersubtype recombinants (Renjifo et al., 1999). The virus that caused the first major epidemic in Asia is CRF01_AE, which apparently originated in the region of the Central African Republic (Gao et al., 1996). Although HIV-1B, from the west, was the first virus detected in injection drug-users in Bangkok, it was rapidly overtaken by CRF01_AE, which now predominates in Thailand, Myanmar, and the Kunming region of China. Another recombinant, CRF02_AG, is the second most common virus in the world, predominating in the countries of West and West Central Africa (Essex & Mboup, 2002). The viruses that are most important in China at present are CRFs made as recombinants of HIV-1B and HIV-1C. The two that are most common are designated CRF07_BC and CRF08_BC (Piyasirisilp et al., 2000; Su et al., 2000; Qiu et al., 2005). Unlike CRF01_AE, these viruses have not been reported outside Asia and so they presumably originated from B and C parental viruses that were already present in the region.

Clinical Significance of Genomic Variation

The elevated mutation rates characteristic of HIVs are responsible for the rapid emergence of drug resistance, especially in HIV-infected people treated with only one or two drugs rather than the three-drug combinations often called highly active antiretroviral therapy (HAART). The use of only one or two drugs happened more often in earlier stages of the epidemic, when fewer drugs were available, but it is also widely practiced when chemoprophylaxis is used to reduce the transmission of HIV from infected mothers to their infants.

Antiretroviral drugs have been very effective for treating clinical AIDS and for chemoprophylaxis in all parts of the world. However, when drug resistance develops, fewer options may be available for switching to new drug combinations in the developing world. The first drugs available were nucleoside analogue reverse transcriptase inhibitors, such as zidovudine, or non-nucleoside reverse transcriptase inhibitors, such as nevirapine. Such drugs have become less expensive and more readily available in developing countries. However, the drug resistance mutations they elicit are often shared by other drugs of their class. Newer drugs that do not share the same patterns of drug resistance, such as the protease inhibitors, the fusion inhibitors, and the integrase inhibitors, are much more expensive and less likely to be available as back-up regimens for patients who become resistant to the first-line drugs in developing countries. For this reason, monitoring for adherence or compliance during therapy is extremely important, particularly in sites where limited drug regimens and highly experienced therapy specialists may not be available.

Some drug resistance mutations may develop more readily with certain viruses. This has been observed, for example, as (1) higher rates of resistance in HIV-1C-infected people, such as pregnant women given nevirapine during labor (Eshleman et al., 2005), (2) faster development of resistance to tenofovir through K65R when selected in vitro in HIV-1C-infected cell cultures (Brenner et al., 2006), and (3) faster development of the resistance mutation D30N when HIV-1C AIDS patients were given nelfinavir (Doualla-Bell et al., 2006).

The high rates of genetic variation observed with HIVs also provide the largest hurdle to the development of vaccines. Antibodies directed at the V3 (i.e., 3rd variable region) of the outer envelope glycoprotein (gp120) can be quite effective for neutralizing the virus. However, with rapid mutation and selection, variant viruses that are not neutralized by the same antibodies soon occur in the same individual. This pattern of immunoselection and immune evasion also occurs with immunodominant epitope targets used by the cytolytic T-cell response, and probably represents the single greatest impediment to the development of an effective vaccine. Current approaches to overcoming this problem involve the targeting of immune responses, through immunogen design, to selected conserved regions. These include structural determinants in gp120 that are exposed as conformational epitopes when the virus unfolds to attach to a co-receptor, and cytolytic T-cell epitopes that contain highly conserved residues for virus survival.

Infection Rates in Asia

According to UNAIDS (2006), infection rates in Asia range from less than one per thousand, for countries such as Japan or Korea, to almost 2% for countries such as Papua New Guinea or Cambodia (See Table 1). Thailand has an estimated rate of 1.4%, and India 0.4% (UNAIDS, 2007). Because it is a very large country, this translates to a total number of about 2,500,000 HIV-infected people in India (UNAIDS, 2007). This is the largest number of total infections for any country in Asia, although

Table 1 Estimated rates of HIV infection in adults in selected countries (UNAIDS, 2006,2007)

Country	HIV in adults		Ratio of infection (men/women)
	Rates	Numbers	
Asia	0.2	4,875,000	2
Australia	0.1	16,000	15.0
Cambodia	1.6	130,000	1.2
China	0.1	650,000	2.6
India	0.4	2,500,000	2.5
Indonesia	0.1	170,000	4.9
Japan	<0.1	17,000	0.7
Myanmar	1.3	350,000	2.2
Papua New Guinea	1.8	57,000	0.7
Thailand	1.4	560,000	1.5
Europe	0.3	760,000	2.3
France	0.4	130,000	1.9
Germany	0.1	49,000	2.3
Spain	0.6	140,000	3.4
North America	0.6	1,300,000	2.6
United States	0.6	1,200,000	3.0
Sub-Saharan Africa	5.0	22,500,000	0.6
Nigeria	3.9	2,600,000	0.6
Senegal	0.9	56,000	0.7
South Africa	18.8	5,300,000	0.7
Swaziland	33.4	210,000	0.8
Uganda	6.7	900,000	0.7

South Africa has a larger number of total infections (5,100,000) with a very small fraction of the population. China has an estimated rate of one per thousand, but because it is such a large country, this comes to about 560,000 people.

In western countries, such as the United States, France, or Spain, rates of infection (0.4–0.6%) are similar to those in India. Some countries, such as Germany or Poland, are estimated to be as low as China. However, the epidemic in the west appears to have plateaued, while it probably has not plateaued in China. In most places in Asia, the HIV epidemic began a decade or more later than it began in the West or in Africa.

In sub-Saharan Africa, HIV infection rates are about 20-fold higher than in Asia, although in southern Africa, which has the most severe epidemic, rates are about 60-fold higher. In Swaziland, for example, it was estimated that about one-third of all adults are infected.

Another major difference between the epidemics of the world is the ratio of infection in men versus women. In Asia, as in the US and Europe, substantially more men are infected than women. In Africa, women are infected significantly more often than men. Considerable variation may occur in selected countries in Asia, however, and Papua New Guinea has a sex ratio that is similar to that of sub-Saharan Africa. Higher ratios in men are generally indicative of transmission by homosexual sex and/or injection drug use, whereas higher rates in women, as in Africa, are generally indicative of an epidemic spread by heterosexual contact.

Conclusions: Lessons from the Newly Emerging Epidemics of HIV/AIDS

One key lesson from HIV/AIDS that seems very common to other infectious disease threats such as SARS and avian influenza is that new human pathogens often enter from other animal species. In the case of HIV/AIDS, this probably occurred when people butchered subhuman primates and, covered with infected blood, perhaps exposed their arms through open wounds. As with other diseases, such cross-species transmissions were rare events rapidly amplified by urbanization and travel. HIV is not spread by inhalation or ingestion, and was harder to identify as compared with the etiologic agents of other new epidemics because of the very long incubation period before disease development.

Another lesson from HIV is that the ability of the organism to rapidly evolve may pose major complications for treatment, vaccination, and even detection. For HIV, as with influenza, genetic change occurs both through the accumulation of mutations and by the exchange of entire genes (recombination in the case of HIV, reassortment in the case of influenza). With both viruses, large genetic changes occur most rapidly when individuals are co-infected with two different parental viruses.

In conclusion, many infectious disease agents have entered the human population from lower animals and we should expect such events to continue to occur in the future. With the numerous opportunities to spread rapidly in people due to modern travel, an increased surveillance of infections in both animals and people may be important.

References

Barre-Sinoussi, F., Chermann, J. C., Rey, F., Nugeyre, M. T., Chamaret, S., Gruest, J., Dauguet, C., Axler-Blin, C., Vezinet-Brun, F., Rouzioux, C., Rozenbaum, W., & Montagnier, L. (1983). Isolation of a T-lymphotropic retrovirus from a patient at risk for acquired immune deficiency syndrome (AIDS). *Science, 220*(4599), 868–871.

Brenner, B. G., Oliveira, M., Doualla-Bell, F., Moisi, D. D., Ntemgwa, M., Frankel, F., Essex, M., & Wainberg, M. A. (2006). HIV-1 subtype C viruses rapidly develop K65R resistance to tenofovir in cell culture. *AIDS, 20*(9), F9–13.

Clumeck, N., Mascart-Lemone, F., de Maubeuge, J., Brenez, D., & Marcelis, L. (1983). Acquired immune deficiency syndrome in Black Africans. *Lancet, 1*(8325), 642.

Curran, J. W., Lawrence, D. N., Jaffe, H., Kaplan, J. E., Zyla, L. D., Chamberland, M., Weinstein, R., Lui, K. J., Schonberger, L. B., & Spira, T. J. (1984). Acquired immunodeficiency syndrome (AIDS) associated with transfusions. *The New England Journal of Medicine, 310*(2), 69–75.

Daniel, M. D., Letvin, N. L., King, N. W., Kannagi, M., Sehgal, P. K., Hunt, R. D., Kanki, P. J., Essex, M., & Desrosiers, R. C. (1985). Isolation of T-cell tropic HTLV-III-like retrovirus from macaques. *Science, 228*(4704), 1201–1204.

Doualla-Bell, F., Avalos, A., Gaolathe, T., Mine, M., Gaseitsiwe, S., Ndwapi, N., Novitsky, V., Brenner, B., Oliveira, M., Moisi, D., Moffat, H., Thior, I., Essex, M., & Wainberg, M. A. (2006). Impact of human immunodeficiency virus type 1 subtype C on drug resistance mutations in patients from Botswana failing a nelfinavir-containing regimen. *Antimicrobial Agents and Chemotherapy, 50*(6), 2210–2213.

Duesberg, P. (1988). HIV is not the cause of AIDS. *Science, 241*(4865), 514, 517.

Eshleman, S. H., Hoover, D. R., Chen, S., Hudelson, S. E., Guay, L. A., Mwatha, A., Fiscus, S. A., Mmiro, F., Musoke, P., Jackson, J. B., Kumwenda, N., & Taha, T., (2005). Nevirapine (NVP) resistance in women with HIV-1 subtype C, compared with subtypes A and D, after the administration of single-dose NVP. *The Journal of Infectious Diseases, 192*(1), 30–36.

Essex, M., & Mboup, S. (2002). Regional variations in the epidemic. In M. Essex, S. Mboup, P. Kanki, R. Marlink, & S. Tlou (Eds.), *AIDS in Africa*, 2nd ed. (pp. 629–638). New York: Kluwer Academic/Plenum.

Essex, M., Hardy, W. D., Jr., Cotter, S. M., Jakowski, R. M., & Sliski, A. (1975). Naturally occurring persistent feline oncornavirus infections in the absence of disease. *Infection and Immunology, 11*(3), 470–475.

Essex, M., McLane, M. F., Lee, T. H., Falk, L., Howe, C. W., Mullins, J. I., Cabradilla, C., & Francis, D. P. (1983a). Antibodies to cell membrane antigens associated with human T-cell leukemia virus in patients with AIDS. *Science, 220*(4599), 859–862.

Essex, M., McLane, M. F., Lee, T. H., Tachibana, N., Mullins, J. I., Kreiss, J., Kasper, C. K., Poon, M.-C., Landay, A., Stein, S. F., Francis, D. P., Cabradilla, C., Lawrence, D. N., & Evatt, B. L. (1983b). Antibodies to human T-cell leukemia virus membrane antigens (HTLV-MA) in hemophiliacs. *Science, 221*(4615), 1061–1064.

Essex, M. E., McLane, M. F., Tachibana, N., Francis, D. P., & Lee, T. H. (1984). Seroepidemiology of human T-cell leukemia virus in relation to immunosuppression and the acquired immunodeficiency syndrome. In R. C. Gallo, M. Essex, & L. Gross (Eds.), *Human T-Cell Leukemia/Lymphoma Viruses* (pp. 355–362). Cold Spring Harbor: Cold Spring Harbor Laboratory.

Francis, D. P., Curran, J. W., & Essex, M. (1983). Epidemic acquired immune deficiency syndrome: epidemiologic evidence for a transmissible agent. *Journal of the National Cancer Institute, 71*(1), 1–4.

Gallo, R. C., Sarin, P. S., Gelmann, E. P., Robert-Guroff, M., Richardson, E., Kalyanaraman, V. S., Mann, D., Sidhu, G. D., Stahl, R. E., Zolla-Pazner, S., Leibowitch, J., & Popovic, M. (1983). Isolation of human T-cell leukemia virus in acquired immune deficiency syndrome (AIDS). *Science, 220*(4599), 865–867.

Gao, F., Robertson, D. L., Morrison, S. G., Hui, H., Craig, S., Decker, J., Fultz, P. N., Girard, M., Shaw, G. M., Hahn, B. H., & Sharp, P. M. (1996). The heterosexual human immunodeficiency virus type 1 epidemic in Thailand is caused by an intersubtype (A/E) recombinant of African origin. *The Journal of Virology, 70*(10), 7013–7029.

Gelmann, E. P., Popovic, M., Blayney, D., Masur, H., Sidhu, G., Stahl, R. E., & Gallo, R. C. (1983). Proviral DNA of a retrovirus, human T-cell leukemia virus, in two patients with AIDS. *Science, 220*(4599), 862–865.

Gottlieb, M. S., Schroff, R., Schanker, H. M., Weisman, J. D., Fan, P. T., Wolf, R. A., & Saxon, A. (1981). Pneumocystis carinii pneumonia and mucosal candidiasis in previously healthy homosexual men: evidence of a new acquired cellular immunodeficiency. *The New England Journal of Medicine, 305*(24), 1425–1431.

Kanki, P. (1997). Epidemiology and natural history of human immunodeficiency virus type 2. In V.T. DeVita, Jr., S. Hellman, S. A. Rosenberg, J. Curran, M. Essex, & A. S. Fauci (Eds.), *AIDS: Etiology, Diagnosis, Treatment and Prevention*, 4th ed. (pp. 127–135). Philadelphia: Lippincott.

Kanki, P. J., McLane, M. F., King, N. W., Jr., Letvin, N. L., Hunt, R. D., Sehgal, P., Daniel, M. D., Desrosiers, R. C., & Essex, M. (1985). Serologic identification and characterization of a macaque T-lymphotropic retrovirus closely related to HTLV-III. *Science, 228*(4704), 1199–1201.

Kanki, P. J., Travers, K., Mboup, S., Hsieh, C.-C., Marlink, R. G., Guèye-NDiaye, A., Siby, T., Thior, I., Hernandez Avila, M., Sankalé, J.-L., NDoye, I., & Essex, M. E. (1994). Slower heterosexual spread of HIV-2 than HIV-1. *Lancet 343*, 943–946.

Keele, B. F., Van Heuverswyn, F., Li, Y., Bailes, E., Takehisa, J., Santiago, M. L., Bibollet-Ruche, F., Chen, Y., Wain, L. V., Liegeois, F., Loul, S., Ngole, E. M., Bienvenue, Y.,

Delaporte, E., Brookfield, J. F., Sharp, P. M., Shaw, G. M., Peeters, M. & Hahn, B. H. (2006). Chimpanzee reservoirs of pandemic and nonpandemic HIV-1. *Science, 313*(5786), 523–526.

Korber, B., Muldoon, M., Theiler, J., Gao, F., Gupta, R., Lapedes, A., Hahn, B. H., Wolinsky, S., & Bhattacharya, T., (2000). Timing the ancestor of the HIV-1 pandemic strains. *Science, 288*(5472), 1789–1796.

Marlink, R., Kanki, P., Thior, I., Travers, K., Eisen, G., Siby, T., Traore, I., Hsieh, C.- C., Dia, M. C., Gueye, E.-H., Hellinger, J., Guèye-Ndiaye, A., Sankalé, J.-L., Ndoye, I., Mboup, S., & Essex, M. (1994). Reduced rate of disease development after HIV-2 infection as compared to HIV-1. *Science 265*, 1587–1590.

Masur, H., Michelis, M. A., Greene, J. B., Onorato, I., Stouwe, R. A., Holzman, R. S., Wormser, G., Brettman, L., Lange, M., Murray, H. W., & Cunningham-Rundles, S. (1981). An outbreak of community-acquired Pneumocystis carinii pneumonia: initial manifestation of cellular immune dysfunction. *The New England Journal of Medicine, 305*(24), 1431–1438.

Piyasirisilp, S., McCutchan, F. E., Carr, J. K., Sanders-Buell, E., Liu, W., Chen, J., Wagner, R., Wolf, H., Shao, Y., Lai, S., Beyrer, C., & Yu, X. F. (2000). A recent outbreak of human immunodeficiency virus type 1 infection in southern China was initiated by two highly homogeneous, geographically separated strains, circulating recombinant form AE and a novel BC recombinant. *The Journal of Virology, 74*(23), 11286–11295.

Poiesz, B. J., Ruscetti, F. W., Gazdar, A. F., Bunn, P. A., Minna, J. D., & Gallo, R. C. (1980). Detection and isolation of type C retrovirus particles from fresh and cultured lymphocytes of a patient with cutaneous T-cell lymphoma. *Proceedings of the National Academy of Sciences USA, 77*(12), 7415–7419.

Qiu, Z., Xing, H., Wei, M., Duan, Y., Zhao, Q., Xu, J., & Shao, Y. (2005). Characterization of five nearly full-length genomes of early HIV type 1 strains in Ruili city: implications for the genesis of CRF07_BC and CRF08_BC circulating in China. *AIDS Research and Human Retroviruses, 21*(12), 1051–1056.

Renjifo, B., Gilbert, P., Chaplin, B., Vannberg, F., Mwakagile, D., Msamanga, G., Hunter, D., Fawzi, W., & Essex, M. (1999). Emerging recombinant human immunodeficiency viruses: uneven representation of the envelope V3 region. *AIDS, 13*(13), 1613–1621.

Rogers, M. F., Morens, D. M., Stewart, J. A., Kaminski, R. M., Spira, T. J., Feorino, P. M., Larsen, S. A., Francis, D. P., Wilson, M., & Kaufman, L. (1983). National case–control study of Kaposi's sarcoma and Pneumocystis carinii pneumonia in homosexual men: Part 2. Laboratory results. *Annals of Internal Medicine, 99*(2), 151–158.

Siegal, F. P., Lopez, C., Hammer, G. S., Brown, A. E., Kornfeld, S. J., Gold, J., Hassett, J., Hirschman, S. Z., Cunningham-Rundles, C., Adelsberg, B. R., Parham, D. M., Siegal, M., Cunningham-Rundles, S., & Armstrong, D. (1981). Severe acquired immunodeficiency in male homosexuals, manifested by chronic perianal ulcerative herpes simplex lesions. *The New England Journal of Medicine, 305*(24), 1439–1444.

Su, L., Graf, M., Zhang, Y., von Briesen, H., Xing, H., Kostler, J., Melzl, H., Wolf, H., Shao, Y., & Wagner, R. (2000). Characterization of a virtually full-length human immunodeficiency virus type 1 genome of a prevalent intersubtype (C/B') recombinant strain in China. *The Journal of Virology, 74*, 11367–11376.

UNAIDS. (2006). Report on the Global AIDS Epidemic. Geneva: UNAIDS, Available online at http://www.unaids.org/en/HIV_data/2006GlobalReport/default.asp. Accessed on 9 February 2007.

UNAIDS. (2007). AIDS Epidemic Update: December 2007. Available Online at http://www. unaids.org/en/KnowledgeCentre/HIVData/EpiUpdate/EpiUpdArchive/2007/default.asp. Accessed on 28 January 2008.

AIDS in China

Gui Xien and Zhuang Ke

AIDS Discovery and Epidemic in China

In June of 1985, an Argentine–American tourist was hospitalized in Beijing's Xiehe Hospital with a pulmonary infection and subsequent respiratory failure. During his hospitalization, he was diagnosed with PCP and AIDS, thereby becoming the first person to be diagnosed with HIV in China (First AIDS case, 2001).

In the same year, four hemophiliacs in Zhejiang province tested positive for anti-HIV antibodies (Zhejiang HIV/AIDS patients, 2005). After ruling out other risk factors such as risky sexual contact, intravenous drug use, and mother-to-child transmission, it was determined that all four people had received Factor VIII treatment in which imported HIV-contaminated products were used. This revelation raised the likelihood that HIV had entered China before 1985.

The Spread of AIDS in China is Marked by Three Periods

1. *1984–1988: Sporadic period

   • During this period, 19 HIV/AIDS cases were identified throughout China. With the exception of the four hemophiliac patients who had acquired HIV infection from imported Factor VIII products, all of the infected people were either foreigners or Chinese people living overseas.

2. *1989–1994: Localized epidemic period

   • In October of 1989, 146 HIV-infected intravenous drug users (IDUs) were found in Ruili, a border town in southwestern Yunnan province, thus marking the first finding of HIV in drug users and in remote rural areas in China. HIV/AIDS was later found in cities and counties throughout the Dehong prefecture in Yunnan and in other provinces as well. The occurrence of HIV infections among commercial sex workers (CSWs), persons with sexually transmitted diseases (STDs), and persons returning home from other countries increased annually.

Y. Lu et al. (eds.), *Emerging Infections in Asia.*
© Springer Science+Business Media, LLC 2008

3. *1995–present: Rapid growth period

- The number of reported HIV-infected persons in China has increased rapidly since 1995, spreading among IDUs throughout Yunnan and reaching other regions in China, including Xinjiang, Guangxi, and Sichuan. Additionally, a new risk group for HIV has been identified in the population of former plasma donors (FPDs) in central China. The high level of mobility of both IDUs and FPDs gives these groups a dangerous potential for transmitting HIV. As in the previous period, HIV infections among STD patients and CSWs continue to increase; moreover, this period has shown increasing numbers of HIV infections among men who have sex with other men (MSM) (Zheng, 1999).

What should be aware of is that HIV is spreading from high-risk populations, such as IDU and sex workers, to the general population. HIV infections have been found in people taking pre-marital exams, pregnant women, children, and college students.

Current Status of the HIV/AIDS in China

By October 2006, there were 183,733 confirmed HIV cases in China, of which 40,667 led to a diagnosis with AIDS. The Chinese Ministry of Health estimates that there are currently 650,000 HIV infections in China (Ministry of Health, 2006).

1. Different areas of China have different major transmission routes of AIDS.

Border regions such as Yunnan, Guangxi, and Xinjiang have the highest HIV incidence among IDUs, while in Henan, Anhui, Hubei, and Shanxi in central China, HIV infections mainly occur among FPDs and recipients of contaminated blood or blood products. In coastal areas such as Guangdong and Fujian, most HIV infections are sexually transmitted.

According to the 2005 Update on the HIV/AIDS Epidemic and Response in China, estimation results indicate that among people currently living with HIV/AIDS, 44.3% were infected through injection drug use, 43.6% were infected through sexual transmission, 10.7% were infected through blood/blood products, and 1.4% were infected through mother-to-child transmission (Ministry of Health People's Republic of China, 2006).

Drug users are found in all 31 provinces, autonomous regions, and municipalities of China, 53.8% of total drug users in China are IDUs. Among all the IDUs, 45% share needles. Up to 89% of IDUs in Yili Xinjiang are infected with HIV, while in Yunnan and parts of Guangxi, the infection rate is over 20%. Nationwide, the prevalence of HIV infection among IDUs is estimated to be 5%–8% (A Joint Assessment of HIV/AIDS prevention, 2004).

2. There are many HIV infections in China due to paid plasma donation and transfusion.

In the early 1990s, paid blood donors were common in some areas of the provinces of Henan, Anhui, Hubei, and Shanxi. Because of poor management at that time, a large group of paid plasma donors, as well as blood or blood product recipients, were infected with HIV. By January 2006, it was estimated that there are 55,000 former paid blood and plasma donors infected with HIV in China (Ministry of Health People's Republic of China, 2006).

3. High prevalence of HIV-MTCT in China.

The rate of HIV infection among women in China has significantly increased in the past 8 years, females account for a large percentage of plasma donors and sex workers, and the number of female IDUs is increasing. Furthermore, the increase in the number of HIV infections among women is reflected in the increased risk of MTCT of HIV. Li Guanha et al. reported that of 80 children born to 73 HIV-infected women, 28 were HIV-positive making the MTCT rate 35% (2002). Another investigation (conducted by the author of this essay) added to Li Guanhan's calculation of the MTCT rate, showing that of 192 children born to 149 HIV-positive mothers, 69 tested positive for HIV (MTCT rate 35.9%). These studies show that, without intervention, the rate of HIV MTCT in China is over 35%.

WHO estimated that through December of 2004, the global number of HIV-positive females was 17.8 million and that of HIV-positive children under age 15 was 2.2 million. Globally, 12.4% of the total HIV infections in women were transmitted to children. The author conducted a study on groups of the HIV-infected population in three provinces. In a total of 9,462 HIV-infected patients in the study, women accounted for 4,588 infections while children made up 402 of the infections. HIV-positive children were 8.3% of the number of HIV-infected women. However, the author estimates the actual number of HIV-infected children in China could greatly exceed the number which has been found.

4. Molecular epidemiology of HIV-1 in China

HIV molecular epidemiology studies have shown that HIV-1 is the main circulating strain in China, although HIV-2 has been reported (Graf et al., 1998; Piyasirisilp et al., 2000; Shao et al., 1999; Su et al., 2000; Xing et al., 2004; Xing et al., 1999). HIV-1 subtypes of A, B (B'), C, D, F and G, recombinant subtype CRF01-AE, and two other different B/C recombinants (CRF07-BC and CRF08-BC) have been detected in China. Of these, the two B/C recombinant strains are only found in China. B', CRF-BC, and CRF01-AE account for approximately 95% of all circulating subtypes (Piyasirisilp et al., 2000; Shao et al., 1999; Su et al., 2000). The distribution of various HIV-1 genotypes is closely related to the mode of transmission of the viruses in distinctive high-risk populations (Zhang Linqi et al., 2004).

Intravenous drug use is a major route of HIV-1 transmission in China (China UN theme group on HIV/AIDS for the UN country team in China, 2001). As early as 1989, HIV was found among IDUs in Yunnan, during which time the predominant circulating strains were HIV-1 subtype B from North America and B' from Thailand (Graf et al., 1998). Subtype B' strain YN.RL42, highly similar to HIV-1 B' in Thailand, was found for the first time among IDUs in the DeHong prefecture of

Yunnan province in 1991 (Cassol et al., 1996) and has been increasing as a circulating strain, making up 20% of all infections in 1990 and up to 90% of all infections in 1996 (Graf et al., 1998; Zhang Linqi et al., 2004). Meanwhile, subtype C from India has also started to spread among IDUs in Yunnan (Li et al., 1996; Luo et al., 1995). Multiple subtypes thus coexisted in the population, offering an ideal site for recombination of distinctive subtypes.

From 1999 to 2000, recombinant forms of CRF07-BC and CRF08-BC derived from subtypes B' and C were found in IDUs in Sichuan, Xinjiang, Yunnan, and Guangxi at different times. By the time they were detected, these recombinants had been spread widely among IDUs (Piyasirisilp et al., 2000; Shao et al., 1999; Su, et al., 2000). Since HIV-1 had first been discovered in Yunnan, as had the current circulating B and C subtypes, which were similar to those later found in Guangxi and Sichuan, it was inferred that the two recombinant subtypes had likewise originated in Yunnan. The circulation of the two recombinant viruses coincided with the two drug trafficking routes stemming from Yunnan: one to the north and one to the east. The first route started from Yunnan, heads northwest through Sichuan, Gansu, Ningxia, Xinjiang, and beyond Chinese boards. The circulation region of CRF07-BC was consistent with this route. The second stretched from Yunnan east through Guangxi and Guangdong to Hong Kong, becoming CRF08-BC (Su et al., 2000). A nationwide molecular epidemiology study in 2002 showed that CRF-BC ranked first in terms of estimated constituent ratio of all subtypes around China, becoming the predominant HIV recombinant form in China. The study also showed that the recombinant virus was more overwhelming in regards of prevalence. At present, the circulating HIV-1 in Yunnan still undertakes the ongoing recombination (Yang et al., 2002).

Paid plasma donation is the second highest route of HIV transmission in China (Su et al., 2003; Wu et al., 1995; Zheng et al., 2000a,b). For more than a decade, Henan served as the nucleus for paid plasma donation in China. This practice spread throughout central China to nearby provinces including Anhui, Hubei, and Shanxi, thereby infecting a large number of paid plasma donors with HIV-1. (Wu et al., 1995; Kaufman and Jing, 2002; Zhuang et al., 2003). This mode of iatrogenic transmission resulted in a single HIV-1 subtype B' strain circulating in central China. DNA sequencing analysis shows that the HIV-1 subtype B' strain circulating among paid blood donors and their spouses shared great similarities with the HIV-1 subtype B' strain in Yunnan. It is therefore likely that the subtype B' strain circulating in central China originated in Yunnan before the recombinant forms appeared in Yunnan. The substitution of recombinant viruses with subtypes B and B' began in the mid-1990s (Graf et al., 1998). In this sense, subtype B' strain may have been introduced into Henan in the early 1990s, earlier than the introduction of recombinant viruses CRF07-BC and CRF08-BC into Guangxi and Xinjiang (Zhang Linqi et al., 2004).

Individuals infected via sexual contact can be found in all regions of China, with the number of infections increasing each year. Various virus subtypes – primarily recombinant virus CRF01-AE – were observed in this sexually infected population (Xing et al., 2004). Initially derived from Thailand, CRF01-AE circulates in southeastern Asia as the main HIV-1 genotype (Robertson et al., 1995; Carr et al., 1996; McCutchan et al., 1996). Prevalent on the southwestern border and southeast coastal regions of China, CRF01-AE recombinant HIV-1 strain was transmitted sexually in 60% of the cases and through intravenous drug use in less than 30% of transmissions. Molecular evolution analysis indicates that CRF01-AE in China primarily comes from Thailand (Xing et al., 2004; Laeyendecker et al., 2005; Kato et al.,1999; Yu et al.,1999) and the percentage of IDUs infected with CRF01-AE increases every year (Xing et al., 2004).

The newest date revealed that the discovery of many sexually transmitted CRF01-AE cases is new in Yunnan and CRF01-AE may lead to a new epidemic in general Chinese population (Yong Zhang et al., 2006).

Opportunistic Infections of AIDS That Need to be Addressed in China

Common blood-borne pathogens include HIV, HBV, HCV, HGV, etc. Because the route of transmission is the same, paid plasma donors or blood transfusion and blood product recipients are often infected with multiple viruses.

Some coinfections, such as HIV-1 and HCV (Hepatitis C virus) coinfection, mutually accelerate disease progression (Soriano et al., 2002) while others, such as HIV and HGV (Hepatitis G virus) coinfection, can prolong disease progression (Tillmann et al., 2001; Tillmann and Manns, 2001).

In China, 38 million people – 3.2% of the total population – are infected with HCV, the most common viral hepatitis among IDUs, paid blood donors, and unsafe blood transfusion recipients (Zhuang Hui, 2004). This high rate of HCV infection, in conjunction with an increasing incidence of HIV, has led to a significant increase in HIV/HCV coinfection in China. As much as 86.9% of HIV-infected plasma donors are tested positive for antibodies against HCV (Luo Jiala et al., 2003).

There are multiple HCV genotypes circulating in China. In regions such as Henan and Anhui, where HIV-1 was acquired primarily through blood transmission, HCV genotypes 1b and 2a and HIV-1 subtype B' are most common, whereas among HIV-infected IDUs, HCV genotypes are 1b, 3a, and 3b, and HIV-1 circulating recombinant form 07 to 08 (Zhang Linqi et al., 2004). More knowledge of the HCV genotype and HIV subtypes will be helpful in treatment and vaccine development.

Some anti-retrovirus (ARV) treatments for HIV/AIDS are associated with hepatotoxicity and should therefore be used cautiously for HIV-HCV coinfected persons. HCV infection has been shown to increase the risk of severe hepatotoxicity associated with Highly Active Anti-Retrovirus Therapy (HAART) (Tori et al., 2005).

Most individuals coinfected with HIV-HCV in China are unable to access interferon and ribavirin because of their cost and the distance to health care facilities with knowledgeable hepatologists. Furthermore, because of the few choices of ARV medication in China, most HIV-infected persons must take nevirapine (NVP).

Further study is needed to determine the impact of NVP-containing regimens on HIV-HCV coinfected persons in China.

Because much is still unknown about the viral interaction and related pathogenesis in the coinfections of HIV/HCV (Graham and Koziel, 2003), there is an urgent need for China to adopt new AIDS prevention and treatment strategies that address the seriousness of this particular coinfection.

The rate of positive Hepatitis B virus surface antigen (HBsAg) among paid blood donors and blood recipients is 4.1% (Luo Jiala et al., 2003) – lower than the average HBsAg-positive rate in the general Chinese population (9.75%) (Liu Chongbai, 1998). Although the interrelation between HIV, HCV, and HBV requires further study, the lower rate of HBsAg may be partially accredited to the effective screening of blood donors in the 1980s.

Like HIV, HCV, and HBV, HGV (Hepatitis G virus) can be transmitted by unsafe blood collection and transfusion. A group led by Luo Jiala reports in 2003 that, of 314 HIV-positive plasma donors, 206 (65.6% of the total) were positive also for HGV-Ab. A follow-up study found that those coinfected with HIV and HGV underwent a slower HIV disease progression to death than those who were HGV-Ab negative (10.7% vs. 27.8%, $p < 0.01$). Determining whether HGV infection interferes with HIV replication or HIV immune damage warrants further research (Luo Jiala et al., 2003).

Tuberculosis (TB) is one of the most common opportunistic infections among AIDS patients (Li Zhenmin, 2004). AIDS and TB mutually accelerate disease progression, which can result in the death of patients. Some anti-TB drugs have overlapping side effects and toxicity profiles with ARVs and can potentially inflict more damage to the liver, thereby generating further difficulty in treatment.

There are over two billion individuals infected with TB worldwide (Li Zhenmin, 2004). Second only to India, China is home to more than 500 million TB-infected individuals, accounting for one-third of China's total population (Li Zhenmin, 2004). China has a high incidence of MDR-TB (Multiple Drug Resistant TB). Following the trend of HIV-1 patients, many of those infected with TB are young, in their prime, and often living in rural areas. Both TB and AIDS are critical public health and social issues for China. The prevention and treatment of HIV-TB coinfection has become an important issue that China must confront.

The incidence rates of TB-HIV coinfection vary significantly by region from 6.1% to 45.4% (Li Bingxi et al., 2003; Song Jianxin et al., 2003; Li Xinghua et al., 2001). The reasons for these differences may be distinctive to the epidemic but may also be related to the varying levels of knowledge of HIV and TB coinfection among health care workers, to workers' diagnostic capabilities, or to the conditions of the medical facilities.

Investigations need to be conducted to clarify whether active TB in coinfected TB-HIV patients in China is caused by endogenous recurrence, exogenous reinfection, or primary infection. Issues such as the clinical features of double infection, diagnostic methods, drug–drug interactions, therapy regimens, and prevention methods all require further study. Additionally, careful observations must be made on whether HIV will promote or accelerate TB prevalence in China.

As HIV infection progresses and damages the immune system, individuals develop opportunistic infections and tumors. As is the case in the rest of the world, the incidence of some opportunistic infections in China varies geographically.

Candida, *Pneumocystis jiroveci*, *Cryptococcus*, *Aspergillus*, *Mucor* fungus, *Penicilliosis marneffei*, and histoplasmosis are among the common deep fungal infections found in HIV-infected persons in China.

Histoplasmosis has been found in individuals with HIV infection and is prevalent along the Yangtze River and southern China (Chen XieJiu et al., 2003; Li Xiaolin and Xu Jingya, 2004).

Penicilliosis marneffei was initially discovered in Vietnam and Thailand and has subsequently been found in China – perhaps because southern China borders these two countries and has similar geography and climate. HIV-infected persons with *Penicilliosis marneffei* have been found in Guangxi, Guangdong, and Hong Kong (Wan Haizhu et al., 2003; Jin Wei, 2004). Some migrant laborers bring *Penicilliosis marneffei* back to their hometowns after contracting the infection in Guangxi or Guangdong, thus accounting for observed cases of *Penicilliosis marneffei* in inland China.

Unfavorable Conditions for Effective HIV-1 Control in China

1. Increasing incidence of HIV in resource-limited rural areas

The rural nature of the epidemic is evident from the site of the 1989 discovery of the first HIV cases in China: Ruili, a rural town in Yunnan, where 146 IDUs were found infected with HIV. In the 1990s, the paid plasma collection industry was active in regions of central China. Because of ineffective regulatory management, thousands of paid blood donors and recipients – mostly farmers – were infected by HIV-1. Among the mobile population in cities, 75% come from villages and may have extramarital relationships or work in the sex industry and subsequently become exposed to HIV and other STDs.

Some estimate that 80% of all HIV infected persons in China live in rural areas (Jin Wei, 2004). The economy and education in rural areas are not as well developed as they are in major cities; sanitary conditions are poor and medical resources are insufficient, facilitating the transmission of HIV in such areas. Over time, these unfavorable conditions will continue to fuel the HIV epidemic.

2. Every year China has 120 million mobile people.

The mobile population generally flows from rural areas to cities in search of better employment opportunities. Most in this group are young and in the prime of their sexually active period, but lack information about HIV and other STDs. For many reasons, healthcare services for mobile population in cities do not and cannot meet the people's needs. One survey found that the HIV infection rate for people returning to their village after working away from home is higher than for those who remain in their hometown (China Ministry of Health, 2003; Sun Jie, 2003).

In addition to the mobile and migrant population within China, there are a number of Chinese tourists going abroad reaching several million each year. This high number of Chinese tourists, in combination with foreign tourists visiting China, facilitates the AIDS epidemic, for although mobility in itself is not a risk factor, it exacerbates the consequences of behavior that puts traveling people at risk for HIV and other STDs. Developing effective prevention strategies for a large, diverse, mobile population remains a challenge for China today.

3. Sexual contact is the major route of HIV transmission globally.

Worldwide, sexual contact accounts for over 80% of infections among HIV-infected adults and with sexually transmitted cases rising each year due to premarital sex (mostly among young people) and an increasing number of extramarital affairs. More young people are having premarital sex than their parents.

In China, national sentinel surveillance sites found in 2004 that the overall rate of HIV infection among commercial sex workers was 1.0%, but the rate in some areas of Yunnan and Xinjiang ranged from 3.3% to 6.7%. The risk of HIV transmission increases due to intravenous drug usage among some commercial sex workers and the reportedly low rate of consistent condom usage (A Joint Assessment of HIV/AIDS prevention, 2004).

The effects of social stigma and discrimination have rendered men who have sex with men (MSM), a population with an increased risk of acquiring HIV and other STIs. MSM in China often conceal their sexual histories and avoid HIV testing out of fear of discrimination. Zhang Baichuang, a well-known scholar in China, estimates that the number of MSM in China is between 10.18 million and 25.45 million (17.82 million on average) in 2002. During his research, Zhang found that approximately 70% of MSM have families with female partners. Zhang estimates that around eight million MSM may engage in high-risk behaviors that put them and their estimated 5.4 million female sexual partners at risk for HIV and other STIs (Zhang Beichuan et al., 2002).

Unprotected sex with multiple sexual partners among MSM occurs widely in China. The HIV prevalence rate in MSM is 2.5–5.5% (Zhang Beichuan et al., 2002). The targeted HIV prevention to the MSM population is important to slow the overall HIV transmission rate in China.

4. Increasing number of illegal drug users.

The number of drug users in China is growing; with registered IDU in 72.7% (2,084) of all counties in China (Sun Jie, 2003), the number now exceeds one million (although some experts estimate the actual number of drug users to be closer to six million), 53.8% of them are IDU and 37% of whom share syringes. The HIV prevalence rate among the IDU population is approximately 5–20%. The relapse rate after quitting drugs is over 95% among drug users. Common among IDUs is low condom usage and the exchange of sex for drugs or money – both high risk behaviors for HIV transmission. Effective harm reduction and drug treatment methods need to be employed in order to control HIV transmission in this high-risk group.

5. Some local governments have not implemented HIV prevention and treatment policies seriously.

Although the central Chinese government and higher level officials have attached a great importance to HIV prevention and treatment, some local officials do not keep pace with the central government. Some officials worry that disclosing information of the real HIV epidemic could affect new investments, economic growth, and their own political performance and achievements.

HIV infections in paid plasma donors were found as early as 1995 at which time the government leaders made the critical decision to shut down unqualified blood banks; however, they did not explain their reasoning or reveal the true problem to the public. As a result, paid plasma donors went directly to the hospitals, thereby eliminating the middleman and supplying HIV-infected blood products directly to patients. If the lessons learned from illegal blood collection and subsequent death from HIV/AIDS were not taken, control of HIV might not have shown such great achievement. Epidemics must be disclosed, policies developed, and prevention and treatment plans seriously implemented.

6. Few types of ARV drugs and difficulty in managing HIV drug resistance

Since 2003, the Chinese government has offered free antiviral drugs to HIV/AIDS patients who are unable to afford them. ARV treatment can drop HIV mortality rates and prolongs the lives of HIV patients, as evidenced in the Hubei province. According to Author's data, the rate of HIV/AIDS-related mortality has dropped from 49.3% in 2002 to 14% in 2005 due to ARV treatment. ARVs therapeutic efficacy is notable, but as time goes by, the drug resistance becomes more frequent. At present, NVP resistance is most common because, in addition to the inherent biochemical and physiological aspects of NVP, it is the cheapest NNRTI (Non-nucleoside analog reverse transcriptase inhibitor) and most commonly administered drug in China, and is also an important measure to prevent MTCT; however, these aspects of the NVP may increase drug resistance. NVP and EFV (Efavirenz) are cross-resistant, and China has no real second line ARV options yet. Traditional Chinese medicine is being researched and is used either as primary treatment or as treatment for patients who cannot take ARVs due to the drugs' side effects or toxicities such as allergy or liver toxicity and anemia, etc. If new approaches for preventing and managing drug resistance are not developed or adopted, HIV/AIDS-related mortality may increase and likely adversely affect HIV prevention efforts.

Main Measures That China Has Taken to Prevent and Control AIDS

1. Law on Blood Donation in the People's Republic of China began to be enforced on October 1998.

The Blood Donation law of People's Republic of China clearly states that all blood donations should be uncompensated and undertaken under safe and hygienic conditions, strictly adhering to operational procedures for the physical safety of all blood donors and blood recipients; that all blood from illegal blood banks should be confiscated; and that the sale of blood is strictly prohibited (China Ministry of Health, 1997). In 2001, central governments allocated 1.25 billion RMB for efforts to reinforce the infrastructure of blood banks, update their facilities, offer training and monitoring of staff in blood banks, and adopt the institutional practice of qualifying blood banks (National debt, 2002). As a result of these efforts, transfusions of blood-borne pathogens are now a rare occurrence in China.

2. Prevention of HIV mother to child transmission

Without intervention, the MTCT rate in China is about 35% (Li et al., 2002). With funding from UNICEF, a PMTCT (prevention of mother to child transmission) trial was conducted in 2002 in Shangcai County, Henan. One year later, the Ministry of Health launched HIV MTCT prevention trials in eight cities (counties) in Henan, Xinjiang, Yunnan, Guangxi, and Shenzhen city. Thus, as of 2005, a total of 15 provinces had developed PMTCT interventions including the use of ARVs during pregnancy and labor, obstetrical interventions, and breast-feeding alternatives. The primary PMTCT intervention used in China is the practice of administering 200 mg NVP at the onset of labor to a woman and then administering $2 \, \text{mg} \, \text{kg}^{-1}$ of NVP to the newborn within 72 h of delivery. This short-course treatment is convenient and inexpensive, but NVP's protective effects and drug resistance require further investigation. The preliminary results of research done on the effectiveness of other ARVs in pregnant women and newborns showed that the intervention reduced the MTCT (Mother to Child Transmission) rate and their subsequent drug resistances are still unclear.

3. Encourage high-risk population to use condoms

Currently most HIV infections in China are caused by blood transmission (IDU, paid plasma donation, blood transfusion); however, sexual transmission is causing an increasing number of infections and henceforth will likely be the key route of transmission. Therefore, the containment of sexual transmission of HIV is of critical importance.

Although the Chinese government is cracking down on illegal activities such as prostitution, its policies have had limited success. The government has realized that the promotion of condom use is an effective measure that requires few resources and is highly efficient in preventing HIV transmission. The plan of "Action on Containment, Prevention and Treatment of AIDS in China" (Jin Wei, 2004) calls for a 50% increase in condom usage in the high-risk population by the end of 2005. Great effort must be put forth to reach this goal.

4. Gradually increase needle exchanges and methadone substitution

Although the Chinese government has been strictly prohibiting on illegal activities such as drug trafficking and drug usage, the number of drug users is still increasing, as is the HIV prevalence among drug users. For drug users who cannot quit using drugs, the HIV prevention tool of harm reduction is implemented, including, among other interventions, methadone substitution and needle exchange. Although some methods are controversial – (there are ongoing trials testing the effectiveness of these harm reduction interventions) – it is predicted that methadone substitution and needle exchange will continue in China.

5. The government proposed the "Four frees and one care" policy in 2003

In detail, the policy provides for (a) free antiviral therapy for AIDS patients of the farmer population and for those facing financial difficulty in cities and towns; (b) free consultation and primary screening for those who voluntarily go for HIV consultation and testing; (c) free MTCT prevention drugs and infant testing reagents for infants born to HIV-infected women; (d) waivers of tuition for AIDS orphans; and (e) incorporate AIDS patients in financial difficulty into the government's aid circle. "Four frees and one care" reflects humanitarianism and is beneficial to PLWHA (people living with HIV/AIDS) as well as preventing MTCT. Free anti-HIV therapy does not only prolong patients' lives, but its use also decreases the chances of infecting others, thereby making it one of the most important policies in HIV prevention and treatment in China.

Urgent Needs and Action Steps

1. The prevention and treatment of HIV has drawn the awareness and attention of Chinese leaders and various social sectors. Why, then, is HIV still rapidly spreading? Until now, many have believed that HIV prevalence in China is still low <0.1% and that Chinese moral sensibilities and traditions are far different from those of other countries, from which they infer that HIV will not become a critical and threatening issue in China.

Since 1985, when the first HIV patient was identified in China, people have maintained the belief that HIV is exclusively a foreigners' disease. The government responded by reinforcing customs management, attempting to ban "AIDS" outside the doors of China. Even when hundreds of HIV-infected drug users were found along China's southwestern borders despite the government's actions, people assumed it was a local problem. Within a short time, HIV had spread across the nation. When attention was given to HIV-infected drug users, new HIV infections were found among paid plasma donors in central China, leading to the discovery of a large number of HIV-infected men, women, and children.

Programs to prevent and treat HIV/AIDS have yet to meet needs, and it is likely that HIV will continue to spread in China. The number of IDUs and those who share syringes continues to increase; the number of commercial sex workers, few of whom consistently use condoms, is large; risk behaviors among MSM, most of who have been shown to have sexual relationships with both men and women, are common; moreover, MTCT and blood transmission have not been prevented completely. If we do not learn from past experiences and thereby let the epidemic continue with inadequate or poor prevention and treatment programs, the consequences will be devastating. This is a critical time for China as HIV is increasingly being transmitted from high-risk populations to the general population. Governments at various levels should carry out HIV prevention and treatment programs with openness and practicality. Healthcare workers and related personnel should actively participate in HIV prevention and treatment and develop a positive environment so that everyone joins the efforts.

2. Serious infectious diseases, including HIV, TB, Hepatitis B, Schistosomiasis, avian flu, and pig streptococcal infection, are most prevalent in rural areas in China.

China has one of the world's largest gaps between rural and urban areas. Because of poverty, many farmers can make a living only by means that may harm their physical health – means such as blood-selling, sex work, and drug trafficking. Currently, 30% of all pregnant women deliver at home, and 70% of severely ill patients die at home as opposed to in hospitals. Each year, hundreds of millions of farmers in search of work flock to cities, where their living conditions are poor and their medical care is not guaranteed. Some PLWHA discontinue ARV therapy because they have to leave home to earn a living; some of them even take HIV back to their villages. Infectious diseases such as HIV are easy to spread in rural areas due to impoverishment, insufficient medical and health knowledge, and inadequate medical resources.

It is urgently requested that HIV prevention and treatment be intensified in rural areas, and moreover, that the efforts be combined with efforts towards improving rural hygiene conditions and updating levels of rural medical teams. Otherwise, HIV and other infectious diseases (including emerging ones) may be free to spread widely from rural areas to cities and thereby spread nationwide.

3. HIV prevention and treatment have to attach importance to science and rely on science.

HIV prevention and treatment in China has not been standardized, and scientific research in this field was launched later than in developed countries. There are many problems that require further study.

Currently, six ARVs are offered free of charge in China: four NRTIs and two NNRTIs. Optimal ARV therapy strategies need to be researched so that the limited medications can be used to their utmost effectiveness. China has witnessed how free ARVs have prolonged the lives of those infected with HIV; however, HIV drug resistance has increased as well. It is critical for China to determine how to promptly monitor drug resistance in regions lacking medical resources and how to develop effective strategies to combat resistance. Traditional Chinese medicine for treating HIV is worthy of research, but it should be conducted with a reasonable study design, adhering to GCP (Good Clinical Practice) requirements and regulations.

The current PMTCT policy in China is less advanced than in developed countries. Therefore, different regimens should be comparatively studied so as to more effectively prevent MTCT.

The number of HIV infections occurring by plasma donation and blood transfusion in China is large. The likely infection time is clear, however, which offers favorable conditions for studies on the natural history of HIV and other related issues. People infected with HIV via plasma donation and blood transfusion are often coinfected with other blood-borne pathogens such as HCV, HBV, and HGV. Further investigations on the impact of other blood-borne pathogens on HIV disease progression and therapy response need to be conducted.

China has a high incidence of TB, as well as a high prevalence of histoplasmosis and *Penicilliosis marneffei* in some areas. In-depth explorations should be launched to study clinical features, diagnostic methods, and methods of treatment, prevention, and interaction of coinfection of HIV and TB.

In 2005, China began a Phase I HIV vaccine clinical trial. China should develop a vaccine suited for the HIV molecular epidemiology features of China.

China should seek to develop more cost-effective drugs and testing methods as well as more directed and feasible intervention measures.

4. China lacks sufficient numbers of qualified health care teams for HIV prevention and treatment work. Many health care workers have inadequate HIV knowledge, may miss diagnosing HIV, improperly diagnose and treat opportunistic infections, and may even show prejudice to PLWHA. This has certainly had a negative impact on the public and is one of the root causes of discrimination and prejudice again PLWHA. Although healthcare workers have participated in HIV training for many years, the need for trained healthcare workers is still great. It is tremendously important to intensify training for healthcare workers at all levels, enabling them to master basic HIV/AIDS knowledge, develop the capacity to correctly diagnose and treat HIV and opportunistic infections, and become familiar with prophylaxis of HIV professional exposure. What needs to be adopted now is the formation of medical teams with the compassion and ability to prevent and treat HIV/AIDS.

5. AIDS has robbed the lives of many Chinese people. The majority of AIDS deaths occur in the young or in those in the prime of their lives, leaving AIDS orphans behind. Statistics show that, in China, there are currently 76,000 children who have lost one or both parents to HIV/AIDS (Children on the Brink, 2002).

In China, most AIDS orphans are not HIV-infected as they were born before their mothers were infected. Nevertheless, they lead a hard and poor life in the shadows of HIV/AIDS, often enduring discrimination. Some AIDS orphans quit school and therefore receive no education. Some of them have ideas of revenging society and even go astray.

The policy of "Four frees and one care" enacted by the country exempts AIDS orphans from tuition and additionally offers certain aids. Although some places have established orphanages, all of these efforts have yet to produce a solution to the orphan issue.

Policies to aid orphans are implemented differently in different regions. Care and aid to these orphans are not enough. The policy for free tuition lasts only through junior high school. The environment in orphanages does little to erase the psychological scar in an orphan's mind exacerbated by the social discrimination

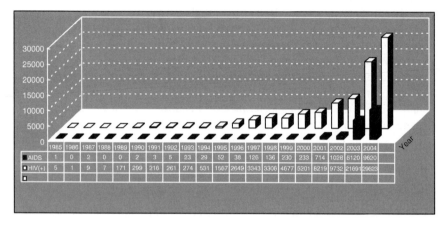

	1985	1986	1987	1988	1989	1990	1991	1992	1993	1994	1995	1996	1997	1998	1999	2000	2001	2002	2003	2004
■ AIDS	1	0	2	0	0	2	3	5	23	29	52	38	126	136	230	233	714	1028	6120	9620
□ HIV(+)	5	1	9	7	171	299	216	261	274	531	1567	2649	3343	3306	4677	5201	8219	9732	21691	29623
□																				

Fig. 1 Cumulative AIDS incidence shows a rising trend in China: Currently, the number of HIV infections in China ranks 2nd in Asia and 14th in the world

HIV/AIDS cases found in two areas in 1985

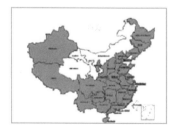

HIV/AIDS cases found in more areas in 1989

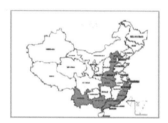

HIV/AIDS cases found in most areas of China in 1995

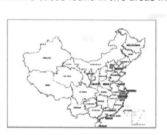

HIV/AIDS cases found in the whole country of China in 1998

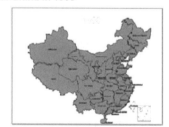

Fig. 2 Increasing HIV incidence every year in China

Cases of HIV/AIDS

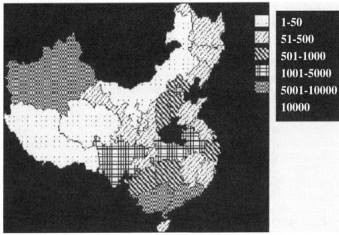

	1-50
	51-500
	501-1000
	1001-5000
	5001-10000
	10000

Fig. 3 AIDS incidence in China varies widely by region

targeted at them. Multiple methods need to be employed to help orphans – establishing orphanages is only one approach. NGOs and individuals should be allowed to run orphanages to add to the number of orphanages organized by the government. Subject to "Adoption Law of People's Republic of China," orphan adoption and help from individuals must be allowed. More mature orphans should be allowed and supported to study in boarding schools (middle school or vocational school).

In areas of high HIV incidence, AIDS orphans have become a real social issue. Caring for and aiding orphans is not only good for humanity but also good for a stable and just society (Figs. 1–3).

References

A Joint Assessment of HIV/AIDS Prevention, Treatment and Care in China. (2004). 12, State Council AIDS Working Committee Office and UN Theme Group on HIV/AIDS in China

Carr, J.K. et al. (1996). Full-length sequence and mosaic structure of a human immunodeficiency virus type 1 isolate from Thailand. J Virol, 70, 5935–5943

Cassol, S. et al. (1996). Detection of HIV type 1 env subtypes A, B, C, and E in Asia using dried blood spots: A new surveillance tool for molecular epidemiology. AIDS Res Hum Retroviruses, 12, 1435–1441

Chen, X.J., Cai, W.P., Chen J.F., et al. (2003). Fungal infection and resistance to antifungal agents in patients with HIV/AIDS. Chin J AIDS/STD, 19, 205–207

Children On The Brink. (2002). A Joint Report on Orphan Estimates and Program Strategies. UNAIDS/UniCEF/USAID

China Ministry of Health. (1997). Blood Donation Law of the People's Republic of China

China Ministry of Health. (2003). A Joint Assessment of HIV/AIDS Prevention, Treatment and Cases in China[R]

China UN Theme Group on HIV/AIDS for the UN Country Team in China, HIV/AIDS. (2001). China's Titanic Peril (2001 update of the AIDS situation and needs assessment report, UNAIDS, Beijing). UNAIDS, Geneva, Switzerland, 1–160

First AIDS Case, How It was Found in China. , The Xinhua News Agency, 30 November 2001

Graf, M., et al. (1998). Cloning and characterization of a virtually full-length HIV type 1 genome from a subtype B -Thai strain representing the most prevalent B-cladeisolate in China. AIDS Res Hum Retroviruses, 14, 285–288.

Graham, C.S., Koziel, M.J. (2003). First things first: Balancing Hepatitis C and human immuno-deficiency virus. Clin Infect Dis, 36, 368–369

Jin Wei. (2004). AIDS is a social problem. In: AIDS in China. International publishing House for Chinese Culture, WA, USA. pp. 90–93

Kato, K., et al. (1999). Genetic similarity of HIV type 1 subtype E in a recent outbreak among injecting drug users in northern Vietnam to strains in Guangxi Province of southern China. AIDS Res Hum Retroviruses, 15, 1157–1168

Kaufman, J., Jing, J. (2002). China and AIDS – the time to act is now. Science, 296, 2339–2340

Laeyendecker, O., et al. (2005). Molecular epidemiology of HIV-1 subtypes in southern China. J Acquir Immune Defic Syndr, 38, 356–362

Li Bingxi, Wang Lin, Zhou Xinhua. (2003). Clinical analysis of 21 cases from pulmonary tuber-culosis related AIDS. Chin J Prev Tuberculosis, 25(1), 21–23

Li, G.H., Chen, H.H., He, Y., et al. (2002). An investigation on HIV-1 transmission from mother to children in selected areas of China. Chin J STD/AIDS Prev Cont, 8(4), 204–208

Li Xiaolin, Xu Jingya. (2004). A case of AIDS complicated Histoplamosis. J Cent South Univ (Med Sci), 29(4), P400, P413

Li Xinghua, Chen He-he, He Yun, et al. (2001). A clinical report on 482 AIDS cases, Chin J Infect Chemother, 1(3), P129–P132

Li Zhenmin. (2004). AIDS and tuberculosis. Chin J AIDS/STD, 10(1), 74–75

Li, D.Q., Zheng, X.W., Zhang, G.Y. (1996). Study on the distribution HIV-1 C subtype in Ruili and other counties, Yunnan, China. Zhonghua Liu Xing Bing Xue Za Zhi, 17, 337–339

Liu Chongbai. (1998). The epidemia features and associated factors of Viral Hepatitis in China. Zhong Hua gan bing zha zhi, 6, 67–70

Luo, C.C., et al. (1995). HIV-1 subtype C in China. Lancet, 345, 1051–1052

Luo Jiala, Gui Xi'en, Zhuang Ke. (2003). A study on the prevalence of anti-HCV, HBsAg and anti-HGV among people infected with HIV. World Chinese J Digestol, 11(11), 1835–1836

McCutchan, F.E., et al. (1996). Diversity of the envelope glycoprotein among human immunode-ficiency virus type 1 isolates of clade E from Asia and Africa. J Virol, 70, 3331–3338

Ministry of Health People's Republic of China. (2006). 2005 Update on the HIV/AIDS Epidemic and Response in China. Joint United Nations Programme on HIV/AIDS, World Health Organization

Ministry of Health reports AIDS epidemic in China. (2006). The China AIDS Prevention. p. 176

National Debt of 1.25 Billion RMB to Support Building Blood Bank. (2002). The Prople's Daily Overseas, p. A1

Piyasirisilp, S. et al. (2000). A recent outbreak of human immunodeficiency virus type 1 infection in southern China was initiated by two highly homogeneous, geographically separated strains, circulating recombinant form AE and a novel BC recombinant. J Virol, 74, 11286–11295

Robertson, D.L., et al. (1995). Recombination in HIV-1. Nature, 374, 124–126

Shao, Y., Zhao, F., Yang, W. (1999). The identification of recombinant HIV-1 strains in IDUs in southwest and northwest China. Zhonghua Shi Yan He Lin Chuang Bing Du Xue Za Zhi, 13, 109–112

Song Jianxin, Xing Mingyou, Tan Mingge, et al. (2003). Analysis on clinical characteristics of 146 cases of HIV-/TB. J HuaZhong Univ Sci Tech (Health Sci), 32(6), 625–627

Soriano, V., Sulkowski, M., Bergin, C., et al. (2002). Care of patients with chronic hepatitis C and HIV co-infection: Recommendations from the HIV-HCV International Panel [J]. AIDS, 16, 813–828

Su, L., et al. (2000). Characterization of a virtually full-length human immunodeficiency virus type 1 genome of a prevalent intersubtype (C/B') recombinant strain in China. J Virol, 74, 11367–11376

Su, B., et al. (2003). HIV-1 subtype B' dictates the AIDS epidemic among paid blood donors in the Henan and Hubei provinces of China. Aids, 17, 2515–2520

Sun jie. (2003). An Analysis of the epidemic of AIDS in China. Chin J Frontier Health Quarantine, 26, 367–368

Tillmann, H.L., Heiken, H., Knapik-Botor, A., Heringlake, S., Ockenga, J., Wilber, J.C., Goergen, B., Detmer, J., Mcmorrow, M., Stoll, M., Schmidt, R.E., Manns, M.P. (2001). Infection with GB virus-C and reduced mortality among HIV-infected patients. N Engl J Med, 345, 715–724

Tillmann, H.L., Manns, M.P. (2001). GB virus-C infection in patients infected with the human immunodeficiency virus. Antiviral Res, 52, 83–90

Tori, C., Lapadula, G., Casari, S., et al. (2005). Incidence and risk factors for liver enzyme elevation during highly active antiretroviral therapy in HIV-HCV co-infected patients: Results from the Italian EPOKA-MASTER Cohort. BMC Infect Dis, 2005, 5, 58. Published online 2005 July 14, doi 10.1186/1471-2334-5-58

Wan Haizhu, Huang Guicai, Gao Hui, et al. (2003). Cases of AIDS co-infection with *Penicilliosis marneffei*. Chin J AIDS/STD, 9(2), 123

Wu, Z., Liu, Z., Detels, R. (1995). HIV-1 infection in commercial plasma donors in China. Lancet, 346, 61–62

Xing, H., et al. (2004). Distribution of recombinant human immunodeficiency virus type-1 CRF01_AE strains in China and its sequence variations in the env V3-C3 region. Zhonghua Yu Fang Yi Xue Za Zhi, 38, 300–304

Xing, H., Qin, G., Feng, Y. (1999). Identification and characterization of HIV-1 subtype D strain in China. Zhonghua Shi Yan He Lin Chuang Bing Du Xue Za Zhi 13, 157–162

Yang, R. et al. (2002). On-going generation of multiple forms of HIV-1 intersubtype recombinants in the Yunnan Province of China. Aids, 16, 1401–1407

Yong Zhang, Lin Lu, et al. (2006). Dominance of HIV-1 subtype CRF01-AE in sexually acquired cases to a new epidemic in Yunnan Province of China. PLOS Med, 3, 0001-0013

Yu, X.F., et al. (1999). Emerging HIV infections with distinct subtypes of HIV-1 infection among injection drug users from geographically separate locations in Guangxi Province, China. J Acquir Immune Defic Syndr, 22, 180–188

Zhang Beichuan, Li Xiufang, Shi Tongxin, Yang Luguang, Zhang Jingtong. (2002) The number of chinese Gay/Bi and HIV infection rate. Chin J STD/AIDS Prev Cont, 8(4), 197–199

Zhang Linqi, Chen Zhiwei, Cao Yunzhen, et al. (2004). Molecular characterization of human immunodeficiency virus type 1 and hepatitis C virus in paid blood donors and injection drug users in china. J Virol, 78(24), 13591–13599

Zhejiang HIV/AIDS patients' number increased 50%. The Youth Times, 1 December 2005

Zheng XW. (1999). The epidemic and control of AIDS in China. Zhonghua Liu Xing Bing Xue Za Zhi, 20, 131–134

Zheng, X., et al. (2000a). Residual risk research of HIV infection after blood screening in one county in China. Zhonghua Liu Xing Bing Xue Za Zhi, 21, 13–14

Zheng, X., et al. (2000b). The epidemiological study of HIV infection among paid blood donors in one county of China. Zhonghua Liu Xing Bing Xue Za Zhi, 21, 253–255

Zhuang Hui. (2004). Towards research on Hepatitis C. Chin J Hepatol, 12(2), 65–66

Zhuang, K., et al. (2003). High prevalence of HIV infection among women and their children in Henan Province, China. J Acquir Immune Defic Syndr, 33, 649–650

Part 4
Other Infections

Enterotoxigenic *Escherichia coli*'s Endemicity in Developing Countries and Its Emergence During Diarrheal Epidemics and Natural Disasters

Tanvir Ahmed and Firdausi Qadri

Enterotoxigenic *Escherichia coli* (ETEC) with Epidemic Potentials During Natural Disasters

Humid and hot climate, high population density, low socioeconomic conditions, poor hygiene and health facilities, and frequent natural disasters of cyclones and floods have made under-developed countries in Asia and elsewhere reservoirs of disease-producing pathogens. Of these factors, contaminated water in densely populated habitats is the single most important cause of many enteric diseases. In Bangladesh, which is a low-lying deltaic region, as well as in other riverine areas in Asia, floods have become more frequent and more devastating. In these regions, waterborne diseases are common, and the ebb and flow of some diseases have a characteristic pattern: increasing exponentially at certain predicted periods of the year, but remaining endemic all year round. If one considers the diarrheal pathogens, a typical pattern has been seen for those which are responsible for over 70% of diarrheal diseases. Of these, the most common is rotavirus, which peaks in the winter, followed by *Vibrio cholerae* and enterotoxigenic *Escherichia coli* (ETEC), both of which have a biannual periodicity and increase tremendously in the spring and autumn seasons (Albert et al., 1999) (Fig. 1). Of the six recognized diarrheagenic categories of *Escherichia coli* (Nataro and Kaper, 1998), ETEC is the most common, particularly in the developing world (WHO, 1999).

Around the end of June 2004, South Asian regions, including Bangladesh, suffered from flooding, the sixth gravely serious case since 1974 (UN-ESCAP, 1999; DER Sub-Group, 2004). It was the worst flood in 15 years – nearly two-thirds of Bangladesh was flooded (Fig. 2a–c). In the three weeks of devastation, the flood affected 30 million of the 140 million people living in this densely populated region, reaching a death toll of 691 (IFRC, 2004); Dhaka city, with a population of 10 million, was worst affected. About 75% of the capital was under water; the sewage system broke down, further contaminating water in the already precarious health and sanitation conditions. The city was like an open sewer; waterborne diseases and diarrheal epidemics shot up. The impact was felt at the hospital of the International Centre for Diarrhoeal Disease Research, Bangladesh (ICDDR,B) where 24,000 people were treated for diarrheal illnesses (ICDDRB, 2004). During the epidemic,

Y. Lu et al. (eds.), *Emerging Infections in Asia.*
© Springer Science+Business Media, LLC 2008

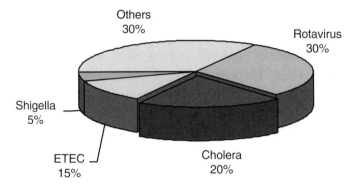

Fig. 1 The relative prevalence (%) of major diarrheal pathogens isolated from patients with diarrhea under the routine surveillance carried out at the ICDDR,B hospital in Dhaka

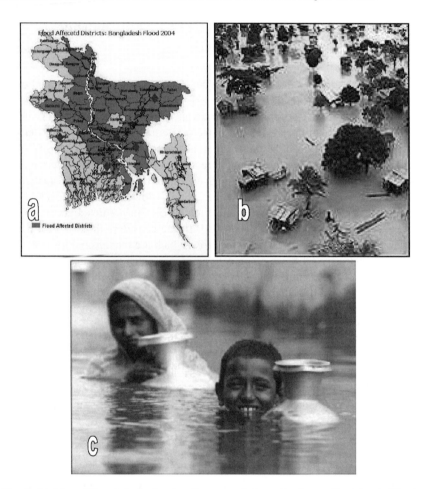

Fig. 2 (a) Map of Bangladesh showing the array of rivers flowing at flood level. Diarrheal epidemics were seen all over the country. The sites where enterotoxigenic *Escherichia coli* has been found to be prevalent during diarrheal epidemics are also shown. (b) Three fourths of Bangladesh was inundated and Dhaka city was the worst affected. (c) Drinking water was the most in demand and people had to obtain these from long distances over 700 patients were admitted every day to the treatment center (Qadri et al., 2005a). Over 77,000 cases of diarrhea and 44 deaths were reported during the peak, although the epidemic continued as expected in the weeks after the water receded.

Although, it is one of the most common bacterial pathogens responsible for acute watery diarrhea, ETEC is often overlooked as a major cause of disease in such natural disasters due to lack of awareness and diagnostic facilities in most laboratories in these regions. We looked at the hundreds of patients with diarrhea severe enough to seek hospital care in the sudden epidemic. Both children and adults were hospitalized with moderate to severe dehydration, with 40% of them requiring intravenous fluid replacement (Qadri et al., 2005a). The facilities at the hospital had to be expanded on an emergency basis and makeshift beds were set up in tents that extended to open areas of the ICDDR,B. It was not unusual to speculate that a large proportion of these patients were also ill with infection due to ETEC. Stools from patients were already being screened for rotavirus and *V. cholerae*, and we started analyzing these specimens for ETEC. As expected, it was found to be the second most common cause of bacterial diarrhea in the epidemic. About 18% of these patients had ETEC infections, following closely behind the *V. cholerae* O1 that was identified in 22% of cases (Qadri et al., 2005a). Of the ETEC strains isolated from patients during the flood, 86% were of the ST (heat stable toxin) phenotype [67% ST and 19% ST/LT (heat labile toxin)] and 75% of isolates were also positive for colonization factors (CFs) – a much higher pathogenic distribution than seen in other periods (Qadri et al., 2000; Rao et al., 2003) (Table 1).

This incident demonstrated that ETEC, which is endemic in Bangladesh with biannual seasonal outbreaks (Qadri et al., 2000), could be further aggravated and propagated during floods in mega cities like Dhaka where the population density is very high ($\sim$8,573 (sq km)$^{-1}$ (SDNP, 2005)). These disasters can thus serve to amplify the spread of ETEC by providing a huge reservoir of bacteria. It is believed that seasonal epidemics of enteric pathogens such as *V. cholerae* are caused by

Table 1 Distribution of toxin types and colonization factors on ETEC isolated from diarrheal patients in Bangladesh

	Routine surveillance	During the 2004 flood
No of patients	628	350
Toxin types (%)		
ST	53%	67%
LT/ST	26%	19%
LT	20%	14%
All ST-ETEC (LT/ST + ST)	79%	86%
CF positive	56%	78%
CF types[b]		
CFA/I	23.5	30%
CS4,CS5,CS6	31	42%
CS1,CS2,CS3	11	14
Others	34.5	14

ecological and environmental changes (Sack et al., 2003) such that the bacterial load in the surface water increases at certain times during the year. Bacteriophages may also modulate the load of pathogens in the environment and the human host and their periodic appearance and disappearance (Faruque et al., 2005a,b). ETEC-specific lytic T4 phages have been isolated from sewers and stools of ETEC patients (Begum et al., 2006; Chibani-Chennoufi et al., 2004) and may also play a role in the survival, endemicity, and epidemic potential of ETEC.

Vulnerable people who ingest contaminated water and food may become ill with diarrhea, infect more people, and continue the viscous cycle of fecal–oral contamination. Once the pathogen passes through the host, it becomes hyperinfective and more virulent (Merrell et al., 2002). During floods, when a large reservoir of the pathogen is present in sewage-contaminated water, a state of hyperinfectivity may already exist and the passage through the host is probably not needed to further augment these infections. This situation of higher infection rates is different from that seen during seasonal epidemic and endemic diarrheal diseases. Thus, this was the point at which it became obvious that ETEC, which has endemic and epidemic potentials, is also a major cause of relatively serious disease during natural disasters. Between July and August 2004, there was a 40% increase in the number of patients compared to that seen in 2003 (ICDDRB, 2004). Equal proportions of children (51%) and adults (49%) seek treatment at the ICDDR,B hospital. Large numbers of patients were more severely dehydrated (39%) and the need for intravenous rehydration therapy increased tremendously (ICDDRB, 2004; Qadri et al., 2005a).

Virulence and Pathogenic Capacity of Enterotoxigenic *E. coli*

ETEC globally causes one billion episodes of diarrhea, of which about 400 million are in children (Sanchez and Holmgren, 2005). It causes over 400,000 deaths – a large proportion of which are in the developing countries of Asia, Africa, and Latin America (WHO, 1999). A single dose (between 10^6 and 10^8 cfu) is sufficient to cause dehydrating diarrhea (Qadri et al. 2005b). Although the most common bacterial pathogen in under 3 year olds, ETEC also causes substantial disease in adults in developing countries as well as in travelers (rev article). These figures may be underestimations because the actual burden of disease due to the pathogen is still not known (Wenneras and Erling, 2004). The bacteria can cause disease of varying scales, ranging from mild to severe secretory diarrhea of such intensity that it has been described as "non *vibrio cholera*" in studies in which it was observed to cause disease (Table 2) (Schwartz et al., 2006; Carpenter et al., 1965). It is also isolated from stools of healthy individuals, but in case of control studies it has been found to be more significantly associated with disease than asymptomatic infection (Wenneras and Erling, 2004).

A regular surveillance for diarrheal diseases all over Bangladesh has shown that ETEC is as common as *V. cholerae*, but is also found in peaks of diarrhea in which no cholera vibrios could be isolated. In some areas, ETEC was more prevalent than *V. cholerae* (Qadri et al., 2005b).

Table 2 Insight into the disease causing potential of ETEC as a pathogen in humans came predominantly from Bangladesh and adjoining regions – aptly described as "non vibrio cholera"

Floods can be a focal point for sparking ETEC diarrheal epidemics
It is the most common bacterial cause of dehydrating diarrhea during flood related epidemics and seasonal outbreaks
A change in proportion of children and adults as well as disease severity is seen during natural disasters
High disease burden due to ETEC results in growth retardation of children and may also impact on future cognitive development
ETEC is a multivalent pathogen and can express a variety of enterotoxin(s) and adhesive antigens and virulent phenotype emerge during natural disasters
Antibiotic resistance is on a steep increase leading to problems in treatment of patients as well as travelers
Immunoprophylaxis is urgently needed for protection against ETEC diarrhea

Although ETEC causes disease in children as well as adults, the clinical features differ in the two age groups. In children, the disease is of a less severe nature, while adults may suffer from severe dehydrating illness requiring intravenous fluid replacement and hospital admission. This may be a dose-related factor since the severity of disease is known to be related to the amount of bacteria ingested (Levine et al., 1979).

Environmental Factors Accentuating the Spread of ETEC Infections

Like *V. cholerae*, ETEC is also prevalent in the environment. Poor public health facilities and a lack of knowledge concerning health and sanitation have led to ETEC's endemicity in less developed regions of the world (Fig. 3); improvement of water and sanitation facilities, however, results in a decrease in infections as is seen in developed countries (Sack, 1978). On a global view, however, the prevalence of ETEC has remained much unchanged over the last 30 years (Qadri et al., 2005a,b). In addition to this, surface water in both urban and rural sites in developing countries has become highly contaminated by ETEC (Begum et al., 2005; Black et al., 1989; Rowland, 1986). This presumably is due to the contamination of surface water with sewage and fecal material (Ohno et al., 1997). ETEC can also be isolated from food, including weaning infant products (Rao et al., 2003; Ohno et al., 1997; Sack et al., 1977; Reis et al., 1980). A comparison carried out on ETEC strains isolated from clinical specimens and environmental water sources in Bangladesh has suggested that the two have a similar distribution of O-antigenic serogroups and phenotypic and genotypic characteristics (Begum et al., 2005). Clones detected in the environment were also isolated from the stools of patients and showed similar antibiotic resistance patterns (Begum et al., 2005, 2006). These results have shown that ETEC is as prevalent in surface water sources in Bangladesh as it is in clinical samples, thus showing the reason for the endemicity of this pathogen in Bangladesh.

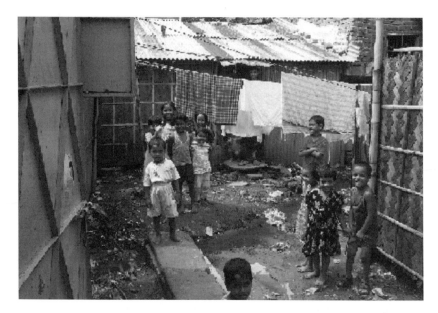

Fig. 3 An area in Dhaka city found to be highly endemic for ETEC diarrhea

Pathogenesis of ETEC

ETEC is a lactose fermenting *E. coli* and is a multivalent pathogen belonging to a variety of serogroups (over 100 O-antigenic serotypes have been identified thus far) (Rao et al., 2003; Wolf, 1997) (Fig. 4). It can express other plasmid encoded factors, including one or two types of enterotoxins (ST, heat stable toxin; LT, heat labile enterotoxin), of which there are a few different subtypes (Steinsland et al., 2003). A single strain of ETEC may express ST, LT, or both (Svennerholm and Holmgren, 1978; Svennerholm et al., 1977). Both ST- and LT-ETEC strains cause clinical disease; however, more severe disease is associated with ST-ETECs (either as ST alone or together with ST and LT) (Qadri et al., 2000; Black et al., 1981; Sack et al., 1975). Over 25 adhesive protein antigens that help anchor the pathogen to receptors on the enterocytes in the gut and then exert their secretory phenotype have been identified (Svennerholm and Savarino, 2004; Rao et al., 2005).

Since ST is not immunogenic, protection from its strains is derived by inhibiting the binding of the CHs to the mucosal enterocytes. It is fortunate that the majority of the CFs that are commonly seen in clinical disease are expressed on ST or ST/LT expressing strains, for this allows protective strategies to be based on CFs for the ST producing strains, which make up roughly 50% of clinical strains (Svennerholm and Steele, 2004) and which can further increase during diarrheal epidemics (Qadri et al., 2005a,b). Although about 50–60% of the ETEC strains isolated from patients with diarrhea express one or more CFs, these have not been identified in all strains. The fact that both CF-positive and negative ETEC strains are able to cause diarrhea

Fig. 4 Electron micrograph of ETEC
(strain H10407) showing colonization
factor antigens (CFs) on the surface
(courtesy: Fleckenstein JM/www.
utmem.edu)

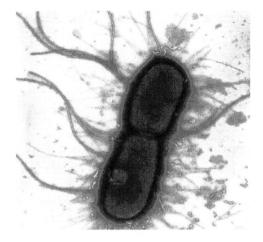

suggests that more unidentified virulence factors may exist. It is also possible that
phenotypic expression is lost on laboratory culture, and genotypic methods that
detect specific virulence genes (Steinsland et al., 2003) may be able to provide a
better understanding of the factors necessary for pathogenesis (Svennerholm et al.,
1977, 1984). New studies are currently striving to achieve a better understanding
of the antigens that are produced during in vivo conditions, but which may be lost
on subculture.

The colonization factors of ETEC are believed to be important antigens contributing to antibacterial immunity. The virulence determinants of pathogenic bacteria
are known not to be necessarily constitutively expressed; thus the identification of
protective immunity cannot solely rely on studies of organisms that have been
grown in vitro (Taylor et al., 1987; Maurelli, 1989). *Vibrio cholerae* O1 has been
shown to express genes and proteins during growth in the adult rabbit intestine
(Jonson et al., 1989, 1991). Comparative genomic analysis by transcriptional
profiling of the pathogen in stool and in vomitus specimens from cholera patients
has shown that passage through the human host leads to an expression of genes
different from that expressed under laboratory condition; this expression also leads
to a hyperinfectious state after passage through humans as well as when it is repli-
cated in the infant mice model (Merrell et al., 2002; Alam et al., 2005). Thus, ETEC
may also express antigens under in vivo growth conditions, which are different
from those expressed under *in vitro, laboratory-cultured* bacteria. There remains a
need to understand the physiology of ETEC during infections, the pathogenic
mechanisms they employ at each stage of infection, and the genes or antigens that
are expressed or down-regulated during this process. Studies are underway to study
mRNA for such antigens using molecular biological techniques including QCRT-
PCR as well as microarray procedures to evaluate whether additional virulence
factors can be detected on ETEC isolated directly from the stool without subcultur-
ing, in comparison to the same bacteria cultured in the laboratory (Qadri and
Svennerholm; ongoing studies).

Disease Burden due to ETEC in Children in Asia

Diarrheal diseases can cause five deaths per 1,000 annually among children below 5 years of age in high endemic regions of the world (Kosek et al., 2003). Although there has been a general decrease in diarrheal disease mortality, overall morbidity and frequent infection remain very high (Guerrant et al., 2005). ETEC morbidity data from developing countries have suggested that the pathogen can be identified in 11–18% of children less than 3 years of age (Huilan et al., 1991). The prevalence of ETEC among children in developing countries has remained consistent over the 30 years since its identification (Qadri et al., 2005b). In Bangladesh, both hospital and community-based surveillance have shown ETEC to be isolated from around 18% of diarrheal stools of young children. The mortality due to ETEC diarrhea in Bangladesh can be estimated to be around 45,000, based on a population of 140 million people of whom about 12% are less than 5 years of age (UNICEF, 2004). Extrapolating this figure to Asia (with a population 30 times larger), one may expect that five million of 400 million children in the under-five age range will suffer from one or more episodes of ETEC diarrhea; figures in other areas of the world such as Africa and South America will be comparable. Mortality figures will also be high. Since ETEC is a pathogen that causes dehydrating disease in adults, these figures can be expected to be higher if all age groups are taken into consideration. These data demonstrate the importance of determining the epidemiology, immunology, and global burden of ETEC disease.

ETEC is the Most Common Cause of Diarrhea in Young Children

It has been estimated that seven to eight episodes of diarrhea may occur annually in children in the developing world; of these, at least two to four attacks may be due to ETEC (Rao et al., 2003; Black, 1993; Qadri et al., 2006). Natural ETEC infection is protective as the incidence of disease decreases by 3 years of age (Qadri et al., 2000). Multiple infections with strains producing different CF antigens are likely needed for a broad protective immunity against ETEC diarrhea (Levine, 1990). In longitudinal studies in communities, ETEC has been found to be the primary cause of diarrhea in infants. In about 50% of children in birth cohorts that have been actively followed, ETEC was the most common cause of disease (Rao et al., 2003; Qadri et al., 2006). In these studies, the incidence of ETEC diarrhea ranged from 1.5 to 2.3 episodes per child-year and has been found to be more common than rotavirus diarrhea, (Anh et al., 2006; Hsu et al., 2005; Unicomb et al., 1997). ETEC infections can also spread within family groups (Black et al., 1981) and not uncommonly from adults to children. Infants can also infect care providers, a transmission factor which may play a role in perpetuating the vicious fecal–oral cycle in households and communities. ETEC infection has been documented to spread to 11% of contacts in a 10-day study period in a household with poor socio-economic status and living conditions (Black et al., 1981). Thus, attempts to decrease transmission of ETEC in the community may also induce herd protection and decrease the prevalence of both disease and asymptomatic infections (Ali et al., 2005).

The frequent episodes of ETEC diarrhea in the first few years of a child's life are not only of short-term consequence, it also leads to faltering growth, growth retardation, and stunting (Ali et al., 2005; Black et al., 1984; Mata, 1992). Frequent diarrheal diseases and infections, as well as the effect of co-morbidity due to other tropical illnesses, have long-term consequences on the protective immune response to pathogens and may also have an impact on the growth, physical, and cognitive development of children (Guerrant et al., 2002).

ETEC as a Causative Agent of Dehydrating Secretory Diarrhea Resembling *Cholera gravis* in Adults

ETEC, although a common cause of childhood diarrhea, also causes acute dehydrating disease in adults (Qadri et al., 2005a,b). It must be considered that ETEC diarrhea in adults has only been reported from a few countries (including India (Sen et al., 1984), Bangladesh (Qadri et al., 2000), and Indonesia (Subekti et al., 2003; Oyofo et al., 2001)) or from adults who travel to ETEC endemic countries. ETEC infection in adults requires medical treatment and is second only to *V. cholerae* in causing severe diarrhea in this age group. It is also particularly common in people 65 years of age and older (Faruque et al., 2004). The basis for the difference in the severity of illness between adults and children is unknown. One reason may be that the dose of bacteria that an adult ingests is much higher than that of a young child, thus leading to the severity of differences which are known to be related to the dosage (Levine et al., 1979). However, during failures in public health facilities, such as those seen during natural disasters, children may also be infected with high doses of bacteria. This may explain why 40% of children with ETEC diarrhea were admitted with more severe dehydrating disease during natural crises than usual (Qadri et al., 2005a,b; Levine et al., 1979).

ETEC Diarrhea in Travelers to Asia

ETEC is the most common cause of travelers' diarrhea and is responsible for one-third to one-half of all episodes among travelers to Asia, Africa, and Latin America (Svennerholm and Steele, 2004). ETEC also causes diarrhea in travelers more often in warm seasons rather than in cool seasons and the rate of disease varies depending on the country visited and its endemicity of ETEC. Furthermore, transmission of ETEC has been reported on cruise ships, suggesting that contaminated food is a potential source of infection (Daniels et al., 2000). Travelers are as susceptible to ETEC infections as children are; however, after residing in ETEC endemic countries for a number of years, travelers develop protective immunity and show decreased attack rates (DuPont et al., 1976).

Treatment for ETEC Diarrhea and Antimicrobial Resistance Pattern

In hospitalized settings in developing countries, it may not be possible to carry out diagnosis for ETEC, in which case treatment for patients is similar to that for cholera caused by *V. cholerae*, since the symptoms in both diseases are similar: patients may suffer from mild to severe dehydration with both vomiting and secretory diarrhea (Black et al., 1981; Sack et al., 1975). Fluid replacement is provided via either intravenous or oral rehydration therapy, depending on the severity of the dehydration status.

Antibiotics are generally used in health centers to decrease the duration of illness, especially during epidemics when limited treatment facilities are available; however, recent data suggest that approximately 82% of the strains are resistant to drugs, including ampicillin, co-trimoxazole, doxycycline, and erythromycin and 25% show multiple antibiotic resistance which are commonly used for treatment of secretory diarrhea (Begum et al., 2005). Reports of resistance to ciprofloxacin and other flouroquinolones are also emerging from India, Japan, (Chakraborty et al., 2001; Matsushita et al., 2001), and Bangladesh (Qadri et al. unpublished data). This is a matter of concern not only for patients who may have better access to rehydration therapy, but also for travelers who use these antibiotics as prophylactic to prevent diarrhea.

The use of ETEC-specific phages as therapeutic agents to control infections and disease is also being considered (Skurnik and Strauch, 2006). Hyperimmune bovine colostrum containing colonization factor-specific antibodies has been tested as an alternative measure for protection from ETEC (Freedman et al., 1998). Therapeutic benefits of such interventions are limited in children with ETEC diarrhea and in human challenge models. These strategies may not be effective as preventive measures (Casswall et al., 2000; Tacket et al., 1999).

Prevention of ETEC Diarrhea

Since ETEC is a multivalent pathogen and can express many different colonization factors, a child can suffer from numerous diarrheal episodes from a variety of ETEC strains in the first 2–3 years of life (Rao et al., 2003; Steinsland et al., 2002; Qadri et al., to be published). This makes the disease problematic to control by immunoprophylactic measures (Svennerholm and Steele, 2004). Intense efforts are being made for the development of ETEC vaccines, which include oral subunit vaccines, attenuated strains produced by recombinant procedures, as well as antigens administered by the transcutaneous route. Among these, the oral whole cell killed heptavalent ETEC vaccine, containing a toxoid antigen together with five strains expressing six different colonization factors, has been tested in Phase I–III trials in various continents and countries with different age groups as well as with adult travelers (Qadri et al., 2005b; Svennerholm and Savarino, 2004). This vaccine was designed based on the observation that the oral whole killed cell cholera vaccine containing the B subunit of cholera toxin provided protection to cholera as well to ETEC diarrhea (Clemens et al., 1988). The ETEC vaccine was immunogenic in clinical trials and provided protection to North American travelers in Mexico and Guatemala from severe or moderate disease, (Svennerholm and Savarino, 2004; Svennerholm and Steele, 2004) but was found not protecting young children in Egypt from diarrhea. New and improved vaccines are under investigation and are being produced based on the experience over the past decade of the requisites for a protective vaccine from the standpoint of both developing and developed country needs.

Conclusions

ETEC is the most common cause of bacteria-induced acute watery diarrhea in children in developing countries, including those in Asia. The pathogen is endemic in these settings and peaks during seasonal epidemics, as well as during natural disasters such as floods. It may be expected that, of 400 million children in the under-five year age range in Asia, five million will suffer from one or more episodes of ETEC diarrhea. The prevalence of ETEC among children in developing countries has remained consistent over the 30 years since it was first studied. The bacteria have multiple virulence attributes, which are primarily plasmid mediated and include enterotoxins as well as different protein adhesion factors that are mostly fimbrial in nature. ETEC can be isolated from diarrheal patients as well as from healthy individuals and is prevalent in surface water samples, suggesting the fecal oral route as a possible source of disease transmission. The bacteria, although a common cause of diarrhea in children under 3 years of age, cause dehydrating cholera-like illness in adults. During floods, ETEC diarrhea in children is of more severe disease intensity than at other times, and has a relatively higher content of colonization factors and ST-enterotoxin phenotype on its strains. Emerging antimicrobial drug resistance elevates the need for prevention of the disease by the use of protective vaccines. Immunoprophylaxis is needed not only to decrease the mortality rate, but more importantly to decrease the overall morbidity related to frequent ETEC infections. An optimal vaccine has yet to be licensed, although intense efforts are being carried out through various strategies.

Acknowledgment This work was supported by the International Centre for Diarrhoeal Disease Research, Bangladesh (ICDDR,B): Centre for Health and Population Research. We acknowledge with gratitude the commitment of the Swedish Agency for Research and Economic Cooperation (Sida-SAREC)) to the Center's research efforts.

References

Alam, A., et al. (2005). Hyperinfectivity of human-passaged *Vibrio cholerae* can be modeled by growth in the infant mouse. *Infect Immun*, 73, 6674–6679

Albert, M.J., et al. (1999). Case–control study of enteropathogens associated with childhood diarrhea in Dhaka, Bangladesh. *J Clin Microbiol*, 37, 3458–3464

Ali, M., et al. (2005). Herd immunity conferred by killed oral cholera vaccines in Bangladesh: A reanalysis. *Lancet*, 366, 44–49

Anh, D.D., et al. (2006). The burden of rotavirus diarrhea in Khanh Hoa Province, Vietnam: Baseline assessment for a rotavirus vaccine trial. *Pediatr Infect Dis J*, 25, 37–40

Bangladesh Disaster & Emergency Response DER Sub-Group, UNDP Bangladesh. (2004). *Monsoon Floods 2004 – Draft Assessment Report*. 28 July 2004, Dhaka, Bangladesh

Begum, Y.A., et al. (2005). Enterotoxigenic *Escherichia coli* isolated from surface water in urban and rural Bangladesh. *J Clin Microbio*, 43, 3582–3583

Begum, Y.A., Talukder, K.A., Nair, G.B., Khan, S.I., Svennerholm, A.M., Sack, R.B., Qadri, F. (2007). Comparison of enterotoxigenic *Escherichia coli* isolated from surface water and diarrheal stool samples in Bangladesh. *Can J Microbiol*, 53, 19–26 (submitted)

Black, R.E. (1993). Epidemiology of diarrhoeal disease: Implications for control by vaccines. *Vaccine*, 11, 100–106

Black, R.E., et al. (1981). Enterotoxigenic *Escherichia coli* diarrhoea: Acquired immunity and transmission in an endemic area. *Bull World Health Organ*, 59, 263–268

Black, R.E., Brown, K.H., Becker, S. (1984). Effects of diarrhea associated with specific enteropathogens on the growth of children in rural Bangladesh. *Pediatrics*, 73, 799–805

Black, R.E., et al. (1989). Incidence and etiology of infantile diarrhea and major routes of transmission in Huascar, Peru. *Am J Epidemiol*, 129, 785–799

Carpenter, C.C., et al. (1965). Clinical and physiological observations during an epidemic outbreak of non-*Vibrio cholera*-like disease in Calcutta. *Bull World Health Organ*, 33, 665–671

Casswall, T.H., et al. (2000). Treatment of enterotoxigenic and enteropathogenic *Escherichia coli*-induced diarrhoea in children with bovine immunoglobulin milk concentrate from hyperimmunized cows: A double-blind, placebo-controlled, clinical trial. *Scand J Gastroenterol*, 35, 711–718

Chakraborty, S., et al. (2001). Concomitant infection of enterotoxigenic *Escherichia coli* in an outbreak of cholera caused by *Vibrio cholerae* O1 and O139 in Ahmedabad, India. *J Clin Microbiol*, 39, 3241–3246

Chibani-Chennoufi, S., et al. (2004). Isolation of *Escherichia coli* bacteriophages from the stool of pediatric diarrhea patients in Bangladesh. *J Bacteriol*, 186, 8287–8294

Clemens, J.D., et al. (1988). Cross-protection by B subunit-whole cell cholera vaccine against diarrhea associated with heat-labile toxin-producing enterotoxigenic *Escherichia coli*: Results of a large-scale field trial. *J Infect Dis*, 158, 372–377

Daniels, N.A., et al. (2000). Traveler's diarrhea at sea: Three outbreaks of waterborne enterotoxigenic *Escherichia coli* on cruise ships. *J Infect Dis*, 181, 1491–1495

DuPont, H.L., et al. (1976). Comparative susceptibility of latin American and United States students to enteric pathogens. *N Engl J Med*, 295, 1520–1521

Faruque, A.S., et al. (2004). Diarrhoea in elderly people: Aetiology, and clinical characteristics. *Scand J Infect Dis*, 36, 204–208

Faruque, S.M., et al. (2005a). Seasonal epidemics of cholera inversely correlate with the prevalence of environmental cholera phages. *Proc Natl Acad Sci USA*, 102, 1702–1707

Faruque, S.M., et al. (2005b). Self-limiting nature of seasonal cholera epidemics: Role of host-mediated amplification of phage. *Proc Natl Acad Sci USA*, 102, 6119–6124

Freedman, D.J., et al. (1998). Milk immunoglobulin with specific activity against purified colonization factor antigens can protect against oral challenge with enterotoxigenic *Escherichia coli*. *J Infect Dis*, 177, 662–667

Guerrant, R.L., et al. (2002). Magnitude and impact of diarrheal diseases. *Arch Med Res*, 33, 351–355

Guerrant, R.L., et al. (2005). Global impact of diarrheal diseases that are sampled by travelers: The rest of the hippopotamus. *Clin Infect Dis*, 41 Suppl 8, S524–S530

Hsu, V.P., et al. (2005). Estimates of the burden of rotavirus disease in Malaysia. *J Infect Dis*, 192 Suppl 1, S80–S86

Huilan, S., et al. (1991). Etiology of acute diarrhoea among children in developing countries: A multicentre study in five countries. *Bull World Health Organ*, 69, 549–555

ICDDRB. (2004). Documenting effects of the July–August floods of 2004 and ICDDR,B's response, vol. 2

Jonson, G., Holmgren, J., Svennerholm, A.M. (1991). Epitope differences in toxin-coregulated pili produced by classical and El Tor *Vibrio cholerae* O1. *Microb Pathog*, 11, 179–188

Jonson, G., Svennerholm, A.M., Holmgren, J. (1989). *Vibrio cholerae* expresses cell surface antigens during intestinal infection which are not expressed during in vitro culture. *Infect Immun*, 57, 1809–1815

Kosek, M., Bern, C., Guerrant, R.L. (2003). The global burden of diarrhoeal disease, as estimated from studies published between 1992 and 2000. *Bull World Health Organ*, 81, 197–204

Levine, M.M. (1990). Modern vaccines. Enteric infections. *Lancet*, 335, 958–961

Levine, M.M., et al. (1979). Immunity to enterotoxigenic *Escherichia coli*. *Infect Immun*, 23, 729–736

Mata, L. (1992). Diarrheal disease as a cause of malnutrition. *Am J Trop Med Hyg*, 47, 16–27

Matsushita, S., et al. (2001). Increasing fluoroquinolone low-sensitivity in enterotoxigenic *Escherichia coli* isolated from diarrhea of overseas travelers in Tokyo. *Kansenshogaku Zasshi*, 75, 785–791

Maurelli, A.T. (1989). Temperature regulation of virulence genes in pathogenic bacteria: A general strategy for human pathogens? *Microb Pathog*, 7, 1–10

Merrell, D.S., et al. (2002). Host-induced epidemic spread of the cholera bacterium. *Nature*, 417, 642–645

Nataro, J.P., Kaper, J.B. (1998). Diarrheagenic *Escherichia coli*. *Clin Microbiol Rev*, 11, 142–201

Ohno, A., et al. (1997). Enteropathogenic bacteria in the La Paz River of Bolivia. *Am J Trop Med Hyg*, 57, 438–444

Oyofo, B.A., et al. (2001). Toxins and colonization factor antigens of enterotoxigenic *Escherichia coli* among residents of Jakarta, Indonesia. *Am J Trop Med Hyg*, 65, 120–124

Qadri, F., et al. (2000). Prevalence of toxin types and colonization factors in enterotoxigenic *Escherichia coli* isolated during a 2-year period from diarrheal patients in Bangladesh. *J Clin Microbiol*, 38, 27–31

Qadri, F., et al. (2005a). Enterotoxigenic *Escherichia coli* and *Vibrio cholerae* diarrhea, Bangladesh, 2004. *Emerg Infect Dis*, 11, 1104–1107

Qadri, F., et al. (2005b). Enterotoxigenic *Escherichia coli* in developing countries: Epidemiology, microbiology, clinical features, treatment, and prevention. *Clin Microbiol Rev*, 18, 465–483

Qadri, F.S., Ahmed, T., Begum, Y.A., Svennerholm, A.M. (2006). *Enterotoxigenic Escherichia coli (ETEC) is a major cause of acute watery diarrhea in children in Bangladesh*. In Program and Abstract of 8th CAPGAN. Dhaka, Bangladesh

Rao, M.R., et al. (2003). High disease burden of diarrhea due to enterotoxigenic *Escherichia coli* among rural Egyptian infants and young children. *J Clin Microbiol*, 41, 4862–4864

Rao, M.R., et al. (2005). Serologic correlates of protection against enterotoxigenic *Escherichia coli* diarrhea. *J Infect Dis*, 191, 562–570

Reis, M.H., Vasconcelos, J.C., Trabulsi, L.R. (1980). Prevalence of enterotoxigenic *Escherichia coli* in some processed raw food from animal origin. *Appl Environ Microbiol*, 39, 270–271

Rowland, M.G. (1986). The Gambia and Bangladesh: The seasons and diarrhoea. *Dialogue Diarrhoea*, 26, 3

Sack, R.B. (1978). The epidemiology of diarrhea due to enterotoxigenic *Escherichia coli. J Infect Dis*, 137, 639–640

Sack, R.B., et al. (1975). Enterotoxigenic *Escherichia-coli*-associated diarrheal disease in Apache children. *N Engl J Med*, 292, 1041–1045

Sack, R.B., et al. (1977). Enterotoxigenic *Escherichia coli* isolated from food. *J Infect Dis*, 135, 313–317

Sack, R.B., et al. (2003). A 4-year study of the epidemiology of *Vibrio cholerae* in four rural areas of Bangladesh. *J Infect Dis*, 187, 96–101

Sanchez, J., Holmgren, J. (2005). Virulence factors, pathogenesis and vaccine protection in cholera and ETEC diarrhea. *Curr Opin Immunol*, 17, 388–398

Schwartz, B.S., Harris, J.B., Khan, A.I., Larocque, R.C., Sack, D.A., Malek, M.A., Faruque, A. S.G., Qadri, F., Calderwood, S.B., Luby, S.P., Ryan, E.T. (2006). Diarrheal epidemics in Dhaka, Bangladesh during three consecutive floods-1988, 1998, and 2004. *Am J Trop Med Hyg*, 74, 1067–1073.

SDNP, *World Environment Day 2005: SDNP Bangladesh. www.sdnpbd.org/sdi/international_days/wed/2005/bangladesh/index.htm.* 2005.

Sen, D., et al. (1984). Studies on *Escherichia coli* as a cause of acute diarrhoea in Calcutta. *J Med Microbiol*, 17, 53–58

Skurnik, M., Strauch, E. (2006). Phage therapy: Facts and fiction. *Int J Med Microbiol*, 296, 5–14

Steinsland, H., et al. (2002). Enterotoxigenic *Escherichia coli* infections and diarrhea in a cohort of young children in Guinea-Bissau. *J Infect Dis*, 186, 1740–1747

Steinsland, H., et al. (2003). Development and evaluation of genotypic assays for the detection and characterization of enterotoxigenic *Escherichia coli. Diagn Microbiol Infect Dis*, 45, 97–105

Subekti, D.S., et al. (2003). Prevalence of enterotoxigenic *Escherichia coli* (ETEC) in hospitalized acute diarrhea patients in Denpasar, Bali, Indonesia. *Diagn Microbiol Infect Dis*, 47, 399–405

Svennerholm, A.M., Holmgren, J. (1978). Identification of *Escherichia coli* heat-labile enterotoxin by means of a ganglioside immunosorbent assay (GM1-ELISA) procedure. *Curr Microbiol*, 1, 19–23

Svennerholm, A.M., Savarino, S.J. (2004). *Oral inactivated whole cell B subunit combination vaccine against enterotoxigenic Escherichia coli,* 3rd edition. New Generation Vaccines, Levine MM, (ed.). Marcel Decker, New York, pp. 737–750

Svennerholm, A.M., Steele, D. (2004). Progress in enteric vaccine development. *Best Pract Res Clin Gastroenterol*, 18, 421–445

Svennerholm, A.M., Back, E., Holmgren, J. (1977). Enterotoxin antibodies in relation to diarrhoea in Swedish soldiers in Cyprus. *Bull World Health Organ*, 55, 663–668

Svennerholm, A.M., et al. (1984). Local and systemic antibody responses and immunological memory in humans after immunization with cholera B subunit by different routes. *Bull World Health Organ*, 62, 909–918

Tacket, C.O., et al. (1999). Lack of prophylactic efficacy of an enteric-coated bovine hyperimmune milk product against enterotoxigenic *Escherichia coli* challenge administered during a standard meal. *J Infect Dis*, 180, 2056–2059

Taylor, R.K., et al. (1987). Use of phoA gene fusions to identify a pilus colonization factor coordinately regulated with cholera toxin. *Proc Natl Acad Sci USA*, 84, 2833–2837

The International Federation of Red Cross and Red Crescent Societies. (2004). Bangladesh: Floods. (web page: http://www.ifrc.org)

UNICEF, *Bangladesh Statistics. Unicef (Web page: www.unicef.org/infobycountry/bangladesh_bangladesh_statistics.html).* 2004.

Unicomb, L.E., et al. (1997). Anticipating rotavirus vaccines: Hospital-based surveillance for rotavirus diarrhea and estimates of disease burden in Bangladesh. *Pediatr Infect Dis J*, 16, 947–951.

United Nations, Economic and Social Commission for Asia and the Pasific (UN-ESCAP). (1999) *Urban Geology of Dhaka, Bangladesh: Atlas of Urban Geology,* vol. 11

Wenneras, C., Erling, V. (2004). Prevalence of enterotoxigenic *Escherichia coli*-associated diarrhoea and carrier state in the developing world. *J Health Popul Nutr*, 22, 370–382

WHO. (1999). New frontiers in the development of vaccines against enterotoxigenic (ETEC) and enterohaemorrhagic (EHEC) *E. coli* infections. *Weekly Epidemiol Rec*, 13, 98–100; WHO. (2004). Floods Situation Report, 26 July 2004

Wolf, M.K. (1997). Occurrence, distribution, and associations of O and H serogroups, colonization factor antigens, and toxins of enterotoxigenic *Escherichia coli*. *Clin Microbiol Rev*, 10, 569–584

Human Cases of Hemorrhagic Fever in Saudi Arabia Due To a Newly Discovered Flavivirus, Alkhurma Hemorrhagic Fever Virus

Remi N. Charrel, Xavier de Lamballerie, and Ali Mohamed Zaki

Arboviruses in Saudi Arabia

Few studies on arthropod-borne viruses in Saudi Arabia have been published. One study on dengue fever confirmed the circulation of three dengue serotypes in Jeddah in 2001 (Fakeeh and Zaki, 2001). Kadam virus, an atypical tick-borne flavivirus, was discovered in Uganda and then isolated in Saudi Arabia from Ixodidae ticks, but so far has not been associated with human or animal diseases (Henderson et al., 1970; Wood et al., 1982). Other arboviruses, such as Sindbis virus, Crimean-Congo hemorrhagic fever virus, Rift Valley fever virus, Bluetongue virus, and Akabane virus, have been reported on several occasions. Because of the studies conducted during the last decade on a novel virus that causes hemorrhagic fever in humans, Alkhurma hemorrhagic fever virus (AHFV) has become the most intensely studied arbovirus in Saudi Arabia. Nonetheless, many aspects of the ecology, epidemiology, and human and veterinary impact of AHFV remain to be determined and merit further study.

Discovery of Alkhurma Hemorrhagic Fever Virus (AHFV)

The genus *Flavivirus* includes 70 viruses, of which 40 have been reported to infect humans. Flavivirus infections in humans cause a wide array of clinical syndromes, including encephalitis, severe hepatitis, and hemorrhagic fevers. Hemorrhagic fevers are caused by yellow fever virus in Africa and South America; dengue virus in Central and South America, Africa, India, Southeast Asia, and the Western Pacific; Omsk hemorrhagic fever virus in Russia; and Kyasanur forest disease virus in India. A novel flavivirus, causing hemorrhagic fever with a mortality rate around 30% (Charrel et al., 2005), was discovered in September 1995 in Saudi Arabia by Dr. Ali Mohammed Zaki and his colleagues with the help of scientists at the U.S. Centers for Disease Control and Prevention (CDC) in Atlanta. The virus, initially named Alkhurma virus [and later Alkhurma hemorrhagic fever virus (AHFV)], was first isolated at the virology laboratory of Dr. Suleiman Fakeeh Hospital in Jeddah, Saudi Arabia, from the blood of a man who experienced fatal viral hemorrhagic fever.

Y. Lu et al. (eds.), *Emerging Infections in Asia.*
© Springer Science+Business Media, LLC 2008

179

The patient, a 32-year-old male butcher, worked in Mecca, which is 50 miles from Jeddah. The patient was initially diagnosed by another laboratory as having Crimean-Congo hemorrhagic fever (CCHF) based on the results of an indirect immunofluorescence assay (IFA). However, in Dr. Zaki's laboratory CCHF virus-specific IgM was not detected using an IgM capture enzyme-linked immunosorbent assay (ELISA), indicating a possible past but not acute CCHF virus infection. Subsequently, the patient's serum was used to inoculate adult mice intraperitoneally and Vero cells. The adult mice died in about 1 week with spastic paralysis. At autopsy, the brain tissue of the mice was very congested and macroscopically hemorrhagic. The brain tissue was suspended in 10% cell culture medium and injected into suckling mice after filtration through 0.22 μm filters; the suckling mice in turn died with tremors and convulsions. Mouse brain suspension was prepared and used to infect Vero cells. A cytopathogenic effect characterized by rounding, shrinkage, and floating cells was observed within 5–10 days, although only part of the monolayer was involved. Infected cells were tested by indirect IFA with monoclonal antibodies specific for Rift Valley fever virus, CCHF virus, dengue virus, yellow fever virus, and a monoclonal antibody reacting with all flaviviruses. Only the latter provided positive results. Sequencing with primers located in the NS5 region of the genome resulted in a sequence that was most closely related to, but distinct from, Kyasanur Forest disease virus – a tick-borne flavivirus, identified in 1957, causing hemorrhagic fever in certain regions of India (Work et al., 1957).

Subsequently, several blood samples collected from patients who died of hemorrhagic fever that was assumed to be caused by dengue virus were inoculated into mice and processed as aforementioned. These samples yielded additional AHFV isolates, identified by either the generic *Flavivirus* monoclonal antibody or polyclonal mouse sera induced by the prototype isolate.

An IgM capture ELISA was developed using inactivated crude mouse brain antigen (prepared from the first AHFV isolate) and *Flavivirus* monoclonal antibody peroxidase conjugate. AHFV-infected Vero cells were used for ELISA detection of specific IgG. Both ELISA assays were subsequently used for serological diagnosis of AHFV. ELISA analysis of 200 human sera referred by the veterinary laboratory at the Ministry of Agriculture resulted in the detection of 20 IgM-positive samples and 40 IgG-positive samples. Storage at inappropriate temperature precluded virus isolation from this material. A seroconversion (rise in IgM titer and IgG appearance in the second specimen) was observed in samples from a worker at the Jeddah Zoo who presented with hemorrhagic fever and encephalitis. At the present time, a total of 16 cases have been confirmed by virus isolation (of which 11 were reported (Charrel et al., 2005)), and 24 probable cases detected by serology (IgM or seroconversion) (Zaki, personal data).

The full-length genome of the prototype strain of AHFV was sequenced (Charrel et al., 2001). Large regions of the envelope, NS3 and NS5 genes, were sequenced from 11 human isolates and one tick isolate, and aligned with reference sequences from closely related flaviviruses (Fig. 1). Based on these alignments, a semi-nested reverse transcription polymerase chain reaction (RT-PCR) was developed. This RT-PCR assay is now routinely used to diagnose AHFV infection in serum or whole blood from patients presenting with hemorrhagic fever.

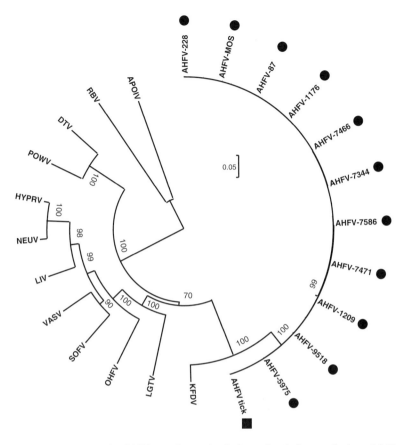

Fig. 1 Phylogenetic analysis of Alkhurma hemorrhagic fever virus isolates and selected tickborne flaviviruses based on a 2097-nucleotide (nt) sequence constituted by the colinearization of Envelope, NS3, and NS5 sequences (699, 713, and 685 nt, respectively). Flavivirus acronyms as determined by the International Committee on Taxonomy of Viruses: AHFV, Alkhurma Hemorrgaic fever virus; KFDV, Kyasanur Forest disease virus; LGTV, Langat virus; OHFV, Omsk Hemorrhagic fever virus; SOFV, Tick-borne encephalitis virus strain Sofin; VASV, Tick-borne encephalitis virus strain Vasilchenko; HYPRV, Tick-borne encephalitis virus strain Hypr; NEUV, Tick-borne encephalitis virus strain Neudorfl; LIV, Louping ill virus; POWV, Powassan virus; DTV, Deer-tick virus; RBV, Rio Bravo virus; APOIV, Apoi virus. Distances and groupings were determined by the Jukes–Cantor algorithm and neighbor-joining method with the MEGA 2.1 software program. Bootstrap values are indicated and correspond to 500 replications. *Closed circle*, strains isolated from human samples; *closed square*, strain isolated from tick

Routes of Transmission and Risk Factors for AHFV Infection

Tick-Vectored Transmission

Until recently, evidence of tick-mediated transmission of AHFV to man was scarce. Clues that the virus could be tick-vectored were based on (1) the report of two cases, in which the patients (one engineer and one student) reported a history of tick

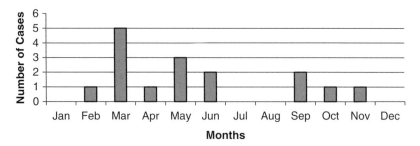

Fig. 2 Monthly distribution of 16 laboratory-confirmed cases of AHFV

bite before the onset of clinical symptoms (Charrel et al., 2005); (2) the topology of the phylogenetic tree with AHFV clustering together with the flaviviruses vectored by ticks (Charrel et al., 2001, 2005; Lin et al., 2003); and (3) two peaks of frequency corresponding to tick activity (Charrel et al., 2005, 2006) (Fig. 2). More recently, AHFV was isolated from a tick collected in Saudi Arabia near Jeddah; the tick was identified as *Ornithodoros savignyi* by morphologic keys (Charrel et al., 2007). This finding constitutes the first direct evidence of the tick-borne nature of AHFV. More extensive studies of ticks in Saudi Arabia are needed to determine the range of tick species hosting AHFV, the prevalence of infected ticks, and the geographic and seasonal distribution of potential AHFV vectors.

Occupational Exposure to AHFV

A majority of AHFV cases that required admission to the hospital have occurred in patients occupationally exposed to sheep and camel blood during butchering activities. This risk factor for AHFV has been documented in multiple studies (Zaki, 1997; Charrel et al., 2005; Madani, 2005; Zaki, 2002, 2004). Whether sheep or camels can be considered natural viral reservoirs is unknown. No new disease affecting sheep and camels has been reported in Saudi Arabia, and inoculation of AHFV into sheep did not cause any overt disease (Zaki, unpublished data). To date, direct contact with infected blood appears to be associated with a high risk of AHFV infection in humans. This route of infection has been reported for another tick-borne flavivirus, the Omsk hemorrhagic fever virus, which is principally transmitted to man through direct contact with muskrats (*Ondatra zibethica*), and usually occurs during the hunting season from September to October (Belov et al., 1995). Of 165 cases of Omsk hemorrhagic fever virus recorded between 1988 and 1997, only 10 were possibly transmitted by the classic route (tick bite) (Busygin, 2000).

Consumption of Raw Milk

Interviews with 11 AHFV-infected patients revealed three cases that may be associated with drinking raw milk from camels (Charrel et al., 2005). Consumption of raw milk has been associated with the transmission of tick-borne encephalitis virus (TBEV) to humans (Gritsun et al., 2003; Gresikova et al., 1975). TBEV was repeatedly isolated from the milk of infected goats up to 25 days after collection, and TBEV can be maintained in unpasteurized milk products, such as yogurt, butter, and cheese. TBEV has been observed in gastric juice for up to 2 h after ingestion of such products (Pogodina, 1958), while pasteurization prevents milk-borne TBEV infection (Dumpis et al., 1999). Further studies should be conducted to confirm whether AHFV can also be transmitted via the consumption of unpasteurized milk products.

Other Hypothesized Routes of Transmission

There is no evidence of airborne transmission of AHFV. However, an airborne route of infection was demonstrated in animals with two flaviviruses that are typically mosquito borne: St. Louis Encephalitis and Japanese Encephalitis (Phillpotts et al., 1997; Larson et al., 1980).

Many mosquito-borne flaviviruses have been isolated in ticks, even though ticks do not play any significant role in the ecological cycle of these viruses in nature. Conversely, only Powassan virus, a tick-borne flavivirus, has been isolated in mosquitoes. The hypothesis that AHFV may be a mosquito-borne virus has been proposed (Madani, 2005), and merits investigation, but is not supported by strong scientific evidence at this stage (Charrel et al., 2006).

No cases of secondary human-to-human transmission of AHFV have been reported to date.

Hadj Pilgrimage

A sudden increase in population size can increase the risk of an outbreak of a transmissible viral disease. Tick-borne flavivirus infections are generally considered not transmissible from man to man. However, direct contact with the blood of an infected patient during the viremic stage could be a risk factor for transmission. Annually, some 2.5 million pilgrims congregate in the city of Mecca in Saudi Arabia to perform the Hajj (pilgrimage), a religious duty for all adult Muslims who are physically and financially able. The Hajj consists of several ceremonies, meant to symbolize the essential concepts of the Islamic faith, and to commemorate the trials of prophet Abraham and his family. During Hajj, the pilgrims sacrifice a sheep, reenacting the story of Abraham, who, in place of his son, sacrificed a sheep that God had provided as a substitute. The meat from the slaughtered sheep is distributed for consumption to family, friends, and poor and needy people in the community. Another rite of the Hajj is for males to shave their heads, although trimming the hair is also acceptable. Most will choose the former, often in make-shift shops run by opportunistic barbers. A razor blade is commonly used, and may be used on several scalps before ultimately being discarded. These practices pose obvious risks for blood-borne infections, such as HIV, and hepatitis B and C, especially considering that many pilgrims come from regions of the world where such infections are endemic. However, the risk of AHFV transmission by shaving a patient with recently acquired and viremic infection is lower than that for chronic infections such as HIV or hepatitis B and C.

Cattle Movements

Geographic displacement of cattle may also represent a risk for expanding the area of dissemination of AHFV through either animal-to-animal transmission or dissemination of ticks to a region previously unharmed by the virus. A similar scenario was shown to disseminate TBEV from Eastern to Western Europe. In addition, the large Saudi Arabian Rift valley fever virus outbreak in 2000 appears to have involved virus introduction from East Africa, based on the close ancestral relationship of a 1998 East African virus (Bird et al., 2006).

Clinical, Epidemiological, and Laboratory Characteristics of AHFV

To date, cases of AHFV infection in humans are characterized by severe to fatal disease. However, in the absence of large-scale studies, it is not possible to evaluate the range of disease caused by the virus. The clinical characteristics of 16 RT-PCR-confirmed cases of AHFV in Saudi Arabia are shown in Table 1 (11 of 16 cases were reported in Charrel et al. (2005) and the other five cases were reported by Dr. Zaki (unpublished data)). A substantial proportion of patients had both neurological and hemorrhagic manifestations. Central nervous system manifestations (encephalitis, convulsions, or coma) were recorded in the fatal cases. Since CNS manifestations have been reported to occur during AHF, it is necessary to perform clinical studies in patients presenting with CNS infections (meningitis, encephalitis) to determine the role of AHFV in these syndromes. Similar studies should be planned to address the role of AHFV in hemorrhagic fevers.

Epidemiological characteristics of the 16 cases are shown in Table 2. Of all pathogenic flaviviruses, AHFV has the highest mortality rate, estimated around 30%.

Table 1 Clinical and laboratory characteristics of 16 cases[a] of AHFV

Symptoms or signs	Number of patients	%
Fever	16	100
Headache	16	100
Malaise	16	100
Myalgias	16	100
Retro-orbital pain	16	100
Generalized body ache	16	100
Anorexia	16	100
Vomiting	10	62.5
Hypotension	5 (fatal cases)	31.25
Central nervous system manifestations (convulsions, coma)	5 (fatal cases)	31.25
Sore throat	5	31.25
Disseminated intravascular coagulation	5 (fatal cases)	31.25
Death	5	31.25
Diarrhea	4	25
Hemorrhagic manifestations	4	25
Encephalitis	4	25
Cough	2	12.5
Skin rash	2	12.5
Hematemesis	2/	12.5
Leukopenia	16	100
Thrombocytopenia $<100 \times 10^9$ L^{-1}	16	100
Elevated transaminases	16	100
Highly elevated Creatine phosphokinase	16	100

[a] Infection was confirmed by viral isolation in all cases

Table 2 Epidemiological characteristics of 16 laboratory-confirmed[a] AHFV-infected patients in Saudi Arabia

Date of isolation	Nationality	Origin	Profession	Age	Sex	Source of infection	Outcome
May 1994	Egyptian	Mecca	Butcher	27	Male	Wound	Death
May 1994	Egyptian	Mecca	Butcher	35	Male	Wound	Recovery
September 1995	Egyptian	Mecca	Butcher	32	Male	Wound	Death
September 1995	Egyptian	Jeddah	Butcher	32	Male	Wound	Recovery
October 1995	Saudi	Jeddah	Soldier	32	Male	Raw camel's milk	Recovery
June 1997	Saudi	Jeddah	Driver	31	Male	Raw camel's milk	Death
March 1998	Saudi	Jeddah	Engineer	58	Male	Tick bite	Recovery
March 1998	Egyptian	Jeddah	Butcher	27	Male	Wound	Recovery
March 1998	Egyptian	Jeddah	Butcher	44	Male	Wound	Recovery
April 1998	Saudi	Jeddah	Student	15	Male	Tick bite	Death
March 1999	Saudi	Jeddah	Unknown	36	Male	Tick bite	Recovery
June 1999	Eritrian	Jeddah	Poultry worker	52	Male	Raw camel's milk	Recovery*
November 1999	Egyptian	Mecca	Butcher	47	Male	Wound	Recovery
March 2001	Saudi	Jeddah	Student	12	Male	Tick bite	Recovery
May 2001	Yemeni	Jeddah	Butcher	38	Male	Tick bite	Recovery
February 2004	Saudi	Al Taief	Housewife	46	Female	Wound	Death

[a] Infection was confirmed by viral isolation in all cases

As is the case for other flaviviruses, there is no specific treatment for AHFV infection to date. Therapeutic efforts are purely symptom-based and supportive.

Diagnosing AHFV

In addition to dengue virus, CCHF virus, and Rift Valley fever virus, AHFV must be included in the test panel for patients who present with hemorrhagic fever in Saudi Arabia. Patients presenting with hemorrhagic fever after traveling in Saudi Arabia or neighboring countries should also be tested for AHFV. In addition to the other flaviviruses that are known to circulate in Saudi Arabia, such as dengue virus, it is likely that other unrecognized flaviviruses also circulate. For instance, West Nile virus has been isolated in countries around Saudi Arabia, and may also be present in Saudi Arabia. AHFV has been isolated and reported in Saudi Arabia, but there is limited data available regarding its occurrence in neighboring countries. Therefore, diagnostic algorithms based on geography or clinical signs most likely will not be useful. A diagnosis of AHFV infection must therefore be considered in cases of dengue-like or influenza-like illness. Biological samples from such cases should be collected and sent to the laboratory for confirmation by virus isolation, PCR assays, or serology.

Virus Isolation

Virus isolation is the most developed method for identifying the recently described AHFV in the Middle East. Therefore, efforts should be undertaken to collect and store biological material that is suitable for virus isolation to allow for further investigation into the ecology and epidemiology of AHFV. Serum or heparinized plasma must be collected during the acute febrile stage of the disease and frozen at −70°C. AHFV can be isolated through viral propagation after serum and/or cerebrospinal fluid (CSF) inoculation onto Vero cell cultures (other cells such as BHK-21, PK, RH, 293, A549 are used for TBEV and are also probably appropriate for AHFV) or into the brains of suckling mice.

To date there is no information concerning the diagnostic value of CSF since all patients have been diagnosed either by virus isolation from blood specimens or by demonstration of seroconversion. Since other tick-borne flaviviruses can be detected in CSF, it would be useful to address the utility of testing CSF for AHFV viral RNA.

Detection of AHFV Sequence by PCR

Direct diagnosis of AHFV may also be achieved with an RT-PCR based assay. Serum or heparinized plasma must be collected during the acute febrile stage of

Table 3 Primers used for diagnosis of AHFV

Primer name	Sequence	Position, per AHFV prototype sequence	PCR product size (bp)
ALK-ES1	CTAATGAGTCCCACAGCAATC	1415–1435	487
ALK-ER	TTCCAAGCAAACTTTGATCCC	1901–1881	
ALK-ES2[a]	ACACGAGGGCGCCCATGAA	1641–1659	261

[a] Combined with ALK-ER for second-round

the disease and frozen at −70°C. Different combinations of oligonucleotide primers have been designed to amplify AHFV genomic RNA (Table 3). The nested system located in the envelope gene is routinely used at Dr. Suleiman Fakeeh Hospital for AHFV diagnosis on patient serum. PCR performed on serum yielded positive results in all 16 cases that were confirmed by viral isolation. To date, the usefulness of PCR on CSF is unknown because this type of specimen has not been tested.

In contrast with TBEV, it is important to underline that viral isolation and molecular techniques play a significant role in the routine diagnosis of AHFV.

Serology

For serologic diagnosis, blood samples should be collected early in the course of disease and a second sample should be obtained 1 or 2 weeks later. When a four-fold rise in antibody titre has not occurred with the second sample, it may be useful to test a third serum sample collected 4–6 weeks later. Samples collected for serologic diagnosis can be stored at 20°C. AHFV-specific antibodies can be detected by ELISA or IFA tests. ELISA is the method of choice for serological diagnosis on paired sera. ELISA may be performed on serum or CSF. Rapid diagnosis is performed by detecting IgM through capture ELISA, which avoids false-positive results due to the interference of rheumatoid factor or heterophilic antibodies (Gunther et al., 1997). However, the suitability of IgM for early diagnosis is questionable since IgM antibodies can persist for up to 10 months in vaccinated individuals (as is the case for TBEV) or in persons who acquired the infection naturally (shown with West Nile virus in Roehrig et al., 2003). Therefore, confirmation of infection through detection of specific IgG through ELISA or a seroneutralization test is recommended. During the early phase of infection, antibody test results may be negative and should therefore be repeated 1–2 weeks later. Interpretation of the results of an antibody test should include consideration that AHFV is a flavivirus and therefore shares several antigenic determinants with other tick- (TBEV, Langat virus) and mosquito-borne viruses (dengue virus, Japanese encephalitis virus, or West Nile virus). Specific identification can usually be achieved by neutralization tests.

AHFV Diagnosis at Dr. Suleiman Fakeeh Hospital Virology Laboratory in Jeddah, Saudi Arabia

Diagnosis of AHFV is routinely performed at the virology laboratory of Dr. Fakeeh hospital. To our knowledge, this is to date the only laboratory that performs specific diagnosis of AHFV in Saudi Arabia. Thus, it is instructive to relay the daily experience of this laboratory in screening and confirming suspected AHFV cases at a hospital within the endemic area. Three tubes of blood are collected from the patient for diagnostic procedures: one EDTA tube for RT-PCR assay, one whole blood tube for serology, and one whole blood tube for virus isolation.

Semi-nested PCR is performed with primer pairs ALK-ES1/ALK-ER and ALK-ES2/ALK-ER for first and second round, respectively (Table 3). PCR products are loaded onto a 2% agarose gel and analyzed by transillumination under UV light. These primers were designed to specifically amplify AHFV but not other tick-borne flavivirus, particularly Kyasanur Forest disease virus. The alignment of the 11 AHFV sequences located in the envelope gene together with homologous sequences from other tick-borne flavivirus was used to design the primers.

IgM capture ELISA is performed using crude mouse brain antigen inactivated by formalin and a flavivirus peroxidase conjugated monoclonal antibody. IgG are detected through IFA using Vero cells infected with the prototypic AHFV strain.

Virus isolation is attempted in Vero cells incubated at $37°C$ (5% CO_2) for 10–15 days for primary isolation and/or by intracerebral or intraperitoneal inoculation into suckling mice. Detection of AHFV in inoculated mice is achieved through RT-PCR and by indirect IFA using locally prepared mouse immune sera raised against the prototypic AHFV strain.

Biosafety Regulations for Handling AHFV

AHFV is classified as a Biosafety-Level-3 or -4 infectious agent depending on country regulations. In the United States, all tick-borne encephalitis flaviviruses are classified as BSL-4 agents and included in the list of Health and Human Services Select Agents and U.S. Department of Agriculture High Consequence Livestock Pathogens and Toxins (www.umich.edu/ oseh/Select_Agents_Appendix_A.pdf). All procedures involving biological samples must be performed according to the safety rules of the country in which specimens are sent, manipulated, or received.

Tools Available for the Detection of AHFV in Field Specimens

Field studies often result in the collection of ticks, which can be analyzed for the presence of AHFV. To date, AHFV has been detected and isolated in *Ornithodoros savignyi* (eyed tampan or sand tampan), collected from a camel resting place northeast of Jeddah (Charrel et al., 2007). Whether other tick species can be infected and/or play a significant role in the ecological cycle of AHFV remains unknown. Answering this question requires tick collection and virus isolation studies to determine ticks' role as vectors of AHFV.

The appropriate method is to test ticks for the presence of the AHFV genome by RT-PCR techniques; real-time RT-PCR techniques are recommended since large samples can be tested in short periods of time and with high sensitivity. Classically, ticks are crushed in 600 μL of PBS medium enriched with 20% fetal bovine serum; an aliquot (100–200 μL depending upon the technique) is used for total RNA extraction and subsequent RT-PCR; the remaining mixture is stored at −80°C, and is available for attempting virus isolation in those cases where the AHFV genome is detected. A detailed protocol is available upon request from the corresponding author. This protocol has been routinely used in the Unité des Virus Emergents for the last 2 years, and has been validated by detection and viral isolation of AHFV in ticks, Lymphocytic choriomeningitis virus in *Mus musculus* kidneys, and Toscana virus in sand flies.

Sending Samples to Fakeeh Hospital for AHFV Testing

Serology and RT-PCR assays can be performed either locally in the virology laboratory at Dr. Suleiman Fakeeh Hospital in Jeddah (contact Dr. A.M. Zaki at azaki53@hotmail.com to arrange for shipping material) or sent to the Virology laboratory in Marseilles (contact Dr. Rémi Charrel at Remi.Charrel@medecine. univ-mrs.fr or Xavier.de-Lamballerie@medecine.univ-mrs.fr).

Evolution of AHFV and Closely Related Viruses

It has been shown that divergence between AHFV and Kyasanur forest disease virus occurred relatively recently, most likely in the twentieth century. Therefore, AHFV is a good candidate for study to understand the evolutionary processes of tick-borne flaviviruses.

Nature of the Reservoir

Arthropod-borne viruses, and specifically flaviviruses, are usually maintained in nature through a cycle involving the vector (arthropod) and a reservoir/amplifying host (usually a vertebrate, mammal, or bird). In the case of tick-borne flaviviruses, reservoirs are represented by large (e.g., sheep) or small (e.g., rodents) mammals. Sheep and camels are good candidates for the AHFV reservoir. However, this hypothesis is mainly based on indirect epidemiological evidence. AHFV has not yet been investigated in sheep and camels.

Urgent Next Steps and Future Studies

Although AHFV was identified a decade ago and it has since been shown to cause severe flavivirus infection in humans, information about the virus remains limited by the absence of large-scale studies.

Different vaccines against TBEV have been developed by commercial companies and made available on the public market. Because of antigenic proximity, it is possible that antibodies directed against TBEV will confer a certain level of protection against AHFV. However, no laboratory studies have been conducted to address this important question. The conduct of these studies represents a priority because vaccination programs for susceptible populations, such as butchers and slaughterhouse workers, could provide immediate assistance.

To evaluate the impact of AHFV in Saudi Arabia, large-scale studies on blood donors should be conducted. Confirmation tests of ELISA-positive sera must be done through plaque reduction neutralization to eliminate the risk of false positive due to cross-reactivity within tick-borne flaviviruses.

The distribution of AHFV in Saudi Arabia's neighboring countries of the Middle East, the Eastern coast of Africa, and the Indian peninsula should be established. Studies should be conducted with techniques that distinguish AHFV from other tick-borne flaviviruses: virus isolation from arthropods (ticks) and detection of AHFV by PCR, with sequencing for confirmation. We advocate the use of PCR assays that are generic for flaviviruses instead of assays specific for AHFV. The reason for that is the absence of knowledge of the genetic heterogeneity within AHFV. In this view, serology based studies should be avoided because of the cross-reactivity within tick-borne flaviviruses or systematically confirmed by neutralization test. The potential of AHFV to spread within and outside of the Middle East, especially to Asian countries, needs a better knowledge of the current distribution and eco-epidemiology of both virus and disease to be anticipated. Given its potential to cause harm in human populations, AHFV emergence should stimulate research towards the discovery of new drugs. To date there is no drug active against Flavivirus infections although this genus comprises at least 40 viruses that can infect humans, including dengue and Japanese encephalitis, which are among the major public health problems in certain regions of the world.

While AHFV is a candidate agent for bioterrorism, it has remained neglected. In Saudi Arabia as in neighboring countries, few laboratories possess an appropriate diagnostic arsenal. Nonetheless, there is an urgent need for studies directed at better understanding of this virus, its natural history, ecology and epidemiology, and the spectrum of disease it causes in humans. It is also necessary for Saudi Arabian authorities to promote and encourage research programs directed at better understanding of AHFV.

References

Belov, G. F., Tofaniuk, E. V., Kurzhukov, G. P., Kuznetsova, V. G. (1995). The clinico-epidemiological characteristics of Omsk hemorrhagic fever in 1988–1992. *Zh Mikrobiol Epidemiol Immunobiol, 4*, 88–91

Bird, B. H., Khristova, M. L., Rollin, P. E., Ksiazek, T. G., Nichol, S. T. (2007). Complete genome analysis of 33 ecologically and biologically diverse Rift Valley fever virus strains reveals widespread virus movement and low genetic diversity due to recent common ancestry. *J Virol,* Mar;81(6):2805–2816

Busygin, F. F. (2000). Omsk hemorrhagic fever—current status of the problem. *Vopr Virusol, 45*, 4–9

Charrel, R. N., Zaki, A. M., Attoui, H., Fakeeh, M., Billoir, F., Yousef, A. I., de Chesse, R., De Micco, P., Gould, E. A., de Lamballerie, X. (2001). Complete coding sequence of the Alkhurma virus, a tick-borne flavivirus causing severe hemorrhagic fever in humans in Saudi Arabia. *Biochem Biophys Res Commun, 287*, 455–461

Charrel, R. N., Zaki, A. M., Fakeeh, M., Yousef, A. I., de Chesse, R., Attoui, H., de Lamballerie, X. (2005). Low diversity of Alkhurma hemorrhagic fever virus, Saudi Arabia, 1994–1999. *Emerg Infect Dis, 11*, 683–688

Charrel, R. N., Zaki, A. M., Fagbo, S., de Lamballerie, X. (2006). Alkhurma hemorrhagic fever virus is an emerging tick-borne flavivirus. *J Infect, 52*, 463–464

Charrel, R. N., Fagbo, S., Moureau, G., Alqahtani, M. H., Temmam, S., de Lamballerie, X. (2007). Alkhurma hemorrhagic fever virus in *Ornithodoros savignyi* ticks. *Emerg Infect Dis* Jan;13(1):153–155

Dumpis, U., Crook, D., Oksi, J. (1999). Tick-borne encephalitis. *Clin Infect Dis, 28*, 882–890

Fakeeh, M., Zaki, A. M. (2001). Virologic and serologic surveillance for dengue fever in Jeddah, Saudi Arabia, 1994–1999. *Am J Trop Med Hyg, 65*, 764–767

Gresikova, M., Sekeyova, M., Stupalova, S., Necas, S. (1975). Sheep milk-borne epidemic of tick-borne encephalitis in Slovakia. *Intervirology, 5*, 57–61

Gritsun, T. S., Lashkevich, V. A., Gould, E. A. (2003). Tick-borne encephalitis. *Antiviral Res, 57*, 129–146

Gunther, G., Haglund, M., Lindquist, L., Skoldenberg, B., Forsgren, M. (1997). Intrathecal IgM, IgA and IgG antibody response in tick-borne encephalitis. Long-term follow-up related to clinical course and outcome. *Clin Diagn Virol, 8,* 17–29

Henderson, B. E., Tukei, P. M., McCrae, A. W., Ssenkubuge, Y., Mugo, W. N. (1970). Virus isolations from Ixodid ticks in Uganda. II. Kadam virus—a new member of arbovirus group B isolated from Rhipicephalus pravus Dontiz. *East Afr Med J, 47*, 273–276

Larson, E. W., Dominik, J. W., Slone, T. W. (1980). Aerosol stability and respiratory infectivity of Japanese B encephalitis virus. *Infect Immun, 30*, 397–401

Lin, D., Li, L., Dick, D., Shope, R. E., Feldmann, H., Barrett, A. D., Holbrook, M. R. (2003). Analysis of the complete genome of the tick-borne flavivirus Omsk hemorrhagic fever virus. *Virology, 313*, 81–90

Madani, T. A. (2005). Alkhumra virus infection, a new viral hemorrhagic fever in Saudi Arabia. *J Infect, 51*, 91–97

Phillpotts, R. J., Brooks, T. J., Cox, C. S. (1997). A simple device for the exposure of animals to infectious microorganisms by the airborne route. *Epidemiol Infect, 118*, 71–75

Pogodina, V. V. (1958). Resistance of tick-borne encephalitis virus to gastric juice. *Vopr Virusol, 3*, 271–275

Roehrig, J. T., Nash, D., Maldin, B., Labowitz, A., Martin, D. A., Lanciotti, R. S., Campbell, G. L. (2003). Persistence of virus-reactive serum immunoglobulin M antibody in confirmed West Nile virus encephalitis cases. *Emerg Infect Dis, 9*, 376–379

Wood, O. L., Moussa, M. I., Hoogstraal, H., Buttiker, W. (1982). Kadam virus (Togaviridae, Flavivirus) infecting camel-parasitizing Hyalomma dromedarii ticks (Acari: Ixodidae) in Saudi Arabia. *J Med Entomol, 19*, 207–208

Work, T. H., Trapido, H., Murthy, D. P., Rao, R. L., Bhatt, P. N., Kulkarni, K. G. (1957). Kyasanur forest disease. III. A preliminary report on the nature of the infection and clinical manifestations in human beings. *Indian J Med Sci, 11*, 619–645

Zaki, A. M. (1997). Isolation of a flavivirus related to the tick-borne encephalitis complex from human cases in Saudi Arabia. *Trans R Soc Trop Med Hyg, 91*, 179–181

Zaki, A. (2002). Tick-borne flavivirus—Saudi Arabia. ProMEd. Archive number 20020509.4144, May 7, 2002. Available at: http://www.promedmail.org. Accessed October 17, 2006

Zaki, A. (2004). Alkhurma virus, human death—Saudi Arabia. ProMED. Archive number 20040302.0631, March 1, 2004. Available at: http://www.promedmail.org. Accessed October 17, 2006

Disease Outbreaks Caused by Emerging Paramyxoviruses of Bat Origin

Lin-Fa Wang, John S. Mackenzie, and Bryan T. Eaton

Introduction

Newly emerging and re-emerging infections are recognized as a global problem and 75% of these are potentially zoonotic (Woolhouse & Gowtage-Sequeria, 2005). Emergence of a new "killer" disease in any part of the world is likely to be a threat world wide in today's society with very rapid means of transportation of both human and animal/animal products. Recent examples include the global outbreaks of severe acute respiratory syndrome (SARS), H5N1 avian influenza, and the outbreaks of West Nile virus in United States. The rapid economic development in the Asian region during the last few decades was accompanied by massive urbanization and environmental changes, which are believed to be one of the triggers leading to the emergence of new zoonotic diseases. Wildlife animals play an ever-increasing role in the emergence of zoonotic diseases, and bats have been identified as natural reservoir host of several lethal zoonotic viruses that emerged in recent times. This review will focus on the disease outbreaks caused by emerging bat viruses in the family *Paramyxoviridae*.

Viruses and Natural Hosts

Viruses in the family *Paramyxoviridae* are well-known due to their ability to cause a variety of severe diseases affecting humans (measles, mumps, and respiratory and encephalitic illnesses) and livestock animals (Newcastle disease, distemper, and rinderpest). Paramyxoviruses contain a nonsegmented negative strand (NNS) RNA genome and share similar genomic features with three other NNS RNA virus families, *Rhabdoviridae* (which contains rabies and vesicular stomatitis viruses), *Filoviridae* (Ebola and Marburg viruses), and *Bornaviridae* (Borna virus). These four families are grouped taxonomically in the order *Mononegavirales* (Pringle, 1991). Members of the family *Paramyxoviridae* are further divided into two subfamilies, *Paramyxovirinae* and *Pneumovirinae*. The *Paramyxovirinae* include five genera: *Respirovirus, Morbillivirus, Rubulavirus, Avulavirus,* and *Henipavirus* (Mayo, 2002).

Y. Lu et al. (eds.), *Emerging Infections in Asia.*
© Springer Science+Business Media, LLC 2008

Since 1994, at least three novel paramyxoviruses of bat origin in the subfamily *Paramyxovirinae* have emerged in Australia and south Asia, some of them causing severe diseases in both human and animals. They are Hendra virus (HeV), Nipah virus (NiV), and Menangle virus (MenV), isolated from infected horses and humans in Australia in 1994, humans and pigs in Malaysia in 1999, and pigs in Australia in 1997, respectively (Chua et al., 2000; Murray et al., 1995b; Philbey et al., 1998).

HeV and NiV represent a new group of paramyxoviruses in this subfamily, and are classified in a separate genus named *Henipavirus* (Mayo, 2002; Wang et al., 2000). Several molecular features distinguish henipaviruses from other paramyxoviruses. While most paramyxoviruses have a genome of approximately 15,000–16,000 nt, the genome length of HeV and NiV is over 18,000 nt. The increase in genome size is mainly due to the expansion of noncoding regions located mainly at the 3' ends of the viral genes. The functional significance of these features is not known. Henipaviruses also have unique biological features. They are the only currently recognized zoonotic paramyxoviruses and are highly pathogenic with mortality rates reaching 75% or greater for NiV (Eaton et al., 2006). The wide host range of henipaviruses is also considered uncommon for paramyxoviruses. For example, NiV naturally infects five terrestrial species in four mammalian orders. Experimental infection extends the number of susceptible terrestrial orders to five by including Rodentia. The highly virulent nature of henipaviruses combined with the lack of therapeutic treatments has led to the classification of HeV and NiV as Biosafety Level 4 (BSL4) pathogens.

In contrast, MenV has a genome length of 15,516 nt, typical of most paramyxovirus genomes (Bowden & Boyle, 2005; Bowden et al., 2001). Comparative sequence analyses indicated that MenV is a new member of the genus *Rubulavirus* in the subfamily *Paramyxovirinae*, but is not closely related to any existing members of the genus, which include mumps virus, porcine rubulavirus, human parainfluenza viruses 2 and 4, and simian viruses 5 and 41. Instead, MenV is closely related to another bat paramyxovirus, Tioman virus (TiV), which was discovered during the search for NiV in bats on Tioman island, east of peninsular Malaysia (Chua et al., 2001b; Chua et al., 2002b). TiV is antigenically related to MenV, but its disease-causing potential in humans or animals is unknown.

All these newly emerged viruses are believed to have flying foxes (fruit bats in the genus *Pteropus*) as natural hosts. Bats have been identified or implicated as the natural reservoir host for an increasing number of new and often deadly zoonotic viruses. In addition to the emergence of paramyxoviruses from frugivorous *Pteropus* bats, insectivorous *Rhinolophus* species have been identified as natural hosts of SARS-like viruses (Lau et al., 2005; Li et al., 2005), and Ebola virus has been shown to have fruit bat reservoir hosts (Leroy et al., 2005). Bats typically respond asymptomatically to virus infection and display a capacity to permit persistent virus infections (Sulkin & Allen, 1974). Their wide distribution and abundant status (one mammalian species in five is a bat) makes them prime candidates for reservoirs of viruses, which may cross the species barrier and infect man and other animals.

Hendra Virus Outbreaks in Australia (1994–2004)

In September 1994, a spectacular outbreak of an acute respiratory syndrome occurred in thoroughbred horses in Hendra, a suburb of Brisbane, Queensland, which resulted in the death of 13 horses and their trainer (Murray et al., 1995b). The causative agent was a novel paramyxovirus, later named Hendra virus after the location of the index case. During this outbreak, two human infections were identified. Both patients presented with myalgia, headaches, lethargy, and vertigo. One recovered after a two-week severe flu-like illness, but the other developed pneumonitis, respiratory failure, renal failure, and arterial thrombosis and died from a cardiac arrest. Findings at autopsy were consistent with a viral infection. Histology revealed focal necrotizing alveolitis with many giant cells, some syncytial formation, and viral inclusion bodies (Selvey et al., 1995). HeV was isolated from the lung, kidney, liver, and spleen of the lethal case (Murray et al., 1995b). Sequence analysis indicated that HeV isolates obtained from horses and humans had identical genetic sequences.

A second outbreak of HeV occurred in Mackay, 1,000 km north of Brisbane, which resulted in the death of two horses and one human (O'Sullivan et al., 1997). The horses died of unknown causes in August 1994, and the farmer who assisted with the necropsies developed a mild meningitic illness, but recovered. Thirteen months later, the farmer became ill and died of severe encephalitis, which was confirmed to be caused by HeV (O'Sullivan et al., 1997). Retrospective investigation revealed that the two horses had also died of HeV infection, and the farmer was infected at that time in August 1994 (Hooper et al., 1996; Rogers et al., 1996). Compared with the two human cases involved in the Hendra outbreak, the human case in the Mackay outbreak presented two interesting differences. First, the virus seemed to have remained latent for 13 months before reactivation to eventually kill the patient. Second, the patient died of encephalitis, whereas the other two human cases presented with respiratory symptoms (Selvey et al., 1995). In this regard, it is interesting to note that although paramyxoviruses are mainly known for their ability to cause respiratory diseases, some do have the capability to infect brain and cause encephalitic illness, such as measles viruses in subacute sclerosing panencephalitis (SSPE) patients (Griffin, 2001).

HeV re-emerged in Queensland in Cairns in January 1999 and in Townsville in December 2004. Both occasions resulted in the death of a single horse. The Cairns case involved a 9-year-old thoroughbred, and there was no horse-to-horse or horse-to-human transmission observed. In the Townsville case, a veterinarian involved in the autopsy developed a HeV-related respiratory illness soon after and recovered (ProMed, 2004).

Extensive seroepidemiologic surveillance of wild and domestic animals revealed the presence of HeV antibodies in four species of flying foxes found in Australia (Young et al., 1997; Young et al., 1996). They are the spectacled flying fox (*Pteropus conspicillatus*), the black flying fox (*P. alecto*), and the grey-headed flying fox (*P. poliocephalus)* in which species seroprevalence can be as high as 47% in some areas (Field et al., 2001a). For reasons that are not yet clear, the seroprevalence rate in the fourth species(the most widely distributed of the four species, the little red flying fox (*P. scapulatus*)) is lower, approximately 15% (Field et al., 2001a). HeV was isolated from uterine fluid and a pool of fetal lung and liver from one grey-headed flying fox and from the fetal lung of a black flying fox (Halpin et al., 2000). The bat isolates had almost identical sequences to those of human and horse isolates.

Nipah Virus Outbreaks in Malaysia (1998–1999)

Between September 1998 and April 1999, a major outbreak of disease in pigs and humans occurred in peninsular Malaysia, which resulted in 265 human cases, 105 of them fatal (Chua et al., 2000). In Singapore, 11 cases and one death were reported among abattoir workers who slaughtered pigs imported from affected areas of Malaysia (Paton et al., 1999). The outbreak was controlled by culling of over 1 million pigs and strict quarantine measures on pig movement.

While the disease in pigs was highly contagious and characterized by acute fever mainly with respiratory involvement, mostly without neurological signs, the predominant clinical syndrome in humans was encephalitic rather than respiratory. The major clinical signs included drowsiness, areflexia, segmental myoclonus, tachycardia, hypertension, pin-point pupils, and an abnormal doll's eye reflex (Chua et al., 1999; Goh et al., 2000). The incubation period ranged from 2 to 45 days, but for most patients it was 2 weeks or less (Chua, 2003; Goh et al., 2000). A majority of patients who survived acute encephalitis made a full recovery, but about 20% had residual neurological sequelae, including cognitive difficulties, tetraparesis, cerebellar signs, nerve palsies, and clinical depression (Goh et al., 2000).

A Hendra-like virus, named Nipah virus (NiV) after the village of the index case, was isolated from the CSF of several patients (Chua et al., 2000). Retrospective investigations suggested that the virus was also responsible for previous disease outbreaks in pigs in peninsular Malaysia since late 1996. Knowledge of the similarities between HeV and NiV facilitated the rapid identification of fruit bats as the reservoir host of NiV. Serological sampling of various bats in Malaysia found five species with neutralizing antibodies to NiV (Field et al., 2001a; Yob et al., 2001). They included four fruit bat species, *P. hypomelanus*, *P. vampyrus*, *Cynopterus brachyotis*, *Eonycteris spelaea*, and an insectivorous bat, *Scotophilus kuhlii*. NiV was subsequently identified and isolated from bat urine samples of *P. hypomelanus* and from a partially eaten fruit swab (Chua et al., 2002a). The genome sequences of bat isolates were largely indistinguishable from human NiV isolates (Chua et al., 2002a).

There is very little knowledge available on the treatment of NiV infection. Ribavirin was used during the NiV outbreak in Malaysia in an open-label study in which 140 patients with encephalitis were given the drug, and 54 patients who presented before the drug became available or who refused treatment acted as controls (Chong et al., 2001). Mortality in the treated and control groups was 32%

and 54%, respectively, indicating a significant reduction in the treatment group. *In vitro*, ribavirin has been shown to inhibit replication of HeV (Wright et al., 2004). In the absence of other therapies, ribavirin is an option for treatment of henipavirus infection. Other potential treatment approaches currently being developed include the use of neutralizing monoclonal antibodies (Zhu et al., 2006; Guillaume et al., 2006), soluble receptor or attachment protein molecules, and fusion-inhibiting peptides (Bossart et al., 2005a,b; Bossart & Broder, 2006).

Nipah Virus Outbreaks in Bangladesh (2001–2005)

Five outbreaks of NiV have been recognized in Bangladesh between 2001 and 2005, and each occurred between January and May. The first recorded outbreak occurred between April and May of 2001 in the western Meherpur District and involved 13 cases with nine fatalities (69% mortality). The second outbreak was in January 2003 in the western Naogaon District. Among the 12 patients who met the case definition, eight died (67% mortality). Patients from both outbreaks displayed similar clinical courses, starting with onset of fever, followed by headache and varying degrees of diminishing consciousness. Coughing and difficulty in breathing were also common and half of the patients had vomiting, but seizures and diarrhea were uncommon (Hsu et al., 2004).

The second and third outbreaks occurred in 2004 in two locations with no apparent link between the two outbreaks. Between January and February 2004, a total of 29 laboratory-confirmed or probable cases were identified with 22 fatalities (75% mortality) (ICDDRB, 2004a). Most cases were located in the central Rajbari District. Among the first group of 12 patients, all but two were between the ages of 7 and 15 years old. From February to April, a separate outbreak occurred in the Faridpur District with 36 patients and 27 deaths (75% mortality) (ICDDRB, 2004b). At least six patients from this outbreak developed acute respiratory distress syndrome, which has not been seen in previously documented Nipah patients. Another unique feature of this outbreak was the epidemiologic evidence supporting human-to-human transmission, the first for NiV infection in the human population.

The fifth and the latest outbreak occurred in January 2005 in the central Tangail District, and it involved 12 patients with 11 deaths (92% mortality) (ICDDRB, 2005). The most common clinical symptom was unconsciousness. Death occurred between 2–9 days after the first reported symptom of illness with a median of 4 days. The onset of illness for all patients occurred within two weeks of each other.

NiV was isolated from four patients during the 2004 outbreaks. Complete genome sequence was obtained from one isolate (from the Rajbari outbreak), and partial sequences were obtained from the other three (Harcourt et al., 2005). The overall genome organization of the Bangladesh NiV isolate is very similar to that of the Malaysian isolate. At a genome size of 18,252 nt, the NiV-Bangladesh genome is 6 nt longer than that of the NiV-Malaysian isolates. The overall nucleotide sequence identity between the two isolates is approximately 92%. Phylogenetically, all of the Bangladesh isolates clustered together and can be distinguished from the cluster of Malaysian isolates.

Although no virus isolation has been made from bats in Bangladesh, there is substantial evidence suggesting that the fruit bat (*P. giganteus*) is the likely reservoir of NiV in Bangladesh. During the investigation of the Naogaon outbreak in 2003, two out of 19 *P. giganteus* bats had antibodies to NiV (Hsu et al., 2004). A larger animal study conducted during the investigation of the 2004 Rajbari outbreak also found that *P. giganteus* was the only species with anti-NiV antibodies (ICDDRB, 2005).

Nipah Virus Outbreak in India (2001)

During January to February of 2001, an outbreak of febrile illness with altered sensorium occurred in Siliguri, West Bengal, India, among hospitalized patients, their family contacts, and the medical staff of four different hospitals (Chadha et al. 2006; Kumar, 2003). While epidemiologic features and serological testing excluded the possibility of Japanese encephalitis, initial laboratory investigations failed to identify an etiological agent for the outbreak (Kumar, 2003).

Among the 66 patients who fit the working case definition, the case-fatality ratio was approximately 74%. All patients were greater than 15 years of age, and 75% of the patients had a history of hospital exposure. The outbreak started at a single hospital, and subsequently spread to three other hospitals. There was no definitive information about the possible index case. Clinical symptoms included fever (exhibited by all patients), headache and myalgia (57% of patients), vomiting (19%), altered sensorium (97%), respiratory symptoms (51%), and involuntary movements or convulsions (43%). Death occurred within 1 week of disease onset for 10 patients, within 2 weeks for 5 patients, and on day 30 for 2 patients (Chadha et al., 2006).

Because of the close geographic proximity of Siliguri to the Nipah outbreak regions in neighboring Bangladesh, a retrospective study was conducted to investigate the possibility of NiV as the causative agent. A total of 17 serum samples from 18 patients were analyzed for NiV-specific antibodies by ELISA. Nine out of the 17 sera were positive for IgM and IgG, and one sample was positive for IgG, but negative for IgM. In addition, six urine samples collected from the 18 patients were also tested by PCR and virus isolation. While there was no virus isolated using Vero E6 cells, five of the six urine samples were PCR-positive, four from sero-positive patients and one from a sero-negative patient. Analysis of a partial sequence from the M gene indicated that the etiologic agent was a strain of NiV, which has a close sequence homology with both the Malaysian and Bangladesh NiV isolates (94% and 99% sequence identity, respectively) (Chadha et al., 2006). The reservoir host for NiV in India has not been identified yet, but it is most likely to be the bat species *P. giganteus*, as suspected to be the case for the Bangladesh NiV outbreaks (Hsu et al., 2004; ICCDRB, 2005) or another closely-related flying fox species.

Presence of Henipaviruses in Other Countries in the Region

The identification of fruit bats in the genus *Pteropus* as the reservoir hosts of HeV and NiV in Australia and Malaysia, respectively, prompted searches for related viruses in other nations in the region. Fruit bats are widely dispersed geographically in a range that extends from the east coast of Africa, through the Indian subcontinent and Southeast Asia, north to Okinawa, and south to Australia (Koopman, 1992).

Serological studies carried out on two species of bats from Madang (*Dobsonia moluccense*, and *P. neohibernicus*) on the north coast of Papua New Guinea (Halpin, Field, Mackenzie, Bockarie, Young & Selleck, unpublished data) and four species of bats (*P. capistratus*, *P. hypomelanus*, *P admiralitatum*, and *D. andersoni*) from Port Moresby and New Britain (Field, Hamilton, Hall, Bornacosso, Halpin, & Young, unpublished data) were found to have antibodies to a HeV-like virus (cited in Mackenzie et al., 2003). Similarly, serological studies from fruit bats (*P. vampyrus*) trapped on the Indonesian islands of Sumatra and Java were found to have neutralizing antibodies for a virus more closely related to NiV than to HeV. In these studies, 11 bat sera neutralized NiV only, one serum neutralized HeV only, and 17 sera neutralized both viruses (Sendow et al., 2006).

A study by Olson et al. (2002) sampled 96 Lyle's flying foxes (*P. lylei*) from restaurants in Cambodia and conducted serological tests using ELISA and the neutralization test for henipavirus antibodies. Of the 96 serum specimens examined, 11 sera (11.5%) were positive in ELISA for NiV antibodies and the results were confirmed by serum neutralization. Some of these sera were also tested for their ability to neutralize HeV and were shown to have equivalent titers to both NiV and HeV. The authors concluded that a closely related virus, which might be neither NiV nor HeV, was circulating in the Cambodian bat population (Olson et al., 2002).

A second study in Cambodia was conducted during 2000–2001, in which a total of 1,303 bats were sampled either from restaurants or at their roosts in the wild, covering 35 locations in nine provinces (Reynes et al., 2005). These animals represented 16 species from six of the seven bat families known to be present in Cambodia. Serum samples from 1,072 bats were taken for NiV antibody ELISA testing and positive signals were obtained only in the species *P. lylei* with a seroprevalence of 10.9% (50 out of 458), corroborating the results conducted in the first study (Olson et al., 2002). Sera from other bat species were all negative and so were the limited number of human sera ($n = 8$) tested from individuals who had contact with sero-positive Lyle bats in restaurants. Attempts to isolate live virus from 769 urine samples yielded two virus isolates from urine samples collected at the same time from a roost of *P. lylei* bats in a village. Sequencing of the N and G genes indicated that the two isolates had identical sequences and that they shared a nucleotide sequence identity of 98% and 98.2%, respectively, with their Malaysian counterpart. Phylogenetic analysis based on current available henipavirus sequences suggest that the NiV isolate from Cambodian bats is more closely related to Malaysian isolates of NiV than isolates from Bangladesh.

A similar study was conducted in Thailand and recently reported (Wacharapluesadee et al., 2005). During March 2002 and February 2004, 1,304 bats were sampled from 15 sites covering nine provinces in central, eastern, and southern Thailand. Among the 12 bat species sampled, six were frugivorous and six were insectivorous. In addition to serum samples taken for NiV antibody tests, saliva (1,286 samples) and urine (1,282) swabs were also taken and analyzed by PCR for the presence of NiV-related sequences. From 1,054 sera tested, 82 positive samples (i.e., positive in NiV IgG ELISA) were obtained from four different species: 76 from *P. lylei*, four from *P. hypomelanus*, and one each from *P. vampyrus* and the insectivorous *Hipposideros larvatus*. PCR analysis using NiV N-gene specific primers demonstrated the presence of NiV-related viruses in both saliva and urine samples collected from different sites. While most of the positive samples were collected from *P. lylei* as expected, there was one positive saliva pool sample from *H. larvatus* (Wacharapluesadee et al., 2005). It is interesting to note that sequence analysis based on a 181-nt N gene PCR fragment indicated that the *H. larvatus* isolate was more closely related to the Malaysian NiV isolates, whereas the *P. lylei* isolates were more closely related to the Bangladesh isolates. It remains to be seen whether this pattern of homology will hold when the full-length genome sequences are compared.

In summary, direct isolation or genetic sequence amplification of henipaviruses from flying foxes has been demonstrated in Australia, Malaysia, Cambodia, and Thailand and the sero-prevalence has been observed in these countries and in Bangladesh, Indonesia, and Papua New Guinea. These studies indicate that further henipavirus-related infection can be expected within the area of distribution of flying foxes and highlight the potential of future henipavirus emergence in this wide region.

Menangle Virus Outbreak in Australia (1997)

Menangle virus (MenV) emerged in 1997 as the etiological agent of a severe reproductive disease in a large intensive piggery in Menangle, near Sydney, in Australia (Philbey et al., 1998). The outbreak caused a reduced farrowing rate and stillbirths with deformities and mummified fetuses (Philbey et al., 1998; Love et al., 2001). No disease was observed in postnatal animals of any age. Affected stillborn piglets frequently had severe degeneration of the brain and spinal cord, arthrogryposis, brachygnathia, and occasionally fibrinous body cavity effusions and pulmonary hypoplasia (Philbey et al., 1998). A high proportion (>90%) of serum collected from pigs of all age groups at the affected piggery from May to September 1997 contained high titers of neutralizing antibodies. MenV antibodies were also detected in pigs from two piggeries that received only weaned pigs from the affected piggery. Other than these three piggeries, an extensive serological survey failed to find any sero-positive pigs from other piggeries throughout Australia.

Two human cases associated with the pig disease outbreak were reported (Chant et al., 1998). In early June 1997, Patient 1 from the piggery where the disease outbreak started had a sudden onset of malaise and chills followed by drenching sweats and fever. He was confined to bed for the next 10 days with severe headaches and myalgia, but had no cough, vomiting, or diarrhea. A few days after the onset of illness, he noted a spotty red rash. He returned to work after two weeks' absence and reported a 10 kg weight loss during his illness. Patient 1 had frequent and prolonged contact with birthing pigs, and exposure to splashes of amniotic fluid and blood was common in his job. He often received minor wounds to his hands and forearms.

Patient 2 worked at one of the two other associated piggeries. He also had an onset of illness in early June 1997 characterized by fever, chills, rigors, drenching sweats, marked malaise, back pain, severe frontal headache, and photophobia (Chant et al., 1998). Similar to Patient 1, Patient 2 had no cough, vomiting, or diarrhea. Four days after onset of illness, he noted on the torso a spotty, red, non-pruritic rash, which lasted for 7 days. He recovered after 10 days, noting a 3 kg weight loss.

Serological investigation indicated that both patients had significant levels of convalescent neutralizing antibodies to MenV and showed no alternative cause. Seroepidemiologic testing of more than 250 persons with potential exposure to infected pigs revealed no additional infection other than the two patients described above. This included the partner of Patient 1, who also tested negative. Although the exact mode of transmission from pigs to humans remains unknown, it was almost certain that the two patients became ill following MenV infection (Chant et al., 1998).

A large breeding colony of grey-headed fruit bats as well as little red fruit bats roosted within 200 m of the affected piggery. A serological study indicated the presence of MenV-neutralizing antibodies in at least three fruit bat species collected in New South Wales and Queensland, and positive samples covered the period from 1996 (prior to the outbreak) to November 1997 (post outbreak). These results strongly suggest that MenV originated from fruit bats. This notion was further supported by the isolation of a closely-related paramyxovirus, Tioman virus (TiV), from fruit bats in Malaysia. MenV and TiV have a high level of sequence homology, almost identical genome organization, and strong antigenic cross reactivity (Bowden et al., 2001; Chua et al., 2001b).

Epidemiology

The mechanisms of henipavirus transmission within flying fox populations remain obscure. Horizontal transmission is suggested by the presence of NiV in urine and the observed licking of the ano-genital area, a behavior that occurs during the breeding season, and urination on the fur followed by licking, which occurs in males as part of their grooming behavior (Hall & Richards, 2000). In contrast, vertical transmission is suggested by the transplacental transmission of HeV in experimentally infected flying foxes without apparent harm to the fetus (Williamson et al., 2000).

Human infections in Australia and Malaysia have occurred through transmission from horses and pigs, respectively, and there has been no evidence of direct transfer from bats despite many opportunities for bat carers to be exposed to HeV in Australia (Chua et al., 1999; Parashar et al., 2000; Selvey et al., 1996). Three hypotheses have been proposed for the transmission of henipaviruses from flying foxes to amplifying hosts:

1. Horses and pigs may have been infected in pastures or pigsties through contact with urine of infected bats (Chua et al., 2002a).
2. Viruses may have been transmitted in partially eaten fruit or fruit pulp, spat out by flying foxes (Chua et al., 2002a).
3. The amplifying hosts may have acquired the virus as a result of licking or eating infected placenta or aborted fetal material. HeV outbreaks occurred at the time of year when some species of flying fox are giving birth (Halpin et al., 2000; Field, et al., 2001b).

In Bangladesh, the role of amplifying hosts is equivocal. Each of the five outbreaks seems to have been associated with a different potential mode of transmission. In the Meherpur outbreak in 2001, Nipah cases were significantly more likely to have contact with sick cow and patient's secretions compared to controls (Hsu et al., 2004). In the 2003 outbreak in Naogaon, cases were more likely to have had contact with a herd of pigs that had passed through the area prior to the outbreak (ICDDRB, 2003). In Rajbari in 2004, Nipah cases were more likely to have climbed trees where bats had been and to have contact with patients. In the 2004 Faridpur outbreak, contact with ill persons was the primary risk factor. In the 2005 outbreak in Tangail, drinking fresh date palm juice potentially contaminated with bat secretions was considered the main route of transmission for most of the Nipah infections (ICDDRB, 2005).

Transmission of henipaviruses from bats to amplifying hosts depends on the susceptibility of the latter to oral infection and the titer of virus in urine, partially eaten fruit, or fetal tissues. The minimum infectious dose for horses or pigs is not known, but it is of interest that the minimum oronasal lethal dose of NiV for hamsters is 47,000 plaque forming units (pfu), compared with 270 pfu administered parenterally (Wong et al., 2003). It may also be pertinent that henipaviruses are isolated only rarely and in low titers from the urine of naturally or experimentally infected animals, but are more readily detected in tissues including those of the fetus (Williamson et al., 1998, 2000).

In contrast to the uncertainty concerning the mode of transmission of henipaviruses from bats to horses and pigs, the high titers of virus in the tissues and secretions of these amplifying hosts offer a range of sources for transmission to man during birthing, handling sick and dying animals, slaughtering, necropsy, and carcass handling (Chua et al., 1999; Murray et al., 1995a,b; Parashar et al., 2000). Although HeV generates predominantly respiratory infections, the virus was detected infrequently in the upper respiratory tract of infected horses, suggesting that aerosol transmission to either man or horses is highly unlikely (Hooper et al., 1997). The failure to transmit HeV from experimentally infected to uninfected, in-contact horses is consistent with this suggestion (Williamson et al., 1998). The presence of HeV in equine saliva suggested that manual feeding of the animals may have facilitated horse to human transmission (Selvey et al., 1995). In contrast to the paucity of HeV virions in the upper respiratory tract of horses, NiV was readily observed in the respiratory epithelium of naturally and experimentally infected pigs. Thus the virus probably spread to humans and within the pig population by aerosol or by direct contact with oropharyngeal or nasal secretions (Middleton et al., 2002; Mohd. Nor et al., 2000).

Risk Factors and Disease Control Strategies

An understanding of the epidemiology of henipaviruses is essential for determining the risk factors associated with the transmission of virus from the reservoir host to either a domestic spillover or intermediate host or directly to humans. The destruction of native forest habitats by humans either to clear land for agriculture or to harvest timber has greatly increased the risk of fruit bats encountering spillover hosts as they seek new roosts and alternative food sources, and thus also increased the risk of emergence of epizootic disease.

For HeV, the risk factors are associated with the interaction between infected fruit bats and horses as the spillover hosts, and then from horses to humans. The risk of transmission between bats and horses appears to be a rare event, as is subsequent transmission between horses (Field et al., 2001b), whereas direct transmission from fruit bats to humans probably does not occur despite a high risk of occupational or recreational exposure among some groups (Selvey et al., 1996). Current strategies for controlling or preventing HeV epizootics are built around the three hypotheses for virus transmission from fruit bats to amplifying hosts listed above. They have centered around management strategies for horses rather than fruit bats and include minimizing exposure by stabling horses at night, excluding from horse paddocks, trees that bear fruit favored by fruit bats, and implementing quarantine and stock movement controls (Field et al., 2004; Mackenzie et al., 2003; Mackenzie and Field, 2004).

For NiV, the risk factors for epizootic emergence are essentially similar to those described above for HeV. However, there are important differences in the epidemiological features of NiV in Malaysia and Bangladesh. In Malaysia, NiV was readily transmitted between pigs and from pigs to humans. Human to human transmission of NiV was not a feature in the Malaysian outbreak (Chua et al., 2001a; Mounts et al., 2001). In contrast, the involvement of spillover hosts was not an obvious aspect of the outbreaks in Bangladesh and probably West Bengal (Chadha et al., 2006). In addition there has been epidemiological evidence to suggest that human to human transmission occurred in at least two of the epidemics in Bangladesh (Hsu et al., 2004; ICDDRB, 2005), as well as the outbreak in Siliguri, West Bengal (Chadha et al., 2006). In the latter situation, nosocomial spread was implicated. The major risk factors in Malaysia and Singapore were associated with a close involvement with pig farming or infected pig carcasses, but in Bangladesh and Siliguri where there was no documented involvement with pigs, the risk factors were more difficult to clearly differentiate.

Control strategies in Malaysia have centered around good farm management practices with regular monitoring of herd health and early recognition of disease syndromes, clearly defined protocols for introducing new stock, and an ongoing disease surveillance program (Daniels et al., 2000; Field et al., 2004). In addition, decreasing the potential for fruit bat–pig interactions is also a major strategy to reduce the possibility of spillover events leading to disease emergence, and include simple measures such as removing fruit trees or orchards from the immediate vicinity of pig sheds, wire screening of open-sided pig sheds to prevent fruit bat access, and ensuring that roof run-off does not enter pig pens (Mackenzie et al., 2003; Field et al., 2004). It is also important that a rapid laboratory diagnostic capability is available with experienced veterinarians to interpret test results, and where necessary, to respond to and conduct outbreak investigations. In Bangladesh and West Bengal, the two most appropriate control measures at this time are to ensure all patients with possible NiV infection are barrier nursed with strict prevention of contact with visitors or other patients, and washing of all fruit for human consumption as well as ensuring all fruit juice is kept under conditions which restrict access to fruit bats.

Concluding Remarks

Since the emergence of HeV in 1994 in Australia, the last decade has witnessed multiple disease outbreaks caused by novel paramyxoviruses of bat origin. Of especial concern is the apparent human to human transmission of NiV in Bangladesh and India. Further investigation is warranted to determine the transmission routes of NiV, especially in the nosocomial setting. The possibility of human to human transmission becomes very important in all future control strategies. It also increases the potential for Nipah to become a disease of international significance.

Recent identification of bats as natural reservoir hosts of henipaviruses, MenV, Ebola virus, and SARS coronavirus highlights the importance of bats in emergence of zoonotic diseases. From the genetic diversity observed from limited genome sequences obtained so far, it is almost certain that other related viruses will emerge from *Pteropus* species or other fruit bats sharing the same or similar habitats. What we do not know is how genetically different they will be and whether they will be more or less transmissible to and among the human population. For example, the *Pteropus* sp in the western Indian Ocean are believed to have separated from other *Pteropus* sp more than 60,000 years ago. If one assumes that viruses coevolve with these hosts, one might expect that henipa-like viruses from these bats could be genetically very different from the ones isolated to date. This will undoubtedly have significant impact on our current diagnosis and control/prevention strategies.

It is therefore essential to focus our future research on a better understanding of virus diversity and distribution among fruit bats in different regions and on a better understanding of factors triggering spillover events and routes of transmission to and among human population. Wide international collaboration will be extremely important for such a multidisciplinary and multisite research endeavor.

References

Bossart, K. N., & Broder, C. C. (2006). Developments towards effective treatments for Nipah and Hendra virus infection. *Expert Review of Anti-infective Therapy*, 4, 43–55.

Bossart, K. N., Crameri, G., Dimitrov, A. S., Mungall, B., Feng, Y. R., Patch, J. R., Choudhary, A., Wang, L. F., Eaton, B. T., & Broder, C. C. (2005a). Receptor-binding, fusion inhibition and induction of cross-reactive neutralizing antibodies by a soluble G glycoprotein of Hendra virus. *Journal of Virology*, 79, 6690–6702.

Bossart, K. N., Mungall, B. A., Crameri, G. C., Wang, L. F., Eaton, B. T., & Broder, C. C. (2005b). Inhibition of henipavirus fusion and infection by heptad-derived peptides of the Nipah virus fusion protein. *Virology Journal*, 2, 57.

Bowden, T. R., & Boyle, D. B. (2005). Completion of the full-length genome sequence of Menangle virus: Characterisation of the polymerase gene and genomic 5 trailer region. *Archives of Virology*, 150, 2125–2137.

Bowden, T. R., Westenberg, M., Wang, L. F., Eaton, B. T., & Boyle, D. B. (2001). Molecular characterization of Menangle virus, a novel paramyxovirus which infects pigs, fruit bats, and humans. *Virology*, 283, 358–373.

Chadha, M. S., Comer, J. A., Lowe, L., Rota, P. A., Rollin, P. E., Bellini, W. J., Ksiazek, T. G., & Mishra, A. C. (2006). Nipah virus identified as the agent responsible for an outbreak of encephalitis in Siliguri, India. *Emerging Infectious Diseases*, 12, 235–240.

Chant, K., Chan, R., Smith, M., Dwyer, D. E., & Kirkland, P. (1998). Probable human infection with a newly described virus in the family Paramyxoviridae. *Emerging Infectious Diseases*, 4, 273–275.

Chong, H. T., Kamarulzaman, A., Tan, C. T., Goh, K. J., Thayaparan, T., Kunjapan, R., Chew, N. K., Chua, K. B., & Lam, S. K. (2001). Treatment of acute Nipah encephalitis with ribavirin. *Annals of Neurology*, 49, 810–813.

Chua, K. B. (2003). Nipah virus outbreak in Malaysia. *Journal of Clinical Virology*, 26, 265–275.

Chua, K. B., Bellini, W. J., Rota, P. A., Harcourt, B. H., Tamin, A., Lam, S. K., Ksiazek, T. G., Rollin, P. E., Zaki, S. R., Shieh, W. J., Goldsmith, C. S., Gubler, D. J., Roehrig, J. T., Eaton, B., Gould, A. R., Olson, J., Field, H., Daniels, P., Ling, A. E., Peters, C. J., Anderson, L. J., & Mahy, B. W. J. (2000). Nipah virus: A recently emergent deadly paramyxovirus. *Science*, 288, 1432–1435.

Chua, K. B., Goh, K. J., Wong, K. T., Kamarulzaman, A., Tan, P. S. K., Ksiazek, T. G., Zaki, S. R., Paul, G., Lam, S. K., & Tan, C. T. (1999). Fatal encephalitis due to Nipah virus among pig-farmers in Malaysia. *Lancet*, 354, 1257–1259.

Chua, K. B., Koh, C. L., Hooi, P. S., Wee, K. F., Khong, J. H., Chua, B. H., Chan, Y. P., Lim, M. E., & Lam Sai Kit, K. (2002a). Isolation of Nipah virus from Malaysian island flying-foxes. *Microbes and Infection*, 4, 145–151.

Chua, K. B., Lam, S. K., Goh, K. J., Hooi, P. S., Ksiazek, T. G., Kamarulzaman, A., Olson, J., & Tan, C. T. (2001a). The presence of Nipah virus in respiratory secretions and urine of patients during an outbreak of Nipah virus encephalitis in Malaysia. *Journal of Infection*, 42, 40–43.

Chua, K. B., Wang, L. F., Lam, S. K., Crameri, G., Yu, M., Wise, T., Boyle, D., Hyatt, A. D., & Eaton, B. T. (2001b). Tioman virus, a novel paramyxovirus isolated from fruit bats in Malaysia. *Virology*, 283, 215–229.

Chua, K. B., Wang, L. F., Lam, S. K., & Eaton, B. T. (2002b). Full length genome sequence of Tioman virus, a novel paramyxovirus in the genus Rubulavirus isolated from fruit bats in Malaysia. *Archives of Virology*, 147, 1323–1348.

Daniels, P., Aziz, J., Ksiazek, T., Ong, B., Bunning, M., Johara, B., Field, H., Olson, J., Hoffmann, D., Bilou, J., & Ozawa, Y. (2000). Nipah virus considerations for regional preparedness. In S. Blacksell (Ed.), *Classical Swine Fever and Emerging Diseases in Southeast Asia. ACIAR Proceedings No. 94* (pp. 133–141). Canberra: Australian Centre for International Agricultural Research.

Eaton, B. T., Broder, C. C., Middelton, D., & Wang, L. F. (2006). Hendra and Nipah viruses: Different and dangerous. *Nature Reviews Microbiology*, 4, 23–35.

Field, H., Mackenzie, J., & Daszak, P. (2004). Novel viral encephalitides associated with bats (Chiroptera)–host management strategies. *Archives of Virology Supplement*, 113–121.

Field, H., Young, P., Yob, J. M., Mills, J., Hall, L., & Mackenzie, J. (2001a). The natural history of Hendra and Nipah viruses. *Microbes and Infection*, 3, 307–314.

Field, H. E., L. S. Hall, & Mackenzie, J. S. (2001b). Emerging zoonotic paramyxoviruses: The role of pteropid bats. In *Emergence and Control of Zoonotic Ortho and Paramyxovirus Diseases* (pp. 205–209), Montrouge France: John Libby Eurotext.

Field, H. F., Mackenzie, J. S., & Daszak, P. (2007). Henipaviruses: Emerging paramyxoviruses associated with fruit bats. *Current Topics in Microbiology and Immunology*, 315, 133–159.

Goh, K. J., Tan, C. T., Chew, N. K., Tan, P. S. K., Kamarulzaman, A., Sarji, S. A., Wong, K. T., Abdullah, B. J. J., Chua, K. B., & Lam, S. K. (2000). Clinical features of Nipah virus encephalitis among pig farmers in Malaysia. *New England Journal of Medicine*, 342, 1229–1235.

Griffin, D. E. (2001). Measles viruses. In B. N. Fields, D. M. Knipe, & P. M. Howley (Eds.), *Fields Virolog*, 4th edn, (pp. 1401–1442), Philadelphia: Lippincott-Raven.

Guillaume, V., Contamin, H., Loth, P., Grosjean, I., Georges Courbot, M. C., Deubel, V., Buckland, R., & Wild, T. F. (2006). Antibody prophylaxis and therapy against Nipah virus infection in hamsters. *Journal of Virology*, 80, 1972–1978.

Hall, L., & Richards, G. (2000). *Flying foxes*, Sydney: University of New South Wales.

Halpin, K., Young, P. L., Field, H. E., & Mackenzie, J. S. (2000). Isolation of Hendra virus from pteropid bats: A natural reservoir of Hendra virus. *Journal of General Virology*, 81, 1927–1932.

Harcourt, B. H., Lowe, L., Tamin, A., Liu, X., Bankamp, B., Bowden, N., Rollin, P. E., Comer, J. A., Ksiazek, T. G., Hossain, M. J., Gurley, E. S., Brieman, R. F., Bellini, W. J., & Rota, P. A. (2005). Genetic characterization of Nipah virus, Bangladesh, 2004. *Emerging Infectious Diseases*, 11, 1594–1597.

Hooper, P. T., Gould, A. R., Russell, G. M., Kattenbelt, J. A., & Mitchell, G. (1996). The retrospective diagnosis of a second outbreak of equine morbillivirus infection. *Australian Veterinary Journal*, 74, 244–245.

Hooper, P. T., Ketterer, P. J., Hyatt, A. D., & Russell, G. M. (1997). Lesions of experimental equine morbillivirus pneumonia in horses. *Veterinary Pathology*, 34, 312–322.

Hsu, V. P., Hossain, M. J., Parashar, U. D., Ali, M. M., Ksiazek, T. G., Kuzmin, I., Niezgoda, M., Rupprecht, C., Brese, J., & Brieman, R. F. (2004). Nipah virus encephalitis reemergence, Bangladesh. *Emerging Infectious Diseases*, 12, 2082–2087.

ICDDRB. (2003). Outbreaks of viral encephalitis due to Nipah/Hendra-like viruses, Western Bangladesh. *HSB Health and Science Bulletin*, 1, 1–6.

ICDDRB. (2004a). Nipah encephalitis outbreak over wide area of Western Bangladesh, 2004. *Health and Science Bulletin*, 2, 7–11.

ICDDRB. (2004b). Person to person transmission of Nipah virus during outbreak in Faridpur district 2004. *Health and Science Bulletin*, 2, 5–9.

ICDDRB. (2005). Nipah virus outbreak from date palm juice. *Health and Science Bulletin*, 3, 1–5.

Koopman, K. F. (1992). Order Chiroptera. In D. E. Wilson & D.M. Reeder (Eds.), *Mammal Species of the World: A Taxonomy and Geographic Reference,* 2nd ed., (pp. 137–241), Washington: Smithsonian Institution Press.

Kumar, S. (2003). Inadequate research facilities fail to tackle mystery disease. *British Medical Journal*, 326, 12.

Lau, S. K. P., Woo, P. C. Y., Li, K. S. M., Huang, Y., Tsoi, H., Wong, B. H. L., Wong, S. S. Y., Leung, S., Chan, K., & Yuen, K. (2005). Severe acute respiratory syndrome coronavirus-like virus in Chinese horseshoe bats. *Proceedings of National Academy of Sciences USA*, 102, 14040–14045.

Leroy, E. M., Kumulungui, B., Pourrut, X., Rouquet, P., Hassanin, A., Yaba, P., Delicat, A., Paweska, J. T., Gonzalez, J. P., & Swanepoel, R. (2005). Fruit bats as reservoirs of Ebola virus. *Nature*, 438, 575–576.

Li, W., Shi, Z., Yu, M., Ren, W., Smith, C., Epstein, J. H., Wang, H., Crameri, G., Hu, Z., Zhang, H., Jianhong, Z., McEachern, J., Field, H., Daszak, P., Eaton, B. T., Zhang, S., & Wang, L. F. (2005). Bats are natural reservoirs of SARS-like coronaviruses. *Science*, 310, 676–679.

Love, R. J., Philbey, A. W., Kirkland, P. D., Ross, A. D., Davis, R. J., Morrissey, C., & Daniels, P. W. (2001). Reproductive disease and congenital malformations caused by Menangle virus in pigs. *Australian Veterinary Journal*, 79, 192–198.

Mackenzie, J. S., & Field, H. E. (2004). Emerging encephalitogenic viruses: lyssaviruses and henipaviruses transmitted by frugivorous bats. *Archives of Virology Supplement*, 97–111.

Mackenzie, J. S., Field, H. E., & Guyatt, K. J. (2003). Managing emerging diseases borne by fruit bats (flying foxes), with particular reference to henipaviruses and Australian bat lyssavirus. *Journal of Applied Microbiology*, 94, 59S–69S.

Mayo, M. A. (2002). Virus taxonomy – Houston 2002. *Archives of Virology*, 147, 1071–1076.

Middleton, D. J., Westbury, H. A., Morrissy, C. J., van der Heide, B. M., Russell, G. M., Braun, M. A., & Hyatt, A. D. (2002). Experimental Nipah virus infection in pigs and cats. *Journal of Comparative Pathology*, 126, 124–136.

Mohd. Nor, M. N., Gan, C. H., & Ong, B. L. (2000). Nipah virus infection of pigs in peninsular Malaysia. *Revue Scientific Et Technical Office Internationale Epizootie*, 19, 160–165.

Mounts, A. W., Kaur, H., Parashar, U. D., Ksiazek, T. G., Cannon, D., Arokiasamy, J. T., Anderson, L. J., & Lye, M. S. (2001). A cohort study of health care workers to assess nosocomial transmissibility of Nipah virus, Malaysia, 1999. *Journal of Infectious Disease*, 183, 810–813.

Murray, K., Rogers, R., Selvey, L., Selleck, P., Hyatt, A., Gould, A., Gleeson, L., Hooper, P., & Westbury, H. (1995a). A novel morbillivirus pneumonia of horses and its transmission to humans. *Emerging Infectious Diseases*, 1, 31–33.

Murray, K., Selleck, P., Hooper, P., Hyatt, A., Gould, A., Gleeson, L., Westbury, H., Hiley, L., Selvey, L., & Rodwell, B. (1995b). A morbillivirus that caused fatal disease in horses and humans. *Science*, 268, 94–97.

O'Sullivan, J. D., Allworth, A. M., Paterson, D. L., Snow, T. M., Boots, R., Gleeson, L. J., Gould, A. R., Hyatt, A. D., & Bradfield, J. (1997). Fatal encephalitis due to novel paramyxovirus transmitted from horses. *Lancet*, 349, 93–95.

Olson, J. G., Rupprecht, C., Rollin, P. E., An, U. S., Niezgoda, M., Clemins, T., Walston, J., & Ksiazek, T. G. (2002). Antibodies to Nipah-like virus in bats (Pteropus lylei), Cambodia. *Emerging Infectious Diseases*, 8, 987–988.

Parashar, U. D., Sunn, L. M., Ong, F., Mounts, A. W., Arif, M. T., Ksiazek, T. G., Kamaluddin, M. A., Mustafa, A. N., Kaur, H., Ding, L. M., Othman, G., Radzi, H. M., Kitsutani, P. T., Stockton, P. C., Arokiasamy, J. T., Gary Jr, H. E., & Anderson, L. J. (2000). Case-control study of risk factors for human infection with a new zoonotic paramyxovirus, Nipah virus, during a 1998–1999 outbreak of severe encephalitis in Malaysia. *Journal of Infectious Disease*, 181, 1755–1759.

Paton, N. I., Leo, Y. S., Zaki, S. R., Auchus, A. P., Lee, K. E., Ling, A. E., Chew, S. K., Ang, B. S. P., Rollin, P. E., Umapathi, T., Sng, I., Lee, C. C., Lim, E., & Ksiazek, T. G. (1999). Outbreak of Nipah-virus infection among abattoir workers in Singapore. *Lancet*, 354, 1253–1256.

Philbey, A. W., Kirkland, P. D., Ross, A. D., Davis, R. J., Gleeson, A. B., Love, R. J., Daniels, P. W., Gould, A. R., & Hyatt, A. D. (1998). An apparently new virus (family Paramyxoviridae) infectious for pigs, humans, and fruit bats. *Emerging Infectious Diseases*, 4, 269–271.

Pringle, C. R. (1991). The order Mononegavirales. *Archives of Virology*, 117, 137–140.

ProMed. (2004). Hendra virus – Australia (Queensland). Archive Number 20041214.3307.

Reynes, J., Counor, D., Ong, S., Faure, C., Seng, V., Molia, S., Walston, J., Georges-Coubot, M. C., Deubel, V., & Sarthou, J. (2005). Nipah virus in Lyle's flying foxes, Cambodia. *Emerging Infectious Diseases*, 11, 1042–1047.

Rogers, R. J., Douglas, I. C., Baldock, F. C., Glanville, R. J., Seppanen, K. T., Gleeson, L. J., Selleck, P. N., & Dunn, K. J. (1996). Investigation of a second focus of equine morbillivirus infection in coastal Queensland. *Australian Veterinary Journal*, 74, 243–244.

Selvey, L., Taylor, R., Arklay, A., & Gerrard, J. (1996). Screening of bat carers for antibodies to equine morbillivirus. *Communiccable Diseases Intelligence*, 20, 477–478.

Selvey, L. A., Wells, R. M., McCormack, J. G., Ansford, A. J., Murray, K., Rogers, R. J., Lavercombe, P. S., Selleck, P., & Sheridan, J. W. (1995). Infection of humans and horses by a newly described morbillivirus. *Medical Journal of Australia*, 162, 642–645.

Sendow, I., Field, H. F., Curran, J., Morrissy, C., Meehan, G., Buick, T., & Daniels, P. (2006). Henipavirus infection in *Pteropus* bats flying foxes in the Indonesian archipelago. *Emerging Infectious Diseases*, 12, 711–712.

Sulkin, S. E., & Allen, R. (1974). Virus infections in bats, Vol. 8. In J. L. Melnick (Ed.), *Monographs in Virology*. Basel: Karger.

Wacharapluesadee, S., Lumlertdacha, B., Boongird, K., Wanghongsa, S., Chanhome, L., Rollin, P., Stockton, P., Rupprecht, C. E., Ksiazek, T. G., & Hemachudha, T. (2005). Bat Nipah virus, Thailand. *Emerging Infectious Diseases*, 11, 1949–1951.

Wang, L. F., Yu, M., Hansson, E., Pritchard, L. I., Shiell, B., Michalski, W. P., & Eaton, B. T. (2000). The exceptionally large genome of Hendra virus: Support for creation of a new genus within the family Paramyxoviridae. *Journal of Virology*, 74, 9972–9979.

Williamson, M. M., Hooper, P. T., Selleck, P. W., Gleeson, L. J., Daniels, P. W., Westbury, H. A., & Murray, P. K. (1998). Transmission studies of Hendra virus (equine morbillivirus) in fruit bats, horses and cats. *Australian Veterinary Journal*, 76, 813–818.

Williamson, M. M., Hooper, P. T., Selleck, P. W., Westbury, H. A., & Slocombe, R. F. (2000). Experimental Hendra virus infection in pregnant guinea-pigs and fruit bats (Pteropus poliocephalus). *Journal of Comparative Pathology*, 122, 201–207.

Wong, K. T., Grosjean, I., Brisson, C., Blanquier, B., Fevre-Montange, M., Bernard, A , Loth, P., Georges-Courbot, M. C., Chevallier, M., Akaoka, H , Marianneau, P., Lam, S. K., Wild, T. F., & Deubel, V. (2003). A golden hamster model for human acute Nipah virus infection. *American Journal of Pathology*, 163, 2127–2137.

Woolhouse, M. E. J., & Gowtage-Sequeria, S. (2005). Host range and emerging and reemerging pathogens. *Emerging Infectious Diseases*, 11, 1842–1847.

Wright, P. J., Crameri, G. S., & Eaton, B. T. (2004). RNA synthesis during infection by Hendra virus: An examination by quantitative real-time PCR of RNA accumulation, the effect of ribavirin and the attenuation of transcription. *Archives of Virology*, 150, 521–532.

Yob, J. M., Field, H., Rashdi, A. M., Morrissy, C., van der heide, B., Rota, P., Binadzhar, A., White, J., Daniels, P., Jamaluddin, A., & Ksiazek, T. (2001). Nipah virus infection in bats (order Chiroptera) in Peninsular Malaysia. *Emerging Infectious Diseases*, 7, 439–441.

Young, P., Halpin, K. F. H., & Mackenzie, J. (1997). Finding the wild life reservoir of equine morbillivirus. *Recent Advances in Microbiology*, 5, 1–12.

Young, P. L., Halpin, K., Selleck, P. W., Field, H., Gravel, J. L., Kelly, M. A., & Mackenzie, J. S. (1996). Serologic evidence for the presence in Pteropus bats of a paramyxovirus related to equine morbillivirus. *Emerging Infectious Diseases*, 2, 239–240.

Zhu, Z., Dimitrov, A. S., Bossart, K. N., Crameri, G., Bishop, K. A., Choudhry, V., Mungall, B. A., Feng, Y.-R., Choudhary, A., Zhang, M.-Y., Feng, Y., Wang, L. F., Xiao, X., Eaton, B. T., Broder, C. C., & Dimitrov, D. S. (2006). Potent neutralization of Hendra and Nipah viruses by human monoclonal antibodies. *Journal of Virology*, 80, 891–899.

Multidrug Resistant TB, TB Control, and Millennium Development Goals in Asia

Srikanth Prasad Tripathy and Sriram Prasad Tripathy

Introduction

Tuberculosis is a major communicable disease, which has existed in the world for over two millennia. It affects people from all countries, more in some and less in others. The Asian countries have over 60% of the global TB burden. Specific treatment for tuberculosis was available only after the 1943 discovery of streptomycin. Many other anti-tuberculosis drugs have since been discovered and their efficacies established through controlled clinical trials. Table 1 presents a list of commonly used anti-tuberculosis drugs that are in use currently. Concerted efforts by researchers spread over the globe have provided us the scientific basis of treatment and management of TB patients through carefully conducted, controlled clinical trials in patients in different countries and settings. The World Health Organization was closely associated with most of those trials and has played a key role in the formulation of national tuberculosis programs in most countries adopting a uniform DOTS (Directly Observed Therapy, Short Course) strategy, which now forms the basis of TB control programs in 184 countries in the world (World Health Organization, 2007a). In the early introduction of chemotherapy, the incidence and prevalence of TB was high in many Asian countries. Mortality was high, diagnosis was delayed, and patients presented with advanced disease including some with acute fulminant tuberculosis, which often ended in death. Today, diagnosis is early, incidence and prevalence of tuberculosis have declined, most patients have access to drugs and are successfully treated, mortality has considerably reduced and very few patients present with acute fulminant TB. Currently available regimens under DOTS strategy include highly potent drugs of streptomycin (S), isoniazid (H), rifampicin (R), ethambutol (E), and pyrazinamide (Z), which form the sheet anchor of treatment programs in most countries. While the DOTS regimens have a potential of curing 100% of new cases in program conditions, a success rate of over 85% is acceptable.

The DOTS strategy includes a strong political commitment, uninterrupted supply of anti-TB drugs of assured quality and administration of the drugs under direct observation, provision of diagnostic facilities for sputum smear examination, and standardized documentation and reporting systems. Nearly all Asian countries have adopted the DOTS strategy in their National TB Control Programs and have

Y. Lu et al. (eds.), *Emerging Infections in Asia.*
© Springer Science+Business Media, LLC 2008

Table 1 Commonly used anti-TB drugs

First line	Oral	Isoniazid (H), Rifampicin (R), Ethambutol (E), Pyrazinamide (Z)
	Injectables	Streptomycin (S)
Second Line	Injectables	Kanamycin (Km), Amikacin (Am), Capreomycin (Cm), Viomycin (Vm)
	Oral	Fluoroquinolones (oral), Ciprofloxacin (Cfx), Ofloxacin (Ofx), Levofloxacin (Lvx), Moxifloxacin (Mfx), Gatifloxacin (Gfx)
	Other oral second line drugs	Ethionamide (Eto), Prothionamide (Pto), Cycloserine (Cs), Para amino salicylic acid (PAS), Thiacetazone (T)

Source: Central TB Division, 2007

seen some decline in the incidence of TB in their countries since the introduction of DOTS (World Health Organization 2007a).

Changes in Drug Resistance Scenario Over Time

The formulation of the DOTS regimens is based on the premise that most newly diagnosed TB cases have organisms fully susceptible to all drugs or have monoresistance to one of the four drugs SHRE: some may have polyresistance to two or more drugs but not to H and R together, and a very small number (about 1–2%) have multi-drug resistance, that is, resistance to both rifampicin and isoniazid, with or without resistance to any other drug. This could well change with the continued use of the current short course regimens under DOTS, with possible increase in MDR rates in patients failing on DOTS regimens. Experience with drug regimens in the past has shown an increase in the level of isoniazid resistance with the use of isoniazid containing regimens in country programs over several years before the formulation of the DOTS strategy.

TB Drug Resistance in Asian Countries

The Asian continent has a very large population with the two most populous countries of China and India and many other countries of varying sizes. In the 1950s, Asian countries with limited financial resources belonged to the class of developing countries with large disease burden, mostly communicable diseases. They could afford only inexpensive drug regimens for TB, sometimes isoniazid alone, but mostly two drug regimens, isoniazid with a companion drug PAS or thiacetazone, both of which are bacteriostatic in activity. The continued use of such regimens with a failure rate of at least 15% over several decades resulted in the emergence of isoniazid resistant strains, their transmission in the community, and a rise in the level of isoniazid resistant strains in new cases from 2% to 3% in the initial years of the program to about 15% in India (Table 2) and in most Asian countries by the 1970s. Thereafter, the countries replaced the companion drug PAS or thiacetazone with more potent drugs Ethambutol or Rifampicin, resulting in fewer failures and hence lower proportions of isoniazid resistance. There has also been a gradual increase in two-drug or three-drug resistant strains including MDR strains, since most failures among new cases with initial drug resistance would result in polyresistance or MDR. The proportion of MDR patients among new TB cases would influence the success of the National TB Control Program. In Asian countries, about 80% of the TB cases treated are new cases with a small number of MDR TB patients and hence, high success rates can be achieved by Category I DOTS regimens (Table 3). About 20% of cases are previously treated cases, with higher rates of MDR TB, and hence the success rates are lower with Category II DOTS regimen used for them. Failures among these patients with

Table 2 Trends in H resistance in new cases in Tiruvellore (1971–1986) prior to use of DOTS

Period	Total patients	Isoniazid resistant (%)
1971–73	709	8
1973–75	621	11.8
1976–78	577	7.4
1979–81	520	13.5
1981–83	531	15.0
1984–86	530	13.6

Source: Tuberculosis Research Center, 2003

Table 3 Categories of DOTS Treatment Regimens

TB treatment category	TB patients	Treatment	
		Initial phase	Continuation phase
Cat I	New cases with smear positive PTB; Severe cases with EPTB; New cases with severe smear negative PTB	2HRZE $2H_3R_3Z_3E_3$ $2H_3R_3Z_3S_3$	6HE 4HR $4H_3R_3$
Cat II	Previously treated smear positive PTB; Relapse; Treatment failure; Treatment after default	2HRZES/1HRZE $2H_3R_3Z_3E_3S_3/$ $1H_3R_3Z_3E_3$	5HRE $5H_3R_3E_3$
Cat III	New cases with smear negative PTB or less severe EPTB	2HRZ $2H_3R_3Z_3$	6HE 4HR $4H_3R_3$

Numbers before the letters indicate the duration of treatment in months; numbers in subscript indicate the number of times the drugs can be administered in a week
Source: World Health Organization, Regional Office for South East Asia, 2002
PTB Pulmonary TB, *EPTB* Extrapulmonary TB

Category II regimen have higher MDR rates and these will transmit MDR strains in the community, resulting in a possible increase in MDR levels in future years with an adverse impact on the success of future TB programs.

DOTS and Millennium Development Goals (MDGs)

Encouraged by the highly promising results obtained in many countries following the introduction of DOTS strategies, the United Nations set up specific targets to be achieved in control programs as a part of the Millennium Development Goals (Table 4). These targets are expected to be reached by individual countries through successful implementation of all components of the DOTS strategy.

Drug Resistance Surveillance (DRS) Project

With current levels of MDR in new cases, it is possible to attain the MDG goals but if the levels increase, the success rates will be substantially lower, as in some parts of China and Russia, where the MDR TB rates are high among new cases (World Health Organization, 2004). It is necessary to maintain surveillance of the drug resistance situation to ensure that resistance levels do not increase or if they do, they are detected early and appropriate corrective steps are taken to prevent further increase through successful management of MDR TB.

The WHO/IUATLD Global Project on Anti-tuberculosis Drug Resistance Surveillance – the DRS Project – established jointly by the World Health Organization and the International Union Against Tuberculosis and Lung Disease has been conducting drug resistance surveys in different countries since 1994 using appropriate sampling techniques and employing reliable drug resistance testing (DST) in accredited laboratories and with appropriate quality assurance (World Health Organization, 2004). Three reports published by the project provide valuable information on the prevalence of drug resistance in different countries and the trends in resistance (World Health Organization, 2004). The third report demonstrated

Table 4 Millennium development goal (MDG) targets for TB control

Epidemiological indicator	MDG target	Target year
DOTS case detection (%)	70	2005 (indicator 25)
DOTS treatment success (%)	85	2005 (indicator 25)
Incidence rate (per 100,000 per year)	Falling	2015 (target 8)
Prevalence rate (per 100,000)	Half 1990 level	2015 (indicator 23)
Mortality rate (per 100,000 per year)	Half 1990 level	2015
Incidence rate (per 1,000,000 per year)	1	2050

Source: World Health Organization, 2005, 2007a

Table 5 DRS findings in eight Districts in India 1999–2003

Resistant to	Range (%)
H	2.5–24.5
R	0.7–3.0
HR	0.5–2.8

Source: Tuberculosis Research Center, 2007 unpublished data

that many countries face endemic and epidemic MDR. In patients never previously treated, the median prevalence of resistance to any of the four drugs SHER was 10% (range 0–57%), most commonly to H or S; 27 sites exceeded 20%. The median prevalence of MDR TB was 1.2% (range 0–14%); 11 sites exceeded 6.5% of threshold for extreme values. In patients who had treatment previously, the median prevalence of any resistance was 23.3% (0–82%) and of MDR TB was 7.7% (0–58%). Generally, the prevalence of MDR in new TB cases was low except in the province of Liaoning in China, where the prevalence was about 10%, possibly reflecting the liberal use of rifampicin in an uncontrolled manner in the pre-DOTS era. While rifampicin was expensive in other countries, China produced rifampicin locally without patent restrictions and hence the drug was available in large quantities at low cost for the TB program. The DRS data in eight districts of India showed a wide range (2.5–24.5%) in the prevalence of isoniazid resistance and a low rate of 0.5–2.8% for rifampicin resistance (Table 5).

Role of Asia in Attaining MDG Targets

Efforts to achieve MDG targets for tuberculosis would need to involve all continents and especially Asia by virtue of its large population and high TB burden. The contribution of Asian countries to TB control and research has been substantial and it is expected that the Asian TB control programs will be able to achieve the targets. Success of the program in Asian countries will be vital for achieving the global target for MDG.

Burden of TB in Asia

The Asian continent has the largest TB burden among all continents, contributing to over 60% of the global disease burden and accounting for over 50% of TB mortality. The World Health Organization has identified 22 countries in the world as High Burden Countries (HBCs) and of these, 11 are in Asia (World Health Organization, 2007a). The disease burden in these countries is presented in Table 6. These data

Table 6 TB in high burden countries in Asia (2005)

Country	Pop (million)	Incidence All forms (×1,000)	Incidence Sm+ve (×1,000)	Prevalence (all forms) ×1,000	Deaths (×1,000)	DOTS coverage (%)
India	1,103	1,852	827	3,399	322	91
China	1,316	1,319	593	2,837	205	100
Indonesia	222	533	240	584	100	98
Bangladesh	142	322	145	575	66	99
Pakistan	158	286	129	468	59	100
Phillipines	83	242	109	374	39	100
Vietnam	84	148	66	198	19	100
Thailand	64	91	41	131	12	100
Myanmar	51	86	38	86	8	95
Cambodia	14	71	32	99	12	100
Afghanistan	30	50	23	86	10	81
HBCs (Asia:11)	3,267	5,000	2,243	8,637	842	81–100
HBCs (22)	4,145	7,033	3,117	11,546	1,265	94
Global	6.462	8,811	3,902	14,052	1,577	89

Source: World Health Organization 2007a

have been collected through surveillance as a part of TB control activity in the respective countries, supplemented by findings of DRS projects in the country. The 11 Asian TB HBCs account for over 50% of the global TB incidence, prevalence, and TB mortality and to over 60% of the total burden in the 22 HBCs, with two countries, India and China, leading the group in morbidity and mortality. Successful implementation of TB control in these 11 countries would contribute significantly to the success of the global TB Program. All these 11 HBCs in Asia have been targeted through well-established DOTS strategy and have achieved coverage of 81–100% of the population in all the 11 countries (Table 6).

In a cohort of patients admitted to DOTS in 2004, the overall success rate of DOTs in newly diagnosed cases was 82% in a total of 2.1 million treated globally, with similar achievement in the 11 Asian HBCs (World Health Organization 2007a). The progress of TB control activities in these countries is being monitored regularly by national authorities as well as by international agencies. Because of successful implementation of DOTS, many of these 11 countries have almost achieved the 2005 goal of 100% DOTS coverage in the country and 70% case detection. In addition, there is a WHO Millennium Development Goal of halting the increase and reversing the trend of incidence of TB in these countries by 2015 (Table 6). Furthermore, the Stop TB Program has set up targets of reducing TB mortality by 2015 and incidence by 50% of the levels in 1990. With the current tempo of control activities in these countries, it is likely that the 11 countries would attain the 2015 targets, barring two confounding factors, HIV incidence and MDR TB in the country. The close interaction between TB and HIV poses a great problem – increased incidence of TB and considerably high mortality rates due to TB as well as AIDS. However, with proper management of TB/HIV patients with ATT, stabilization of the HIV epidemic through National AIDS Control Programs, and access of AIDS patients to standard anti-retroviral therapy (ART) in some of these countries as part of the 3 by 5 program of the WHO, HIV epidemic by itself may not be an impediment in achieving the target of halving the TB mortality by 2015 to 50% of the level in 1990 in each country. The magnitude of the adverse impact of MDR in achieving this target, however, is unpredictable and would depend on the trends of MDR in the country in the coming years.

The level of MDR is not a static figure in any country. Data on prevalence of MDR TB in the 11 HBCs are presented in Table 7. The prevalence is low in new cases, ranging from 0% to 5.3%. Understandably, the proportions are higher, 3.1–27%, in previously treated cases. The regimens in the DOTS program are robust enough to tackle single drug resistance such as isoniazid or streptomycin but are totally inadequate if there is multidrug resistance, defined as resistance to at least isoniazid and rifampicin, with or without resistance to any other anti-TB drugs. As many as 80% of such cases would fail on regular DOTS regimens. However, the overall success rate in new cases is still high – indeed over 85% success rates have been achieved – largely because the prevalence of MDR TB in newly diagnosed TB cases is low (Table 7). High success rates with the present regimen in new cases would be dependent upon continued low prevalence of MDR in the countries. Much would depend on the dynamics of transmission of resistant strains in the community.

Evolution of MDR TB During Treatment

During bacterial subdivision, isoniazid resistant mutants occur spontaneously, at a low frequency of about 1 in 10^6 bacilli. The presence of a small number of isoniazid-resistant mutants among predominantly isoniazid-sensitive bacilli in

Table 7 Prevalence of MDR TB in Asian HBCs (2004)

Country	DOTS coverage (%)	New cases		Previously treated cases		HIV in TB cases (%)
		MDR (%)	DOTS success rate (%)	MDR (%)	DOTS success rate (%)	
Afghanistan	91	1.7	86	28	–	0.0
Bangladesh	99	1.8	90	14.0	81	0.1
Cambodia	100	0.0	91	3.1	86	6
China	100	5.3	94	27	89	0.5
India	91	2.5	86	15	73	5.2
Indonesia	98	1.6	90	14	82	0.8
Myanmar	95	4.4	84	16.0	74	7.1
Pakistan	100	1.9	82	28	78	0.6
Philippines	100	1.5	87	14	53	0.1
Thailand	100	0.9	74	20	56	7.6
Vietnam	100	2.3	93	14.0	84	3.0

Source: World Health Organization 2007a

new cases of tuberculosis is of little consequence in a patient undergoing DOTS, since the other three drugs – Rifampicin, Ethambutol, and Pyrazinamide – would eliminate the isoniazid-resistant mutants. Indeed, none of the single drug-resistant mutants is of clinical significance. Mutants resistant to both H and R would not be eliminated by the two most potent drugs, H and R; however, their frequency is so low (about 1 in 10^{14}) that they rarely occur through spontaneous mutation in a bacterial population in a patient with drug sensitive bacilli. The emergence of such HR resistant strains would occur more easily if the patient has primary H-resistant strains to begin with or has acquired H-resistance during treatment; the frequency of occurrence of R-resistance in such populations would be about 1 in 10^7–10^8, and the resulting mutants would be resistant to both H and R. Continued use of rifampicin would eliminate the rifampicin sensitive bacteria, leaving a residual homogenous population of bacilli resistant to both H and R, i.e., multidrug resistant (MDR) TB. Such a person is unlikely to respond to further treatment with H and R containing regimens and is likely to infect contacts with MDR strains. The infection remains latent over several years with reactivation to active disease occurring in some persons. Most cases of TB occur as a result of endogenous reactivation in about 10% of persons with latent infections over a lifetime and hence only about 10% of the persons having latent infection with MDR strains will ever develop active TB with MDR strains, as in the case of persons infected with drug sensitive strains.

Changes in Incidence of MDR TB in the Community

The transmission of infection by patients with acquired MDR-TB would thus lead to an increase in the incidence of MDR-TB in newly diagnosed TB cases in future years. The increase of MDR-TB in new cases would depend on the relative proportions of MDR-TB and drug sensitive TB strains infecting the population. If the program produces a few failures, only a small number of MDR-TB patients will be transmitting infection with MDR strain. If there are more failures and many of them have MDR-TB, there will be more transmission of MDR-TB infection and hence higher incidence of MDR-TB disease in later years. This number will steadily increase, resulting in significant numbers of MDR-TB patients among newly diagnosed TB cases. This increase will be seen after a gap of 5–10 years, since TB disease usually occurs due to endogenous reactivation of latent infection after several years.

Although these sequence of events can be inferred by analysis of surveillance data from the countries and correlating them with changes in the drug sensitivity patterns over the years in each country and with the drug regimens used, comparison of data from different settings becomes difficult since the data on drug resistance are based on different methods of sensitivity tests as well as unstandardized tests. Such a comparison would be possible if the methods of Drug Sensitivity Testing (DST) are standardized and remain unchanged over time. Such reliable data are available from the Indian TB program and research activities, and provide valuable information as to how drug resistance has evolved over the years in the face of ongoing control activities in the country. Lessons learnt from the Indian situation would be equally applicable to the other Asian countries.

TB Control in India

India initiated a control program in 1952 that aimed to provide free treatment to all TB patients diagnosed in the country. The regimens used were PAS plus Isoniazid (PH) or Thiacetazone plus Isoniazid (TH). The regimens were unsupervised, self-medicated, and produced a cure in about 50% of cases under program conditions. Among the failures, many developed H resistance and transmitted H resistant strains to their contacts. Reactivation in about 10% of those having latent infection with isoniazid resistant strains must have produced active disease and thus, this increased the level of isoniazid resistance in newly diagnosed cases in the first four decades of the TB program. Patients with primary and acquired resistance to isoniazid responded poorly to the PH regimen used (Tripathy et al., 1969); this resulted in more failures, and further transmission of H resistant strains. While many countries in the world had H resistance levels of 3–5% in new cases, India had levels of about 15% (Tables 2 and 8).

Rifampicin was not used in the program in these years, and hence MDR was infrequent in such patients. Rifampicin was included as a part of short course regimens in 18 districts (out of about 450 districts) in the eighties, and as DOTS in a pilot project in Delhi in 1993. DOTS was adopted as the Revised National TB Control Program (RNTCP) in 1998 in some districts and has been steadily expanded to cover 67% of the country by 2003 and 100% by 2005. Under DOTS, patients receive four drugs RHEZ for 2 months followed by RH thrice weekly for 4 months (2RHEZ$_3$/4RH$_3$) in newly diagnosed cases (Category I); patients who have been previously treated with at least 1 month of anti-tuberculosis therapy (ATT) are placed in a separate category (Category II) in which they receive RHEZ for 3 months, with a streptomycin supplement in the first two months, plus RHE for 5 months thrice weekly, all under direct observation (Table 3). The four drug combination, HRZE, has been shown in clinical trials to be highly effective in the

Table 8 Drug resistance among TB cases in a DOTS program, Tiruvellore, India, 1999–2003

	Percent resistant	
	New cases (n = 1603)	Previously treated (n = 226)
Fully sensitive	85	59
Any resistance	15	41
Any H resistance	10	37
HR resistance	1.7	12

Source: Santha et al., 2006b

management of TB with low rates of emergence of drug resistance in sputum positive patients (Tuberculosis Research Center, 2001)

India's DOTS program has been a good success story and has served as a model program globally (Dye, 2006; Central TB Division, 2006). The latest report indicates that 86% of new cases have been successfully treated (85% cured, 1% completed) (World Health Organization, 2007a). Only 2.5% of the patients failed, and thus would pose only a small problem regarding transmission of isoniazid resistance or MDR strains. Only 2.4% of the new cases diagnosed in 2004 had MDR (Table 7); among those previously treated the proportion of MDR TB was higher −25% − mostly following the emergence of isoniazid resistance as the first step, followed by subsequent emergence of Rifampicin resistance − i.e., the emergence of MDR-TB.

Can tuberculosis burden decline with DOTS? This issue was addressed hypothetically with a presumed success of 85% and a coverage of 70%. It was seen that at the end of 2 years of successful DOTS implementation, there would be an over 30% reduction in the prevalent TB cases in the community (Frieden, 2002). Of the 5% who fail and have active TB, half are likely to have resistance to R and H, i.e., MDR − a figure no higher than what was prevalent before the start of DOTS.

The Indian data on the results of DOTS under RNTCP provide a strong indication that MDR prevalence in new cases will not increase as a result of the failure of a proportion of patients treated with the Category I regimen and further management of the failures with a Category II regimen containing rifampicin. DST results on a cohort of new patients admitted to a control program in the Model DOTS area in Tiruvellore indicated that in the Program area, the prevalence of MDR in new cases in 2003 was no higher than the level at the start of 1999 when DOTS was introduced there (Table 9).

Can the Category I failures be treated with Category II regimen successfully? The reservations regarding the efficacy of Category II regimens have the basis in the composition of the Category II regimen, which has the same four Category I drugs, RHEZ, with only one more drug, Streptomycin, added and the duration of treatment is extended to 8 months. While prima facie, it would seem that the benefit from the Category II regimen may not be substantial, the regimen indeed proved

Table 9 Trends in drug resistance in 1,603 new cases in a DOTS program (1999–2003)

Year	H resistance	HR Resistance (MDR)
1999	16	3.5
2000	9.8	0.9
2001	9.8	1.1
2002	9.3	1.0
2003	9.7	2.7

Source: Santha et al., 2006b

to be highly effective in the model DOTS project in Tiruvellore in India (Santha et al., 2006a). It is thus expected that by and large, using Category I regimen in new patients and Category II regimen in previously treated cases and in failures of Category I cases would be an appropriate strategy, which would provide very good results (Joseph et al., 2006).

There is, however, a small risk of a high proportion of failure patients having MDR. The present group of patients placed on the Category II regimen is a mixture of failure of patients treated outside DOTS, patients with relapsed disease, bacteriological failure of the Category I regimen under DOTS, and patients who have returned after default. Patients who relapse usually do so with drug sensitive cultures and those who default are less likely to have developed drug resistance and hence both these groups of patients should respond to the Category II regimen. Patients who are treated outside DOTS and had failed generally do so because of inadequate and irregular treatment and the chances of MDR in them may not be high. The only category that may have substantial rates of MDR is the group of bacteriological failures on the Category I regimen. This group, however, currently constitutes only a small proportion of patients placed on the Category II regimen. This may change as the DOTS coverage expands to the entire country, and in future years, most of the Category II failures will be the failures of the DOTS Category I regimen and will have a relatively larger proportion of MDR cases than at present. For this reason it would be desirable to monitor the drug sensitivity patterns in retreatment cases to ensure that the Category II regimen would be adequate, and should the MDR rates increase, modify the composition of the Category II regimen to ensure a high level of efficacy.

The highly encouraging results achieved with Category I and Category II DOTS regimens in India augur well for the TB control programs in other Asian countries which have similar epidemiological TB burden and have adopted DOTS as their national strategy.

Monitoring of Drug Resistance in the Community

The current success of DOTS is largely due to the low prevalence of drug resistance in general and MDR in particular in new TB cases in large parts of the countries in Asia and a presumption that such low levels prevail in future years. With the increasing use of DOTS, most of the failure patients will almost certainly have MDR and will pose problems for current management and future transmission potential. The global DRS program currently in position in several Asian countries including India and China provides for conducting drug resistance surveys using standardized sampling procedures and reliable laboratories with accredited facilities for drug sensitivity testing.

The technical support provided by the DRS project to Asian countries, including India, will help in establishing a large number of peripheral regional and national DST centers and in monitoring the drug resistance patterns in the community.

Management of MDR TB in Asian Countries

According to DRS data, there were about 400,000 MDR TB cases globally in 2004 (Zignol et al., 2006); half of these were new cases and the remaining were previously treated cases. Over 60% were from China, India, and Russia. No adequate data are available on the current MDR TB burden in Asian countries; it is likely to be over 200,000. The management of these cases would pose a formidable task for the MDR TB control program.

Most of the Asian countries do not have adequate human, financial, and technical resources to organize on their own a program for management of MDR TB. With appropriate guidance and assistance of the Green Light Committee (GLC) and support of the Global Fund for AIDS, TB, and Malaria (GFATM), Asian countries have embarked on an ambitious strategy to mount a DOTS-Plus strategy for the management of MDR TB in close coordination with their existing DOTS strategy. Most Asian countries did not have adequate facilities for routine DST for first line drugs and hardly any facilities for DST for second line drugs, but the situation has improved with guidance and support from international agencies. While some Asian countries have established new DST facilities, have strengthened existing DST facilities, and have established regional and national DST laboratories, other countries do not have facilities for DST and need to outsource the testing to supranational laboratories (World Health Organization, 2004).

Currently, DOTS strategies in the Asian countries do not use pretreatment DST in the program. However, there are special situations in MDR hot spots in some provinces of China where a high prevalence of MDR in new cases of TB has been demonstrated (World Health Organization, 2004). In such situations, pretreatment DST would be needed to strengthen the program. Generally, new cases have a low probability of drug resistance in general and MDR in particular, and with a standardized Category I regimen, very high cure rates are achieved. Surveillance of drug resistance in patients on the Category II regimen for previously treated cases has shown low levels of resistance in patients who relapse and in those who return after default, while the group that had failed on the Category I regimen may have a higher probability of MDR. Such failures on the Category I regimen are few and hence the groups of patients on the Category II regimen fare well with a standardized regimen with no dependence on DST. With a well organized DOTS program, only about 5% are bacteriological failures of the Category I regimen and proceed to Category II; failures on Category II are less than 10%, but these patients have a strong probability of having MDR TB. Thus, the failures of patients on Category II will require a Category IV regimen under a MDR TB management program (DOTS Plus strategy) (World Health Organization, 2006).

Asian countries do not have access to rapid DST facilities that can yield sensitivity test results within weeks (Sam et al.; World Health Organization, 2006). Conventional DST has a turn around time of several months. For best results with the Category IV regimen, the failures of the Category II regimen should be identified as early as possible (usually after 4 months of chemotherapy) and prescribed a standardized Category IV regimen without recourse to DST. If DST facilities exist and test results become available, appropriate modifications can be made to the standardized regimen so that the regimens become individualized.

Choice of Drugs for Standardized Regimens for MDR TB

During the formulation of regimens for the DOTS strategy, the program opted to use the best five anti-TB drugs namely SHREZ, which have high bactericidal activity. Since these drugs can no longer be used in patients who have failed on Category I and Category II regimens, the choice for treating MDR TB must be made from among the remaining anti-TB drugs. Almost all such drugs are less effective therapeutically, have more clinical adverse reactions and are much more expensive, and are associated with high levels of patient nonadherance. In principle, the regimens must have four core drugs which are reasonably effective, must be administered daily and under direct observation, and should be administered for a duration of 18–24 months. Many of these patients have a prior history of inadequate compliance. Their treatment should therefore be carefully monitored and special efforts need to be made to ensure maximum compliance. The aim must be to achieve success in almost every patient because any patient who fails on the Category IV regimen will have very few effective drugs to fall back upon. The following are some of the suggested standardized Category IV regimens:

1. 6(9) Km-E-Ofx-Eto-Cs-Z/18 Ofx-Eto-Cs-E
2. 6 Z-Km-Ofx-Eto-Cs/12 Z-Ofx-Eto-Cs
3. 6 Km-Ofx-Eto-Cs-PAS/12 Ofx-Eto-Cs-PAS

The prefix before a regimen indicates the duration of the regimen in months, thus there is an initial intensive phase of 6–9 months with five to six drugs followed by a continuation phase of 12–18 months with four drugs. In general, the initial intensive phase includes an injectable drug such as kanamycin or capreomycin along with a fluoroquinolone (ofloxacin or an alternative) and three or four other oral drugs. Thereafter, the oral drugs are continued for a further period of at least 12 months. The occurrence of adverse reactions must be monitored throughout chemotherapy and appropriate steps need to be taken promptly to provide palliative treatment, to reduce the dosage of the offending drug, to temporarily withhold the drug, or to discontinue the offending drug as may be needed. In the event of discontinuation of a drug, an alternate drug may be substituted.

Cross Resistance Between Drugs

There is cross resistance between (1) amikacin and kanamycin (2) viomycin and capreomycin (3) prothionamide and ethionomide (4) among rifamycin derivatives, and (5) among fluoroquinolones – gatifloxacin, moxyfloxacin, ofloxacin, levofloxacin, and ciprofloxacin. If resistance to a drug is suspected, the use of a drug with cross resistance should be avoided.

Pyrazinamide can be used with the category IV regimen even though the drug may have been used earlier as a part of Category I and Category II regimens, when it may have been used for 2–3 months at a time and the resistance to pyrazinamide may not have appeared. In most Category IV regimens, fluoroquinolones form a key component. In many countries, fluoroquinolones are routinely used for treatment of other acute bacterial infections and sometimes more than one course of treatment. Concurrent undiagnosed TB in such patients may cause the emergence of fluoroquinolone-resistant M tuberculosis in some of them. Not enough data are available on the prevalence of primary fluoroquinolone resistance in new cases of TB. GLC recommends routine DST of all patients who are put on the Category IV regimen. Testing should be done for the first line as well as second line drugs. Such documentation will help in the determination of the sensitivity factor. This will help to discontinue the use of drugs to which the bacilli are resistant thereby reducing the risk of adverse reactions and the cost of regimens.

Availability of Second Line Drugs for MDR TB Management Program

The Green Light Committee assists countries with limited resources to arrange for second line anti-TB drugs for approved MDR TB programs at subsidized rates. The substantially reduced prices make it affordable for these countries to procure these drugs through their own resources or through funding from the GFATM. The list of second line anti-TB drugs included in the WHO model list of essential medicines are Amikacin, Capreomycin, Cycloserine, Ethionamide, Kanamycin, Levofloxacin, Ofloxacin, P-aminosalicylic acid, and Prothionamide. The GLC assists countries with a credible DOTS Plus Strategy to grant access to reduced price, quality assured second line drugs.

The MDR TB Control or DOTS Plus Strategy has the following framework: a well-functioning DOTS program, integration of the MDR TB control program with the main DOTS program, long term political commitment, diagnosis of MDR TB through quality assured culture and DST, treatment strategies that use second line drugs under proper management conditions, uninterrupted supply of quality assured drugs, appropriate monitoring and recording systems, and monitoring and evaluation of program performance and treatment outcome.

Treatment Outcome under MDR TB Control Program

The outcome of treatment with standardized MDR TB regimens (Category IV) will depend on several factors, including prior treatment, new cases of MDR TB (primary

MDR TB), cases of MDR TB previously treated with a first line regimen, and cases of MDR TB previously treated with first line and second line regimens, with successively decreasing rates of treatment success. A recent report of treatment of MDR TB in patients enrolled during 1999–2001 under five MDR TB projects in Estonia, Latvia, Lima (Peru), Manila (Philippines), and Omsk (Federation of Russia) indicated a success rate of 77% in new cases of MDR TB compared to 69% in previously treated MDR TB patients (Table 10). Mortality during treatment was 3% in new cases compared with 14% in previously treated group. Default rates were high with 15% in new cases and 10% in the previously treated group. Thus, the treatment success rates are substantially lower and death rates are significantly higher compared with over 85% cure rate and about 2% death rates in new cases treated with the Category I regimen in patients with predominantly drug sensitive population.

Treatment of MDR TB/HIV

The management of MDR TB in HIV infected subjects provides a major challenge to TB control programs. Co-infection of TB infection with HIV increases the risk of reactivation of latent tuberculosis to active tuberculosis and thus increases the incidence of tuberculosis in the country. The lifetime risk of reactivation of latent TB infection to active TB disease is 10%; however, in patients with concurrent HIV infection, the risk of reactivation is 8–10% each year of over eight million HIV infected persons in Asia (UNAIDS/WHO, 2006), about four million would harbor co-infection with TB. This would mean increasing the TB burden in Asia by additional 650,000 new cases of TB each year. TB/HIV poses diagnostic challenges because sputum smears in pulmonary TB are often negative and cavity formation is less frequent. While this may result in delay in diagnosis, response to treatment with anti-TB drugs is at least as good as in the absence of HIV. The drug sensitivity pattern, including the level of MDR TB, is generally uninfluenced by the HIV status. MDR TB patients with HIV do not differ in their clinical presentation from MDR TB patients who do not have HIV. However, mortality associated with MDR TB/HIV is considerably higher because of rapid progression of TB in the

Table 10 Treatment outcome of MDR TB patients in five centers (Estonia, Latvia, Lima, Manila, and Omsk)v

Treatment outcome	New cases		Previously treated cases		All patients	
	n	%	n	%	n	%
Total	119	100	928	100	1,047	100
Success	92	78	637	69	729	70
Failed	5	4	65	7	70	7
Defaulted	18	15	92	10	110	11
Died	4	3	132	14	136	13

Source: Nathanson et al., 2006

absence of appropriate drugs for successful elimination of bacilli and due to mortality associated with AIDS. In Asian countries such as India, Thailand, Myanmar, and parts of China where HIV prevalence is high, special attention should be paid to the drug sensitivity of infecting TB strains in patients with TB/HIV to detect cases with MDR TB/HIV and to treat them with second line drugs. Many of these MDR TB/HIV patients may need to be provided Anti Retroviral Therapy (ART) concurrently with anti-tuberculosis treatment (ATT) based on their CD4 counts (less than $250 \mu l^{-1}$) and the clinical stage of AIDS (WHO clinical stage IV). Rifamipicin is known to interfere with the metabolism of ART drugs such as Protease Inhibitors and Nevirapine, resulting in reduced serum concentrations of these drugs, thereby reducing their therapeutic efficacy. This is, however, unlikely to be a major issue with the management of MDR TB/HIV since such patients will be on second line anti-TB drugs and will not receive rifampicin because of resistance to the drug.

The management of new cases of TB/HIV can be done along the same lines as TB without HIV, as MDR is infrequent in such patients – 10% in Pune (Pereira et al., 2005) and 4% in Chennai (Table 11) in India. TB/HIV cases on the Category II regimens may have a greater chance of acquiring MDR TB because of large bacterial populations involved in HIV infected patients. For this reason, many Asian countries with high prevalence of HIV have established collaborative activities between TB control and AIDS control programs so that the TB/HIV patients are identified and appropriately managed, their therapeutic needs for TB as well as HIV are adequately taken care of, and MDR TB/HIV patients are managed with DST and prescription of appropriate second line drugs.

While TB patients transmit infection to contacts, HIV positive TB patients often have smear negative pulmonary TB and transmit infection to their contacts less efficiently than HIV negative TB patients (Crampin et al., 2006); this however, may not be true of MDR TB/HIV patients since such patients are likely to have chronic TB, attain large bacterial populations, and hence may transmit TB infection to contacts efficiently.

XDR: Extensively Drug Resistant Tuberculosis

The emergence of drug resistance during treatment under a program indicates a weakness in the tuberculosis management. Inadequate regimens result in selection

Table 11 Drug resistance in HIV/TB patients in Chennai, India

	New cases ($n = 168$)	Previously treated cases ($n = 37$)
Susceptible	83.4	62.2
Any res	15.4	37.8
Res to H	13	27
MDR	4.2	5.9

Source: Swaminathan et al., 2005

of drug resistant strains that proliferate. Continued treatment with the drug regimen thereafter results in sequential emergence of strains resistant to other companion drugs. Thus, many of the bacteriological failures of new patients treated with the Category I regimen are usually resistant to isoniazid and/or rifampicin. Their subsequent management with Category II regimens, though largely successful, leads to the emergence of MDR strains among the failures on Category II regimens. These patients now need to be treated with second line drugs under Category IV regimens as a part of DOTS Plus Strategy. These drugs have substantially lower microbicidal activity, are expensive, and are associated with higher incidence of adverse reactions. They need to be prescribed for 18–24 months or longer, adding substantially to the risk of lower patient compliance, lower success rates, and successive emergence of strains resistant to the second line drugs. Such pan-resistant strains had been encountered in practically all programs where second line drugs had been used for failure cases.

The existence of pan-resistant strains received worldwide attention when exposure of immunosuppressed HIV infected persons to such resistant strains in South Africa resulted in rapid spread of tuberculosis with such resistant strains under nosocomial conditions (Gandhi et al., 2006). Among 1,539 patients tested, MDR TB was detected in 223, of whom 53 had also resistance to second line drugs and were designated as XDR tuberculosis (Extensively Drug Resistant tuberculosis). According to the current accepted definition, the term XDR TB refers to MDR TB strains which, in addition to isoniazid and rifampicin, are also resistant to at least one of the injectable drugs – capreomycin, kanamycin, and amikacin – and to any quinolone drug. An XDR tuberculosis patient has virtually no choice of effective anti-tuberculosis drug and faces imminent death. Of the 53 patients with MDR reported by Gandhi and colleagues (2006), all 44 who were tested for HIV were found to be co-infected with HIV; 52 of the 53 XDR patients died with a median survival time of 16 days from the time of diagnosis.

XDR tuberculosis is untreatable. All possible efforts should therefore be made to prevent their occurrence by efficient and effective management of MDR TB. Most Asian countries would have considerable difficulty in organizing countrywide DOTS Plus Programs. At 1,600 US dollars per patient for a course of treatment for MDR TB (Agarwal, 2006), a countrywide DOTS Plus strategy would stretch the resources – financial as well as infrastructure – considerably in most Asian countries. The emergence of MDR tuberculosis and XDR tuberculosis reflects deficiency in implementing the well established measures recommended by WHO's Stop TB Strategy. To prevent the emergence of MDR and XDR TB, the DOTS Program in each country must be strengthened and implemented to achieve the highest targets of treatment outcome, strengthening all components of the DOTS strategy, addressing HIV associated tuberculosis and drug resistance (Raviglione and Smith, 2007).

There are indications that the global tuberculosis epidemic may be on the decline, as seen from the Global TB incidence data during 2005 (World Health Organization, 2007a). Continued decline in the incidence would eventually result in decreased prevalence and a corresponding decrease in MDR and XDR tuberculosis.

Some indication about the number of XDR tuberculosis cases in Asian countries can be obtained from the estimated incidence of MDR tuberculosis. Globally, about 400,000 cases of MDR tuberculosis were estimated to have occurred in 2004; of these, China, India, and the Russian Federation accounted for about 260,000 (62%) of the MDR TB cases (Zignol et al., 2006). Asian countries (including India and China) may be assumed to have contributed at least to about 200,000 MDR TB cases.

In reality, far less number of retreatment patients were treated in 2004 (World Health Organization 2007a). Globally, about 500,000 retreatment cases were treated, and of these, 73% had treatment success and 7% died, so that in the worst case scenario, about 20% of the cases failed with possible MDR TB, i.e., only about 100,000 globally (as against the estimated 400,000 indicated earlier), including about 60,000 in Asian countries. Most of the 60,000 will have little chance of receiving the second line drugs under the current conditions and hence, only a small number of XDR tuberculosis cases may have occurred among the few who did get treated with second line drugs. DST data from the DRS project showed that XDR strains were prevalent in all the WHO regions; however, only 234 (6.6%) of 3,520 MDR TB patients tested were found to be XDR TB (Shah et al., 2007). The magnitude of the XDR tuberculosis cases is small but may increase in numbers in future years as more and more failures of retreatment cases are treated with second line anti-TB drugs.

Adverse Reactions to Anti-TB Drugs

The incidence of adverse reactions to second line drugs is much higher than to the first line anti-TB drugs. The common adverse reactions associated with the second line drugs are indicated in Table 12.

While in the initial stages, a patient may be hospitalized and treated as an inpatient, thereafter he will be managed on an ambulatory basis drugs and will be provided drugs by the DOTS provider who will observe the consumption of drugs. The DOTS provider should be trained to closely monitor patients and to recognize the adverse effects of drugs in the early stages. They should be trained to recognize adverse reactions like nausea, vomiting, diarrhea, skin rash, ototoxicity, peripheral neuropathy, psychiatric symptoms, and jaundice. The management of the adverse reactions, including modifications of treatment, should be undertaken by the clinician in charge.

Planning and Implementation of MDR TB Control Program

It must be realized that while the number of patients requiring MDR TB management is considerably smaller than those on DOTS, MDR TB Control Program has

Table 12 Adverse reactions to anti-TB drugs

Drug	Adverse reactions
Aminoglycosides – Kanamycin, Amikacin	Ototoxicity, nephrotoxicity, vertigo
Quinolones – Ofloxacin	Diarrhea, vomiting, dizziness, convulsions, ototoxicity, photosensitivity, tendonitis, nephrotoxicity, cardiotoxicity, arthralgia, skin rash
Ethambutol	Visual disturbance
Pyrazinamide	Arthralgia, hyperuricemia, hepatitis, pruritus
Ethionamide	Anorexia, nausea, vomiting, sulphurous smell, hepatitis, mental depression, goiter, peripheral neuropathy
Cycloserine	Convulsions, tremor, insomnia, suicidal tendency, hypersensitivity reaction
PAS	Anorexia, nausea, vomiting, skin rash, hepatic dysfunction, goiter

Source: Central TB Division, 2006

many more aspects of management in addition to all the components of DOTS strategy, such as establishment of DST facilities, need to monitor drug resistance patterns in the community, constant review of progress of treatment, monitoring for a variety of adverse reactions, and the assessment of patient adherence. For this reason, there is need for meticulous planning and preparations including training of staff before starting DOTS Plus Strategy in any country. Appropriate guidelines for DOTS Plus Strategy have been prepared – a global guideline has been prepared by the WHO (World Health Organization, 2006) and India has produced similar guidelines for the Indian program (Revised National Tuberculosis Control Program 2006). Other countries may use these documents as reference for preparing appropriate guidelines for their own countries.

Achievement of Millennium Goals

Contribution of the DOTS Strategy

The attainment of the millennium goal of reducing TB incidence, prevalence, and mortality in Asia by 2015 requires a substantial reduction in the Annual Risk of Infection from its current levels of 1–2% in most of the Asian countries. Reduction in ARI would result in a reduced pool of TB infected population. About 50% of the adult Asian population is currently infected with the bacillus; they contribute to over 80% of the incident cases of clinical TB and help to maintain a substantial pool of infectious patients. Most of the cases in Asia are in the TB high burden countries, all of which have well established DOTS strategies in their national programs. Hopefully, DOTS expansion in these countries would reach an area coverage of nearly 100%, but in addition would ensure that over 90% of all diagnosed patients receive DOTS. TB control measures need to be considerably strengthened to achieve coverage of all patients and to ensure over 85% cure rates in new cases. With assured National and International commitment to DOTS implementation and expansion, the TB Control Programs in the HBCs are well placed to achieve high cure rates and reduced incidence and prevalence of infection and disease.

Contribution of the DOTS Plus Strategy

For reducing prevalence of disease, it is essential to ensure that the frequency of drug resistance, especially of MDR, should be maintained at a low level. Successful implementation of DOTS will ensure reducing the prevalence of monoresistant and polyresistant TB in new cases and in maintaining MDR at low levels. The management of failures of Category I and Category II regimens with a well-organized and efficiently managed MDR TB Control Program would ensure patients to become bacteriologically negative and cease to be a source of transmission of MDR strains.

In the absence of a DOTS Plus Strategy, MDR strains will persist and would transmit infection with MDR strains, resulting in an increase in the MDR levels among new cases of TB in future years. In such an event, the efficacy of the present DOTS regimens will decrease and the progress towards elimination of TB by 2050 will be impeded. With little prospects of discovery of newer anti-TB drugs and establishing their efficacy in the near future, the world will have to manage with the current first line anti-TB drugs under the DOTS strategy. Appropriately implemented, DOTS will be able to keep the failures and the emergence of MDR strains to the minimum and with a good program, and the few MDR cases resulting from the failure of DOTS can be successfully treated. A successful program now can ensure the continued success of the DOTS strategy in future years, resulting in reduced prevalence and incidence rates of TB in Asian countries.

Contribution of AIDS Control Activities

Asian countries with significant levels of HIV infection have established national AIDS control programs, which are functioning reasonably efficiently. Currently, the transmission of HIV infection has been substantially slowed down due to several preventive measures such as health education, condom use, and application of vaginal microbicides. Many Asian countries are now able to offer treatment to HIV patients with ART through international guidance and support, and this in turn will result in reduced transmission of HIV infection. Furthermore, collaborative activities between the TB control and the AIDS control programs in each country will result in identification of dually infected patients and better management of HIV/TB.

AIDS control activities in these countries would ensure that the HIV epidemic will not prove an impediment in our efforts to achieve reduction in the transmission of TB infection and achievement of the millennium goals.

Contribution of Socio-Economic Improvement

The incidence of tuberculosis is linked with socio-economic development of countries. Generally, TB incidence is higher among the poorer segments of the society. Recently, Asian countries have seen considerable socio-economic development with economic growth rates of 4–8% annually. The per capita income has risen and is continuing to rise and poverty levels have been decreasing in these countries in successive years. The improvements in socio-economic conditions including better health care will make a significant contribution to decreased incidence of disease through a reduction in the rates of reactivation of latent TB to active TB.

In summary, TB control programs have made spectacular gains and achievements in recent years and hold great promise of further gains in the coming years. The combined contributions of socio-economic developments, strengthening and expanding the DOTS strategy, introduction and implementation of the DOTS Plus Strategy for MDR TB, and efficient National AIDS Control Programs will help Asian countries to reach the millennium goals of reducing TB incidence, prevalence, and mortality. Most Asian countries have already reached the 2005 target of 70% case detection and 85% cure. Even so, there is considerable scope for further strengthening of the case detection programs to ensure that people from all parts of a country avail of the DOTS facility at the health care centers. There are indications from the 2005 data that the global TB incidence rate is falling, thus meeting the 2015 MDG Target 8 ten years ahead of schedule (World Health Organization 2007a). Continued decline in incidence rate would in due course be reflected in lower prevalence, fewer MDR TB cases, and hence, still fewer XDR TB cases. With the great impetus in implementing the DOTS strategy, including the DOTS Plus component in Asian countries, and with determination, thrust, and assistance from the World Health Organization and other international organizations, the prospects of Asian countries eliminating TB as a public health problem, with an incidence of less than 1 in 1,000,000 population, by 2050 appear to be bright.

References

Agarwal, S.P. (2007). Multidrug resistant tuberculosis. *Ind J Tuberc*, 52, 175–177
Central TB Division. (2006). DOTS – Plus Guidelines. Central TB Division, Directorate General of Health Services, New Delhi, India
Central TB Division India. (2007). TB India 2007: RNTCP Status Report. Directorate General of Health Services, Ministry of Health and Family Welfare, New Delhi

Crampin, A.C., Glynn, J.R., Traore, H., Yates, M.D., Mwaungulu, L., Mwenebabu, M., Chaguluka, S.D., Floyd, S., Drobniewski, F., Fine, P.E.M. (2006). Tuberculosis transmission attributable to close contacts and HIV status, Malawi. *Emerg Inf Dis*, 12, 729–735

Dye, C. (2006). India's leading role in tuberculosis epidemiology and control. *Ind J Med Res*, 123, 481–484

Gandhi, N.R., Mall, A., Sturm, A.W., Pawinski, R., Govender, T., Lalloo, U., Zeller, K., Andrews, J., Friedland, G. (2006). Extensively drug resistant tuberculosis as a cause of death in patients coinfected with tuberculosis and HIV in a rural area of South Africa. *Lancet*, 368, 1575–1580

Frieden, T. (2002). Can tuberculosis be controlled? *Int J Epidem*, 31, 894–899

Joseph, P., Chandraskaran, V., Thomas, A., Gopi, P.G., Rajeswari, R., Rani, B., Subramani, R., Selvakumar, N., Santha, T. Influence of drug susceptibility on treatment outcome and susceptibility profile of failure to category II regimen. Indian J Tuberc, 53, 141–148

Nathanson, E., Lambregts-van Weezenbeek, C., Rich, M.L., Gupta, R., Bayona, J., Blondal, K., Caminero, J.A., Cegielski, J.P., Danilovits, M., Espinol, M.A., Hollo, V., Jaramillo, E., Leimane, V., Mitnick, C.D., Mukherjee, J.S., Nunn, P., Pasechnikov, A., Tupasi, T., Wells, C., Raviglione, M.C. (2006). Multidrug-resistant tuberculosis management in resource limited settings. *Emerg Inf Dis*, 12, 1389–1397

Pereira, M., Tripathy, S., Inamdar, V., Ramesh, K., Bhausar, M., Date, A., Iyyer, R., Acchammachary, A., Mehendale, S., Risbud, A. (2005). Drug resistance pattern of Mycobacterium tuberculosis in seropositive and seronegative HIV-TB patients in Pune, India. *Ind J Med Res*, 121, 235–239

Raviglione, M.C., Smith, I.M. (2007). XDR tuberculosis – implications for global public health. *New Engl J Med*, 356, 656–659

Sam, I.C., Drobniewski, F., More, P., Kemp, M., Brown, T. (2006). Mycobacterium tuberculosis and rifampicin resistance, United Kingdom. *Emerg Inf Dis*, 12, 752–759

Santha, T., Gopi, P.G., Rajeswari, R., Selvakumar, N., Subramani, R., Chandrasekaran, V., Rani, B., Thomas, A., Narayanan, P.R. (2006a). Is it worth treating Category I failure patients with Category II regimen? *Indian J Tuberc*, 52, 203–206

Santha, T., Thomas, A., Chandrasekaran, V., Selvakumar, N., Gopi, P.G., Subramani, R., Rajeswari, N., Rani, B., Paramasivan, C.N., Perumal, N., Wares, F., Narayanan, P.R. (2006b). Initial susceptibility profile of M. tuberculosis among patients under TB programs in South India. *Int J Tuberc Lung Dis*, 10, 52–57

Shah, N.S., Wright, A., Bai, G., Barrera, L., Boulahbal, F., Martin-Casabona, N., Drobniewski, F., Golpin, C., Havelkova, M., Lepe, R., Lumb, R., Metchcock, B., Portaels, F., Rodrigues, M.F., Rusch-Gerdes, S., Van Deun, A., Vincent, V., Laserson, K., Wells, C., Cegielski, J.P. (2007). Worldwide emergence of extensively drug resistant tuberculosis. *Emerging Inf Dis*, 13, 380–387

Swaminathan, S., Paramasivan, C., Ponnuraja, S., Iliayas, S., Rajasekaran, S., Narayanan, P.R. (2005). Antituberculosis drug resistance in patients with HIV and tuberculosis in South India. *Int J Tuberc Lung Dis*, 9, 896–900

Tripathy, S.P., Menon, N.K., Mitchison, D.A., Narayana, A.S.L., Somasundaram, P.R., Stott, H., Velu, S. (1969). Response to treatment with isoniazid plus PAS of tuberculosis patients with primary isoniazid resistance. *Tubercle Lond*, 50, 257–268

Tuberculosis Research Centre. (2001). Low rate of emergence of drug resistance in sputum positive patients treated with short course chemotherapy. *Int J Tuberc Lung Dis*, 5, 40–45

Tuberculosis Research Centre. (2003). Trends in initial drug resistance over three decades in a rural community in South India. *Ind J Tuberc*, 50, 75–86

UNAIDS/World Health Organization. (2006). AIDS Epidemic Update: Geneva, December 2006

World Health Organization. (2004). Anti-Tuberculosis Drug Resistance in the World: Report No. 3. Geneva, WHO

World Health Organization. (2005). Health and the Millennium Development Goals. Geneva, WHO

World Health Organization. (2006). Guidelines for the Management of Drug Resistant Tuberculosis. Geneva, WHO

World Health Organization. (2007a). Global Tuberculosis Control, Surveillance, Planning, Financing. Geneva, World Health Organization

World Health Organization. (2007b). Global Tuberculosis Epidemic Leveling Off. News Release WHO/8. 21 March 2007

World Health Organization Regional Office for South East Asia. (2002). Tuberculosis Epidemiology and Control. Narain J.P., (ed). New Delhi, India

Zignol, M., Hosseini, M.S., Wright, A., Weezenbeek, C.L., Nunn, P., Watt, C.J., William, B.J., Dye, C. (2006). Global incidence of Multi-drug resistant tuberculosis. *JID*, 194, 479–485

Emergence of *Staphylococcus aureus* with Reduced Susceptibility to Vancomycin in Asia

Jae-Hoon Song

Introduction

Staphylococcus aureus is one of the most important bacterial pathogens causing various infections from mild skin and skin structure infections to potentially fatal systemic illnesses such as endocarditis and sepsis. *S. aureus* has developed anti-microbial resistance to various antibiotics since the introduction of modern chemotherapeutic agents in the 1940s. Particularly, the emergence and dissemination of methicillin-resistant *S. aureus* (MRSA) has become a global concern since the first report in 1961. Nowadays, MRSA is the most common nosocomial pathogen in many hospitals. MRSA is also emerging in the community in many countries in recent years. The high rate of MRSA infections has led to an increasing use of vancomycin in clinical practice during the past two decades. Since the early 1990s, there have been some concern about the emergence of *S. aureus* with reduced susceptibility to vancomycin, as vancomycin-resistant enterococci (VRE) has rapidly emerged in many countries. Furthermore, conjugative transfer of the *van*A gene from VRE to *S. aureus* was demonstrated in the laboratory (Noble et al., 1992). This theoretical concern became a reality in 1996 when the first strain of *S. aureus* with intermediate resistance to vancomycin was found from a 4-month-old infant patient who underwent open heart surgery in Japan (Hiramatsu et al., 1997). Subsequently, infections with vancomycin-intermediate *S. aureus* (VISA) strains have been reported in patients from the United States, Europe, and Asia.

Growing concern of vancomycin resistance in *S. aureus* was deepened by the emergence of high-level vancomycin-resistant *S. aureus* (VRSA) strains from the United States since 2002 (CDC, 2002a,b, 2004; Tenover and McDonald, 2005). The third type of reduced susceptibility to vancomycin in *S. aureus* is heterogenous vancomycin-intermediate resistance (hVISA), which had been first reported by Hiramatsu et al. in 1997. These various types of reduced susceptibility to vancomycin could lead to clinical failures of vancomycin treatment. This review will summarize the current epidemiology of *S. aureus* with reduced susceptibility to vancomycin, especially in Asian countries, as well as the resistance mechanism, clinical implications, and infection control measures.

Y. Lu et al. (eds.), *Emerging Infections in Asia*.
© Springer Science+Business Media, LLC 2008

Definitions and Detection of Vancomycin Resistance in *S. aureus*

Vancomycin-resistant S. aureus (VRSA). According to the Clinical and Laboratory Standards Institute (CLSI, formerly NCCLS) guidelines, *S. aureus* isolates for which the MIC of vancomycin is $\leq 2\,\mu$g ml^{-1} are susceptible, and isolates for which the MIC of vancomycin is $4–8\,\mu$g ml^{-1} are intermediate. Vancomycin resistance is defined if the MIC of vancomycin is $\geq 16\,\mu$g ml^{-1} (CLSI, 2006). However, the term "resistant" is used to refer to *S. aureus* isolates for which the MIC of vancomycin is $\geq 8\,\mu$g ml^{-1} in Japan and the UK (Tenover et al., 2001).

Vancomycin-intermediate S. aureus (VISA). The Centers for Disease Control and Prevention (CDC) has proposed three criteria to identify VISA strains: (1) broth microdilution vancomycin MIC of $4–16\,\mu$g ml^{-1}, (2) E-test vancomycin MIC of $\geq 6\,\mu$g ml^{-1}, and (3) growth within 24h on commercial brain heart infusion agar (BHIA) screen plates containing $6\,\mu$g vancomycin ml^{-1} (Tenover et al., 1998).

Heterogeneous vancomycin-intermediate S. aureus (hVISA). The original definition of hVISA by Hiramatsu et al. was an *S. aureus* strain that gave vancomycin resistance at a frequency of 10^{-6} colonies or higher, which could be identified by population analysis (Hiramatsu et al., 1997). Hetero-VISA could be defined as strains of *S. aureus* containing subpopulations of vancomycin-intermediate daughter cells but for which the MIC of vancomycin for the parent strain is $1–4\,\mu$g ml^{-1} (Hiramatsu, 2001). Heterogeneous resistance to vancomycin in *S. aureus* is considered as a precursor stage to intermediate resistance because hVISA could develop into VISA. However, the criteria for identifying VISA strains have not been standardized yet.

Detection of vancomycin resistance. Detection of VISA isolates in the clinical laboratory is often difficult, because VISA isolates sometimes grow slowly with atypical morphology. Quantitative methods of MIC determination including broth dilution, agar dilution, and agar gradient diffusion (Etest) should be used to accurately detect VISA isolates. Broth dilution test in cation-adjusted Mueller–Hinton broth using a 0.5 McFarland standard as the inoculum with incubation at 35°C for a full 24h is currently recommended by CLSI. If *S. aureus* isolates have an MIC of $\geq 4\,\mu$g ml^{-1}, it would be considered as presumptive VISA and should be confirmed by MIC retesting. Screening of *S. aureus* with reduced susceptibility to vancomycin could be done by using a brain–heart infusion agar plate containing $6\,\mu$g ml^{-1} of vancomycin. However, routine screening of hVISA is not recommended in the clinical laboratory.

Mechanism of Vancomycin Resistance in *S. aureus*

VRSA. The mechanisms by which *S. aureus* become resistant to vancomycin are different between VRSA and VISA or hVISA. VRSA showed high-level vancomycin resistance by acquiring the *van*A gene on Tn*1546*-like element from vancomycin-resistant enterococci (VRE) via plasmids or transposons (Weigel et al., 2003). The structure of Tn*1546*-like element including the *van*A gene affects the

MIC and stability of VRSA isolates. The enzyme encoded by the *van*A gene replaces D-alanine-D-alanine residues of *S. aureus* peptidoglycan by D-alanine-D-lactate, to which vancomycin cannot bind. Therefore, the cell wall of *S. aureus* under *van*A gene expression is resistant to vancomycin.

VISA. The most striking feature of VISA strains is cell wall thickening with more peptidoglycan layers (Cui et al., 2003). Because vancomycin binds to the D-alanine-D-alanine residues of murein monomers on the cytoplasmic membrane, thickened peptidoglycan layers outside the cytoplasmic membrane may inhibit the access of vancomycin to the targets (Hiramatsu, 2001; Cui et al., 2003). Unlike VRSA, the vancomycin resistance in VISA is not due to the acquisition of a resistance gene from other bacterial species or by a single-step mutation process. Based on the repeated passage experiments, VISA strains could gradually acquire many mutations from repeated exposure to vancomycin (Hiramatsu, 2001).

Hetero-VISA. The mechanism of hetero-VISA is basically the same as that of VISA. The original strain of hetero-VISA Mu3 strain shares the common phenotypic features with VISA Mu50 strain. Hetero-VISA can be selected in vitro from vancomycin-susceptible *S. aureus* strains either by exposures to vancomycin or by selection with β-lactam antibiotics such as imipenem (Hiramatsu et al., 2005). Heteroresistance to vancomycin can be acquired by multiple steps of genetic mutations through this selection process.

Current Epidemiology of Vancomycin Resistance in Asia

VRSA. All six cases of VRSA infection were reported from the United States. In June 2002, the first clinical VRSA strain (MIC, 1,024 μg ml⁻¹) was isolated from a patient with chronic foot ulcer, diabetes, and chronic renal failure in Michigan (Chang et al., 2003). Two months later, a second VRSA strain was found from a patient with chronic foot ulcer and osteomyelitis in Pennsylvania (CDC, 2002b). This Pennsylvanian strain was different from the first Michigan strain with regard to low vancomycin MIC (32 μg ml⁻¹), modified *Tn*1546 element, and instability (Clark et al., 2005). These two VRSA isolates belonged to the same common MRSA lineage, the New York/Japanese clone, but they showed different PFGE profiles, indicating that the *van*A gene was acquired independently. The third VRSA strain (vancomycin MIC 64 μg ml⁻¹) was isolated from a patient in a long-term nursing facility in New York (CDC, 2004). Also, in early 2005, a fourth strain (vancomycin MIC 256 μg ml⁻¹) was identified from a second patient in Michigan (Tenover et al., 2005). Recently, additional two VRSA strains were also found in the United States (Wang et al., 2006).

VISA. A total of 22 cases of VISA infection have been reported in the literature (Walsh and Howe, 2002; Wang et al., 2006). In Asia, three cases of VISA infections have been reported from Japan (sternal wound infection), Korea (bacteremia), and Taiwan (septic arthritis) (Hiramatsu et al., 1997; Hiramatsu, 1998; Kim et al., 2000; Lu et al., 2005) (Table 1).

Table 1 Reported cases of VISA and hVISA infections in Asian countries

Country	Patient	Underlying diseases	Diagnosis	VAN exposure	Outcome	Reference
VISA						
Japan	4 Mo./M	Pulmonary astresia	Surgical site infection	29 days	Cleared with ABK + AMS	Hiramatsu et al. (1997)
Korea	45/M	Colon cancer	Bacteremia	8 days + 30 days TEI	Died	Kim et al. (2000)
Taiwan	19/M	Left lemur/osteomyelitis	Septic arthritis	3 weeks	Recovered with GEN+CFZ	Lu et al. (2005)
hVISA						
Japan	64/M	Post surgery for lung carcinoma	Pneumonia	12 days	Recovered with AMS+ABK	Hiramatsu et al. (1997)
Hong Kong	78/M	End stage renal disease	Septic arthritis		Died despite VAN+RIF	Wong et al. (1999)
	53/F	Mycosis fungoides	Neutropenic sepsis		Died	
	77/M	Stomach carcinoma	CVC-related sepsis		Recovered after CVC removal	
Thailand	68/F	Diabetes mellitus, post-knee replacement	Surgical site infection	75 days	Died	Trakulsomboon et al. (2001)
	16/F	–	Retroperitoneal infection	14 days	Recovered	
	61/F	Diabetes mellitus, Hepatic cirrhosis	Nosocomial pneumonia		Died	
Taiwan	89/M	Ischemic bowel disease	MRSA bacteremia	14 days	Died	Wang et al. (2004)
	72/M	Coronary artery disease & chronic renal insufficiency	Catheter-related MRSA bacteremia	12 days + TEI, 30 days	Recovered	
Singapore	74/M	Trans-urethral rectal prostactectomy	MRSA bacteremia	2 months	Died	Sng et al. (2005)
	68/M	Chronic renal failure, diabetes, and hypertension	MRSA line-sepsis	2 weeks	Died	

Country	Age/Sex	Underlying condition	Infection	Duration	Outcome	Reference
Korea	63/M	Trauma with tibial fracture	Wound infection	7 days + 7 days TEI	Recovered	Kim et al. (2002)
	58/M	Biliary adenocarcinoma	Pneumonia	9 days	Recovered	
	73/M	Intracranial hemorrhage	Urinary tract infection	25 days	Died	
	31/M	Trauma with femur fracture	Wound infection	63 days	Recovered	
	75/M	Rectal cancer	Pneumonia	28 days	Recovered	
	34/M	Thoracic vertebrae fracture	Wound infection	14 days	Recovered	
	58/F	Schwannoma	C-line site infection	16 days	Recovered	
Japan	2/M	Sustaining flame burns	Wound infection	14 days	Recovered with AMS + ABK	Haraga et al. (2002)

VAN vancomycin, *ABK* arbekacin, *AMS* ampicillin-sulbactam, *GEN* gentamicin, *TEI* teicoplanin, *CFZ* ceftazidime, *RIF* rifampin *hVISA*. Hetero-VISA strains were more frequently reported worldwide than VISA or VRSA. In Asia, hVISA strains were reported from several countries (Table 1). When hVISA is defined by the selection of subpopulations with vancomycin MIC of $8\,\mu g\ ml^{-1}$, the incidence of hVISA among MRSA isolates ranged from 1.3% to 20% in Japan, 2.7% in Hong Kong, and 1.9% in Thailand (Hiramatsu et al., 1997; Wong et al., 1999; Trakulsomboon et al., 2001). Cases of hVISA infections were also reported from Taiwan and Singapore (Wang et al., 2004; Sng et al., 2005).

A recent multinational surveillance study reported that prevalence rates of hVISA strains are relatively high in some Asian countries such as India (6.3%), Japan (8.2%), and Korea (6.1%) (Song et al., 2004). In contrast to these reports, two surveillance studies found no hVISA strains from Japan and Korea, although they have tested 6,625 MRSA isolates and 682 *S. aureus* isolates, respectively (Ike et al., 2001; Kim et al., 2003). However, this discrepancy could be the result of difficulties in defining and detecting hVRSA (Howe and Walsh, 2004). Multilocus sequencing typing showed that VISA and hVISA strains around the world have arisen from five pandemic lineages of MRSA, suggesting that reduced vancomycin susceptibility in *S. aureus* would become a widespread problem in the MRSA population (Howe et al., 2004).

Risk factors of VRSA/VISA. Risk factors associated with VISA infections include prolonged vancomycin use, hemodialysis, and indwelling foreign bodies. According to a recent study on risk factors with 19 patients with VISA infections (Fridkin et al., 2003), patients who are infected or colonized with MRSA and who received vancomycin frequently over several months are at highest risk for subsequent isolation of *S. aureus* with reduced vancomycin susceptibility, and these patients showed higher mortality (63%) compared with control subjects (12%). Interestingly, the second VRSA strain from Pennsylvania was isolated from a patient who had not received vancomycin in the 5 years prior to his VRSA infection due to allergy to the drug (Whitener et al., 2004). Charles et al. (2004) also found that hVISA bacteremia was significantly associated with infections that have high bacteria loads such as endocarditis, longer duration of fever, longer time until clearance of bacteremia, longer hospitalization, and failure of vancomycin treatment. Risk factors for acquisition of VRSA are not well defined because there have been only four reported cases to date.

Clinical Impact of VRSA/VISA/hVISA

The clinical significance of *S. aureus* with reduced susceptibility to vancomycin is difficult to evaluate due to the small number of reported cases. It is obscure whether levels of resistance are responsible for treatment failures. Four VRSA strains that have been isolated to date were susceptible to some available antimicrobial agents, although their MICs of vancomycin were very high. These strains were resistant to vancomycin, aminoglycosides, tetracycline, and some fluoroquinolones, but they were susceptible to quinupristin-dalfopristin, linezolid, trimethoprim-sulfamethoxazole, chloroamphenicol, and minocycline (CDC, 2002a,b, 2004). Cases with VRSA infections were treated with surgical intervention of the infected wound and various antibiotics including trimethoprim-sulfamethoxazole or linezolid with successful control of infections. In addition, they did not appear to be highly virulent and were not transmitted to other patients, family members, or health care workers.

Although the clinical impact of VISA infections is also hard to evaluate based on the current number of cases worldwide, some reports suggested that VISA strains are generally considered to be responsible for the clinical failures to vancomycin treatment (Bert et al., 2003). Several reports indicated that the mortality in patients infected with *S. aureus* with reduced vancomycin susceptibility is very high (Liñares, 2001; Fridkin et al., 2003). Evaluation of the clinical significance of hVISA infections has been hampered by difficulties in detecting them in the laboratory and a lack of confirmatory tests. The original report by Hiramatsu described the re-growth of hVISA strain (Mu3) after the exposure to vancomycin, which correlated with exacerbation of pneumonia after the ninth day of vancomycin therapy in the patient (Hiramatsu, 2001). Some reports have described poor clinical response to vancomycin treatment in patients with hVISA infections (Ariza et al., 1999; Goldstein and Kitzis, 2003; Moore et al., 2003). Recently, Charles et al. (2004) showed that hVISA bacteremia was associated with vancomycin failure. Also in Asia, deaths of patients with hVISA infection have been reported from Hong Kong, Thailand, Taiwan, and Korea (Table 1). However, Schwaber et al. (2003) found no outcome difference between hVISA and VISA infections.

Prevention and Control of VRSA/VISA

The emergence of VISA and VRSA underlines the importance of infection control procedures, because these strains could spread within the hospital like MRSA. Indeed, clonal dissemination of VISA strains within the hospitals has been reported in several countries including Asian countries (Wong et al., 1999; Kim et al., 2002). Recently, CDC has published guidelines for the investigation and control of VISA strains and specific recommendations to reduce the development and transmission of these strains (Cosgrove et al., 2004; CDC, 1997). Effective control of VISA isolates in the hospital depends on all health care workers including clinical microbiologists, infection control practitioners, medical and nursing staff, as well as the patient and the patient's family. Strict isolation of the patient in a private room, contact precautions such as gowns and gloves, proper hand hygiene, environmental control, and education of health care personnel are essentially required for effective control of VISA in the hospital. Surveillance cultures of specimens from the nares of persons with extensive patient contact and decolonization with mupirocin are also recommended for evaluation of the spread. Infection control precautions should remain in place until a defined endpoint, for example, until the patient has been culture-negative three times over 3 weeks or the patient's infection has healed.

Conclusion

S. aureus with reduced susceptibility to vancomycin has become a new threat to the modern antimicrobial chemotherapy in clinical medicine. Although the current number of reported cases with VISA or VRSA is still small, it is anticipated that these strains will become more frequent in all continents in the near future. Particularly, Asian countries, where the prevalence of MRSA is very high and vancomycin is widely overused, would have a higher risk to be a main focus of vancomycin resistance in *S. aureus*. The incidence of VISA, VRSA, or hVISA based on standardized detection methods, risk factors, clinical impact, and treatment options against VISA or VRSA strains is an area of active investigation for the future. Also, strict infection control procedures to prevent the spread of resistant strains should be implemented in hospitals.

Acknowledgements I thank Prof. Keiichi Hiramatsu, who is a pioneer of research on vancomycin resistance in *S. aureus*, and Dr. Kwan Soo Ko for their sincere support and invaluable advice.

References

Ariza, J., Pujol, M., Cado, J., Pena, C., et al. (1999). Vancomycin in surgical infections due to methicillin-resistant *Staphylococcus aureus* with heterogeneous resistance to vancomycin. *Lancet*, 353, 1587–1588

Bert, F., Clarissou, J., Durand, F., et al. (2003). Prevalence, molecular epidemiology, and clinical significance of heterogeneous glycopeptide-intermediate *Staphylococcus aureus* in liver transplant recipients. *Journal of Clinical Microbiology*, 41, 5147–5152

Centers for Disease Control and Prevention. (1997). Interim guidelines for prevention and control of staphylococcal infections associated with reduced susceptibility to vancomycin. *Morbidity and Mortality Weekly Report*, 46, 626–628, 635

Centers for Disease Control and Prevention. (2002a). *Staphylococcus aureus* resistant to vancomycin-United States, 2002. *Morbidity and Mortality Weekly Report*, 51, 565–567

Centers for Disease Control and Prevention. (2002b). Vancomycin-resistant *Staphylococcus aureus*-Pennsylvania, 2002. *Morbidity and Mortality Weekly Report*, 51, 902

Centers for Disease Control and Prevention. (2004). Vancomycin-resistant *Staphylococcus aureus*-New York, 2004. *Morbidity and Mortality Weekly Report*, 53, 322–323

Chang, S., Sievert, D. M., Hageman, J. C., et al. (2003). Infection with vancomycin-resistant *Staphylococcus aureus* containing the *vanA* resistance gene. *New England Journal of Medicine*, 348, 1342–1347

Charles, P. G., Ward, P. G., Johnson, P. D., Howden, B. P., Grayson, M. L. (2004). Clinical features associated with bacteremia due to heterogeneous vancomycin-intermediate *Staphylococcus aureus*. *Clinical Infectious Diseases*, 8, 448–451

Clark, N. C., Weigel, L. M., Patel, J. B., Tenover, F. C. (2005). Comparison of Tn1546-like elements in vancomycin-resistant *Staphylococcus aureus* isolates from Michigan and Pennsylvania. *Antimicrobial Agents and Chemotherapy*, 49, 470–472

Clinical and Laboratory Standards Institute. (2006). Performance standards for antimicrobial susceptibility testing; fifteenth informational supplement. CLSI/NCCLS document M100-S16. CLSI, Wayne, PA

Cosgrove, S. E., Carroll, K. C., Perl, T. M. (2004). *Staphylococcus aureus* with reduced susceptibility to vancomycin. *Clinical Infectious Diseases*, 39, 539–545

Cui, L., Ma, X., Sato, K., et al. (2003). Cell wall thickening is a common feature of vancomycin resistance in *Staphylococcus aureus*. *Journal of Clinical Microbiology*, 41, 5–14

Fridkin, S., Hagman, K. J., McDougal, L. K., Mohammed, J., Jarvis, W. R., Perl, T. M., Tenover, F. C.; and vancomycin-intermediate *Staphylococcus aureus* Epidemiology Study Group. (2003). Epidemiological and microbiological characterization of infections caused by *Staphylococcus aureus* with reduced susceptibility to vancomycin, United States, 1997–2001. *Clinical Infectious Diseases*, 36, 429–439

Goldstein, F. W., Kitzis, M. D. (2003). Vancomycin-resistant *Staphylococcus aureus*: no apocalypse now. *Clinical Microbiology and Infection*, 9, 761–765

Haraga, I., Nomura, S., Fukamachi, S., Ohjimi, H., Hanaki, H., Hiramatsu, K., Nagayama, A. (2002). Emergence of vancomycin resistance during therapy against methicillin-resistant *Staphylococcus aureus* in a burn patient – importance of low-level resistance to vancomycin. *International Journal of Infectious Diseases*, 6, 302–308

Hiramatsu, K., Aritaka, N., Hanaki, H., et al. (1997). Dissemination in Japanese hospitals of strains of *Staphylococcus aureus* heterogeneously resistant to vancomycin. *Lancet*, 350, 1670–1673

Hiramatsu, K. (1998). The emergence of *Staphylococcus aureus* with reduced susceptibility to vancomycin in Japan. *American Journal of Medicine*, 104, 7S–10S

Hiramatsu, K. (2001). Vancomycin-resistant *Staphylococcus aureus*: a new model of antibiotic resistance. *Lancet Infectious Diseases*, 1, 147–155

Hiramatsu, K., Hanaki, H., Ino, T., Yabuta, K., Oguri, T., Tenover, F. C. (1997). Methicilllin-reistant *Staphylococcus aureus* clinical strain with reduced vancomycin susceptibility. *Journal of Antimicrobial Chemotherapy*, 40, 135–136

Hiramatsu, K., Kapi, M., Tajima, Y., Cui, L., Trakulsomboon, S., Ito, T. (2005). Advances in vancomycin resistance: research in Staphylococcus aureus. In White D. G., Alekshun M. N., Hawkins P.F. (Eds.), *Frontiers in Antimicrobial Resistance: A Tribute to Stuart Levy*, Washington DC, ASM Press, pp. 289–296

Howe, R. A., Monk, A., Wootton, M., Walsh, T. R., Enright, M. C. (2004). Vancomycin susceptibility within methicillin-resistant *Staphylococcus aureus* lineages. *Emerging Infectious Diseases*, 10, 855–857

Howe, R. A., Walsh, T. R. (2004). hGISA: seek and ye shall find. *Lancet*, 364, 500–501

Ike, Y., Arakawa, Y., Ma, X., Takewaki, K., Nagasawa, M., Tomita, H., Tanimoto, K., Fujimoto, S. (2001). Nationwide survey shows that methicillin-resistant *Staphylococcus aureus* strains heterogeneously and intermediately resistant to vancomycin are not disseminated throughout Japanese hospitals. *Journal of Clinical Microbiology*, 39, 4445–4451

Kim, H. B., Park, W. B., Lee, K. D., et al (2003). Nationwide surveillance of *Staphylococcus aureus* with reduced susceptibility to vancomycin in Korea. *Journal of Clinical Microbiology*, 41, 2279–2281

Kim, M.-N., Pai, C. H., Woo, J. H., Ryu, J. S., Hiramatsu, K. (2000). Vancomycin-intermediate *Staphylococcus aureus* in Korea. *Journal of Clinical Microbiology*, 38, 3879–3881

Kim, M.-N., Hwang, S. H., Pyo, Y.-J., Mun, H.-N., Pai, C. H. (2002). Clonal spread of *Staphylococcus aureus* heterogeneously resistant to vancomycin in a university in Korea. *Journal of Clinical Microbiology*, 40, 1376–1380

Liñares, J. (2001). The VISA/GISA problem: therapeutic implications. *Clinical Microbiology and Infection*, 7 (Suppl 4), 8–15

Lu, J.-J., Lee, S.-Y., Hwa, S.-Y., Yang, A.-H. (2005). Septic arthritis caused by vancomycin-intermediate *Staphylococcus aureus*. *Journal of Clinical Microbiology*, 43, 4156–4158

Moore, M. R., Perdreau-Remington, F., Chambers, H. F. (2003). Vancomycin treatment failure associated with heterogeneous vancomycin-intermediate *Staphylococcus aureus* in a patient with endocarditis and in the rabbit model of endocarditis. *Antimicrobial Agents and Chemotherapy*, 47, 1262–1266

Noble, W. C., Virami, Z., Cree, R. G. (1992). Co-transfer of vancomycin and other resistance genes from *Enterococcus faecalis* NCTC 12201 to *Staphylococcus aureus*. *FEMS Microbiology Letter*, 72, 195–198

Song, J. H., Hiramatsu, K., Suh, J. Y., et al. (2004). Emergence in Asian countries of *Staphylococcus aureus* with reduced susceptibility to vancomycin. *Antimicrobial Agents and Chemotherapy*, 48, 4926–4928

Sng, L.-H., Koh, T. S., Hsu, L.-Y., Kapi, M. (2005). Heterogeneous vancomycin-resistant *Staphylococcus aureus* (hetero-VISA) in Singapore. *International Journal of Antimicrobial Agents*, 25, 177–184

Schwaber, M. J., Wright, S. B., Carmeli, Y., et al. (2003). Clinical implications of varying degrees of vancomycin suscepbility in methicillin-resistant *Staphylococcus aureus* bacteremia. *Emerging Infectious Diseases*, 9, 657–664

Tenover, F. C., McDonald, L. C. (2005). Vancomycin-resistant staphylococci and enterococci: epidemiology and control. *Current Opinion in Infectious Diseases*, 18, 300–305

Tenover, F. C., Lancaster, M. V., Hill, B. C. (1998). Characterization of staphylococci with reduced susceptibilities to vancomycin and other glycopeptides. *Journal of Clinical Microbiology*, 36, 1020–1027

Tenover, F. C., Biddle, J. W., Lancaster, M. V. (2001). Increasing resistance to vancomycin and other glycopeptides in *Staphylococcus aureus*. *Emerging Infectious Diseases*, 7, 327–332

Trakulsomboon, S., Danchaivijitr, S., Rongrungruang, Y., Dhiraputra, C., Susaemgrat, W., Ito, T., Hiramatsu, K. (2001). First report of methicillin-resistant *Staphylococcus aureus* with reduced susceptibility to vancomycin in Thailand. *Journal of Clinical Microbiology*, 39, 591–595

Walsh, T. R., Howe, R. A. (2002). The prevalence and mechanisms of vancomycin resistance in *Staphylococcus aureus*. *Annual of Review of Microbiology*, 56, 657–675

Wang, G., Hindler, J. F., Ward, K. W., Bruckner, D. A. (2006). Increased vancomycin MICs for *Staphylococcus aureus* clinical isolates from a university hospital during a 5-year period. *Journal of Clinical Microbiology*, 44, 3883–3886

Wang, J.-L., Tseng, S.-P., Hsueh, P.-R., Hiramatsu, K. (2004). Vancomycin heteroresistance in methicillin-resistant *Staphylococcus aureus*, Taiwan. *Emerging Infectious Diseases*, 10, 1702–1704

Weigel, L. M., Clewell, D. B., Gill, S. R., et al. (2003). Genetic analysis of a high-level vancomycin-resistant isolate of *Staphylococcus aureus*. *Science*, 302, 1569–1571

Whitener, C. J., Park, S. Y., Browne, F. A., et al. (2004). Vancomycin-resistant Staphylococcus aureus in the absence of vancomycin exposure. *Clinical Infectious Diseases*, 38, 1049–1055

Wong, S. S. Y., Ho, P. L., Woo, P. C., Yuen, K. Y. (1999). Bacteremia caused by staphylococci with inducible vancomycin heteroresistance. *Clinical Infectious Diseases*, 29, 760–767

Subject Index